A SYSTEM OF
COMPLETE
MEDICAL POLICE

A SYSTEM OF COMPLETE MEDICAL POLICE

Selections from
JOHANN PETER FRANK

Edited with an Introduction
by
ERNA LESKY

The Johns Hopkins University Press
Baltimore, Maryland

TT 72–50095

Prepared under the Special Foreign Currency Program of
The National Library of Medicine,
National Institutes of Health, Public Health Service,
U.S. Department of Health, Education and Welfare,
and published for
THE NATIONAL LIBRARY OF MEDICINE
pursuant to an agreement with
THE NATIONAL SCIENCE FOUNDATION, WASHINGTON, D.C.,
by
THE ISRAEL PROGRAM FOR SCIENTIFIC TRANSLATIONS,
JERUSALEM, ISRAEL

Translated from the third, revised edition of Vienna, 1786
by
E. Vilim

The present translation is one of a series of classics in the history of medicine funded through
the International Programs Division of the National Library of Medicine in collaboration
with the Ad Hoc Committee on Historical Translations of the American Association for
the History of Medicine.

The Johns Hopkins University Press, Baltimore, Maryland 21218

Library of Congress Catalog Card Number 75–39820
ISBN 0–8018–1839–7
IPST 60124 0

Set, printed and bound by Keterpress Enterprises, Jerusalem
PRINTED IN ISRAEL

CONTENTS

Foreword by E. Lesky vii

Introduction by E. Lesky ix

Volume One. Human Procreation and Marriage Institutions. Preservation and
Care of Pregnant Women, their Fetuses, and of Lying-In Women in Each
Community 1

Volume Two. Human Procreation and Marriage Institutions. Preservation and
Care of Pregnant Women, their Fetuses, and of Lying-In Women in Each
Community 87

Volume Three. Food, Drink and Vessels. Laws of Moderation, Unhealthy
Clothing, Popular Amusements. Better Layout, Construction, and Necessary
Cleanliness of Human Dwellings 137

Volume Four. Public Safety Measures as Far as they Concern Public Health 197

Volume Five. Safety Measures as Far as Public Health is Concerned and the
Interment of the Dead 269

Volume Six. Medical Affairs 281
  1. Medical Science and Medical Educational Institutions in General 283
  2. Medical Institutions in Particular 325
  3. Medical Institutions of Learning; the Examination and Confirmation of
     Medical Practitioners 363

Supplementary Volumes to Medical Police, or a Collection of Various Special
Treatises Concerning this Science:

Volume One 377

Volume Two 385

Third and Last Volume 403

Bibliography 453

Index of Personal Names 459

Index of Subjects and Places 461

FOREWORD

Since the 1940's H. E. Sigerist and his disciples, especially George Rosen, have tried to introduce Johann Peter Frank (1745–1821), the 18th century pioneer of social medicine, to the Anglo-Saxon world. In the course of this endeavor Frank's creed of social medicine, his oration *The People's Misery—Mother of Diseases,* delivered in Pavia in 1790, as well as other minor works, was translated into English. His monumental work in six volumes (the sixth volume consisting of two parts and three supplementary volumes) *System einer vollständigen medicinischen Polizey* (*A System of Complete Medical Police*)* with which he established hygiene as a systematic science has not yet been translated into English. It is, however, regarded as a landmark in the history of thought on the social relations of health and disease, and it has been shown that the idea of medical police has had an impact on developments in Great Britain and the United States of America. (G. Rosen, 1953).

One must be all the more grateful that now, through the initiative of the National Library of Medicine, a selection can be presented which, it is to be hoped, will be representative of Frank's monumental work. It was our concern not only to present a well-balanced cross-section of the subjects classically included in *Medical Police,* but above all to shed a new light on their socially relevant aspects. By so doing we hope not only to appeal to the physician, the medical historian, and the social worker, but also to the historian, the sociologist, the cultural historian, and the folklorist. The English edition will have served its purpose if the interest in Frank and his *Medical Police* has hereby been increased.

The present English translation is one of a series of classics in the history of medicine made possible through funds provided by the International Programs Division of the National Library of Medicine in collaboration with the Ad Hoc Committee on Historical Translations of the American Association for the History of Medicine.

---

* L. Baumgartner and E. M. Ramsey ("Johann Peter Frank and His 'System einer vollständigen Medicinischen Polizey'". *Ann. Med. Hist.,* n.s. 5, 525–532, p. 525, 1932) referred to the difficulties of translating the title into modern English. Our translation uses the title chosen by G. Rosen, although we are fully aware of the fact that the modern term 'police' is not as all-encompassing as Frank's meaning.

The editor wishes to express her thanks to Dr. Jeanne L. Brand for her continuing interest in the translation of this work. I am also indebted to the translators of the Israel Program for Scientific Translations, who had an extremely difficult task to fulfill. They had to create a readable English text from a cumbersome 18th century German one. I would especially like to thank my assistant, Dr. Manfred Skopec, and his wife, Margaret Russell Skopec, who helped me in revising the translation.

Vienna, November 1975   Erna Lesky

INTRODUCTION

There are, without a doubt, men in whom the spirit of an epoch is embodied with great purity. We call these men leaders. Frank is such a man from the era of enlightened absolutism. He carried the light of reason, which penetrated all spheres of governmental life during the Enlightenment, into the realm of public health. Frank taught the monarchs that the greatest wealth of a state lies in its subjects, who should be as numerous, healthy, and productive as possible; that it is possible to maintain this precious "fortune" and through rational hygienic measures to increase it, if the power of the state would be combined with the knowledge of the physician. *Servandis et augendis civibus* ("For the Preservation and Increase of the Population") is the motto which precedes the first volume of his monumental work *System einer vollständigen medicinischen Polizey* that appeared in 1779. The work has become a "monument in the field of hygiene to the absolutist state." (H. E. Sigerist)

BIOGRAPHY

We are well informed about Frank's life in his autobiography, the first part of which was published in 1802 and translated into English in 1948 by George Rosen. There he tells us of his youth, his student years, and his works. The second part of his autobiography, which H. Haubold used for his Frank monograph, has only been published in small fragments. (St. Trzebinski, 1928–29.) The autobiographical passages which we find in the introductions to the fifth and sixth volumes of *Medical Police,* as well as in the first supplementary volume, are therefore all the more valuable to us.

Frank was born in 1745 in Rotalben in the Palatinate. He was the son of a trader. There he grew up, in the borderland between French and German civilization. His family was originally French on his father's side (his grandfather was a purveyor to the French army); on his mother's side his family was Palatine-Tyrolese. He inherited his good humor and quickness of tongue from his father's side, which always helped him find the right words at the right moment in his intercourse with emperors and czars—Joseph II, Napoleon, Alexander I. This may also have been the source of his inner restlessness. Frank never stayed long in one place. Even in his student days he often moved from one university to the next: from Pont-à-Mousson in France, where he took his Ph.D., to Heidelberg in Germany, then to Strasbourg, and back again to Heidelberg, where the title of Dr.med. was conferred upon him in 1766.

Even at that time—Frank was 21 years old—he knew what his life's mission was to be. In a memorable conversation with the Dean of the Medical Faculty at Heidelberg Frank said that he wanted to trace the causes of those diseases which "greatly affect the people" ("ins Grosse auf die Völker wirken"), yet which are for the most part preventable, because the causes are rooted in the social conditions of society. At that time also he had already conceived a plan to write a comprehensive book on this subject which was concerned with man's physical and social environment from the cradle to the grave.

Before he could devote himself to these ambitious plans he had to procure a means of living. In 1766 Frank settled in Bitche in the Lorraine and worked as a general practitioner. That he changed his place and position four times within six years typifies the restlessness and career drive in his life. He left Bitche, where he was a country doctor from 1766 to 1768, for a position as district medical officer in Baden. In 1769 he went to Rastatt as physician-in-ordinary to the Margrave of Baden-Baden, only to leave for Bruchsal three years later, where he became personal physician to the Prince-Bishop of Speyer in 1775.

The principality of Speyer became Frank's working model for his concept of health. Within this small region he could try out all the plans and ideas with which his thoughts had been occupied since that decisive conversation in Heidelberg. Here he could study the living and working conditions of the serfs. Here he could show what governmental care could do for the health of the subjects, if the rulers would combine their efforts with medical knowledge. We will give only two examples: Before Frank's arrival in Bruchsal there was only one trained midwife in the entire principality. Of 85 women who were pregnant, one died in labor, or lying-in. In nine years, after the establishment of a school for midwives, only one out of 125 died. A second example: Up to this time the serfs in the 36 towns of the Speyer district were, for the most part, in the hands of crude, ignorant quacks and charlatans. As a result, many perished or were reduced to disabled cripples. Then two hospitals and a school of surgery were established in Bruchsal. Frank himself instructed here with the aid of a surgeon whom he had summoned from Vienna. The population of the whole principality was now well-provided for with surgically-trained physicians.

This is the milieu in which the first volume of his *Medical Police* appeared in 1779. It dealt with such sensitive subjects as marriage, its fertility, pregnancy and childbearing, and also with celibacy of the clergy. It took courage for a Prince-Bishop's personal physician, which indeed Frank was, to criticize premature ordinations. For this reason Frank had asked a Jesuit priest to censor his manuscript. The priest wrote, "This work will bring you great fame, but it is my experience that it will cause you so much unpleasantness that you will regret having it published." (H. Haubold, p. 35.)

Frank, however, did not regret it; otherwise, the Jesuit's prediction was to be correct. The book was much discussed and severely criticized. All of a sudden Frank had become famous. He became even more famous when, in 1780 and 1783, volumes two and three of *Medical Police* appeared, the second dealing with sexual intercourse in general, prostitution, venereal diseases, abortion, and foundling hospitals; the third dealing with nutrition, food control, clothing, and housing.

In the meantime Frank's relationship with the Prince-Bishop had become so unbearable that he decided to leave Bruchsal at the first opportunity. In the spring of 1784 he resigned his position with the Prince-Bishop of Speyer when (the now famous) Frank received three offers: a call to Mainz, one to Göttingen, and another to Pavia. He would have liked to accept the call to Pavia which at that time was under Austrian administration. However, Joseph II, the "traveling emperor," was— as so often—on tour and his carriage difficult to catch. The decision was pressing; so Frank accepted the call to the professorship of clinical medicine in Göttingen. After all, as famous a scholar as Albrecht von Haller had taught there and the University of Göttingen was held in very high esteem.

In spite of everything, his professorship in Göttingen from May 1784 to March 1785 was only an interlude. The post in Pavia was still vacant and Joseph II, of whose medical reforms the papers eloquently reported, attracted Frank. Just then, in 1784, they had reported the opening of a new, huge hospital with 2,000 beds— the Vienna General Hospital. So off to Pavia, to meet Joseph II!

In March 1785, Frank was presented to His Imperial Majesty for the first time. In his autobiography Frank relates his conversation with the Emperor, which took place in the Hofburg. The Emperor, proud of his latest creation, the General Hospital, asked Frank, "Are you satisfied with the hospital?" Of course, the Emperor wanted to hear something complimentary from the famous expert Frank. But Frank had been sceptical of such monstrous hospitals all his life, due to their high mortality rates. The Emperor noted his scepticism and wanted to know the cause of it. "The fact that such a large mechanism rarely operates properly," was my reply. "But it works!" said the ruler, well aware of the infinite care which he bestowed on this institution that he had founded. "Certainly," I replied, full of confidence in this great Prince's love of truth, "it works as long as it has such a great power to set it in motion." (Autobiography, ed. by G. Rosen, p. 283.)

And so it was. After Joseph II's death in 1790 the hospital no longer ran like clockwork. It was to become the task of Frank in 1795 to take over the administration of the General Hospital as Director, and make the star creation of Joseph II operable and efficient once again.

In 1785 Frank was able to become acquainted with the spirit of the Emperor of Reform, as it extended even to Pavia. Joseph II's requests for reform came to the new Professor of Clinical Medicine in rapid succession. A change in the medical curriculum was the first task. Here for the first time Frank was able to realize his conceptions of medical instruction as he later set forth in the sixth volume of *Medical Police* and its second supplementary volume. His foremost principle "that in science the practical aspect not be taught separately from the theoretical aspect" has not lost its impact. Frank acted according to this principle in all places of duty from Pavia to St. Petersburg and in all disciplines of medicine from botany and pathological anatomy to surgery and obstetrics, and of course in his own specialty internal medicine. He made alive the often antiquated instruction which his era of enlightenment demanded. By creating a museum of pathology and anatomy in Pavia and later a pathological institute in Vienna in 1795 he became the great promoter of pathological anatomy. In Pavia and Vienna he introduced practical instruction into the curriculum of surgery and obstetrics, which until then had been primarily taught theoretically at the universities. In internal medicine especially he practiced and intensified the examination and treatment of the patient at the bedside. The medical curriculum was extended to five years. Another fact has to be considered: While Herman Boerhaave was limited to only twelve sick beds in his bedside teaching in Leyden, Frank was able to arrange to have all the in-patient wards of the Pavian hospital and later of the Vienna General Hospital at his disposal for teaching and research purposes. The developments resulting from the curriculum of 1785–1786 established these places as model hospitals of clinical instruction. A great physician and teacher had put into practice the didactic principles of medicine of the Enlightenment.

Equally important to the author of *Medical Police* was that in 1786 Joseph II appointed Frank *Protophysicus,* that is, Director General of Public Health of Austrian Lombardy and the Duchy of Mantua. Frank was well aware of the unique opportunity that this position provided in order to fulfill his life's task. In the fourth volume of *Medical Police* which he published while at Pavia in 1788, he was able to state with great inner satisfaction: "An additional advantage of this work is that I am in a position to put into effect a large part of my medical proposals and I am therefore able to adjudge their consequences and difficulties better than can most writers." And there were numerous difficulties in the hospitals, mental asylums, maternity clinics, in the foundling hospitals, poor houses, and pharmacies, all of which he inspected with expert knowledge on his journeys throughout his district. During these journeys he contacted physicians, surgeons, and midwives, and studied the working and social conditions of the Lombardian peasants as he described so vividly in his oration *The People's Misery—Mother of Diseases* on 5 May 1790.

But only a few months before, on 20 February 1790, Frank's powerful patron and congenial supporter, Joseph II, had died in Vienna. On his deathbed he was forced by revolts in parts of the empire to revoke most of his reforms. Frank, too, had become uneasy in his work as *Protophysicus.* He already felt his enemies at work. Leopold II, Joseph's brother and successor, did uphold his appointment regarding Frank's sanitary reform work in the Lombardy; but this Emperor, too, had died by 1792. In an absolute monarchy everything depends on the personal patronage of the monarch. At first Frank won the favor of Franz II, who had become the new holder of absolute power in Vienna. In 1795 he was appointed Director of the General Hospital in Vienna and Professor of Clinical Medicine. The highest court officials sought his advice. The second supplementary volume of *Medical Police* is full of suggestions for a reform of medical education, for a new law code, for a reform of the Supreme Sanitary Board. It seemed as if he had reached the climax of his career, as if he were to become the medical heir to Gerard van Swieten who, under Maria Theresa, headed the public health system from 1745 to 1772 as *Protomedicus*, that is, Director General of Public Health of the Hapsburg Empire.

Frank always knew how to live in accordance with his rank. After all, he was a Privy Councillor now, which in the army is equivalent to the rank of lieutenant general. In Vienna he lived in a small palace at 20 Alserstrasse, where Billroth was to live later. Like Billroth, Frank liked music and arranged musical soirées at his house. Haydn was a welcome guest at any time. A document written by the Geneva-born physician Jean de Carro, who then practiced in Vienna and met Frank on several occasions, tells us about Frank's years in Vienna: "But I cannot remember one who combined in such a high degree all that we generally imply when we call a man a *great physician*. He possessed an inexhaustible erudition, medical and literary, without being pedantic in any way, an astonishing memory, and he wrote German, Italian, and French in the most elegant way. Whatever subject he touched on he discussed with the greatest clarity. His figure was imposing, his manners most affable. He devoted as much attention to the poor as to the rich when he received and treated them. In one word, he combined all those qualities that we like to find in the physician, the statesman, and what the English call 'a perfect gentleman'."*

One can only call it a tragedy that this great physician failed to climb the very last step of his career and did not become *Protomedicus* of the entire Hapsburg Empire, but fell victim to a paltry intrigue of the physician-in-ordinary to Emperor Franz II, Joseph Andreas Stifft. In 1804, when almost sixty years old, Frank had to leave Vienna and Austria. For just one year he was Professor of Clinical Medicine at the University of Vilna. In 1805 he left for St. Petersburg. There a strange fate awaited him. Once again he was to experience a bitter intrigue involving the physician-in-ordinary, this time of Czar Alexander I. Frank went about his work as Director of the Medicosurgical Academy, drafting a new curriculum in full detail. As he began to instruct, the Czar's personal physician, the Scotsman James Wylie, inter-

---

* Mémoires du Chevalier Jean de Carro. Carlsbad, pp. 75–78, 1855. Quoted after H. E. Sigerist, p. 58, 1956.

fered and deprived Frank of the fruits of his three years' work in St. Petersburg.

In 1808 Frank left St. Petersburg and arrived in July in Vienna. In 1809 we still find him in Vienna. After the battle of Wagram Napoleon occupied Vienna and resided at Schönbrunn Castle. One can easily understand that after the bitter experiences in St. Petersburg and Vienna, Frank declined Napoleon's offer to become his personal physician and to go with him to Paris. "What destiny is mine; I shall always be thrown from one end of Europe to the other without rest unto my grave," (H. Haubold, p. 135) Frank groaned when the decision was forced upon him. But he did not alter his previous decision and, similarly, he turned down an invitation to Berlin which came in the same year and would have made Frank Chief of the Prussian Public Health System.

In November 1809, together with his favorite daughter Caroline, Frank moved to Freiburg (Breisgau). There he finished the first supplementary volume of his *Medical Police* on 19 March 1811. After his daughter's death in the same year he began to take a dislike to Freiburg. He fled, as he wrote in his own words in the preface to the fifth volume of *Medical Police* in 1812, "into the arms of my friendship with Vienna; a friendship that had become gray with me but had always been as strong as an anchor." And the restless Frank lived in Vienna until his death in 1821. Here he found the peace he needed to complete his work. From 1817 to 1819 the sixth and last volume of *Medical Police* appeared in two books. The first deals with 'Medical Science in General and its Influence upon the Welfare of Society.' In the second book he discusses in great detail all problems of medical education. He treats the subject with such clarity and experience as only a person who had spent forty years of teaching at five European universities could.

Vienna also offered to Frank the professional and social stimulation a man of the world and physician like Frank did not want to miss. His house on the Alserstrasse became a kind of medical congress center, particularly during the Congress of Vienna (1814–15). Many foreign physicians accompanying their sovereigns to the Danube metropolis met at Number 20 Alserstrasse. But in the same house every morning, year after year, the poor of Vienna met, for the great physician held free office hours for their treatment.

Frank died in Vienna on 24 April 1821 as a consequence of apoplexy. He was buried in the same cemetery in which Beethoven and Schubert found their final resting places. The epitaph on his gravestone gives evidence of how far his fame as physician reached:

Divis Manibus
D. Joannis Petri Frank
Gottingae Ticini Vindobanae Vilnae Petropoli
Academicarum Quae Per Europam et Americam florent Sodalis.

THE POLITICAL, ECONOMIC, AND PHILOSOPHICAL BACKGROUND OF *MEDICAL POLICE*

Due to the manifold problems caused by the population explosion during the last decades, modern society has to control the birth rate. The motto is 'family planning.' The reader of *Medical Police* is confronted with exactly the opposite attitude. Its motto is *augmendis civibus*. The first two volumes deal exclusively with measures to procure a controlled, steady expansion of the population. Among the physicians and jurists of the latter half of the 18th century Frank is by no means the only representative of this viewpoint. A. Fischer (1933), George Rosen, and E. Lesky (1959–1960) have been able to show in their works that Frank's view is deeply rooted in specific economic and political ideas that have their origins in the 17th century. These ideas are very closely connected with the development of absolutist states in Austria, Prussia, France, and Spain. The rulers of these countries needed money and people, people for the army to support power politics, and people to develop industries and agriculture and thus to produce wealth. While mercantilism developed in France, under Colbert, in the Germanic states its German variation developed, viz., cameralism. The term has its origin in the accounting offices of the monarchs, where cameralists such as Johann Joachim Becher (1635–1682), Philipp Wilhelm von Hörnigk (1640–1714), or Wilhelm von Schröder made calculations on the value of the people and found out that numerous and healthy subjects constitute an almost inexhaustible source of a monarch's wealth and power. Measures had to be taken not only to increase a population but also to keep them healthy and able-bodied. The welfare of the state was therefore considered as being identical to the welfare of the people, even in the 17th century.

In order to systematize and bring these ideas of social medicine into a concrete form within the political and economic concept as represented by cameralism, it became important to establish chairs for *Polizeiwissenschaft,* i.e., the science of the police. These chairs were established by the King of Prussia at the beginning of the 18th century. Here 'police', as a science of administrating a state, was taught to future civil servants. In 1750 Maria Theresa, the enlightened ruler of the Austrian Empire, gave Heinrich Gottlob von Justi (1717–1771) the opportunity to teach the new 'science of police' at the Collegium Theresianum, a school for civil servants. She offered a similar position at the University of Vienna to Joseph von Sonnenfels (1732–1817) in 1765. Joseph von Sonnenfels published his popular textbook *Grundsätze der Polizey, Handlung und Finanz* in 1765. In Chapter V, "On the Security of the Person," he deals expressly with matters of public health such as care of the sick, poor relief, prevention of epidemics, regulation of medical and surgical practice, crimes of violence, cleanliness of cities, methods of procuring abortions, etc. In many passages of his *Medical Police* Frank quotes Sonnenfels, with whom he collaborated to establish the Austrian law code from 1795 to 1804. But it is not

only Frank who is deeply influenced by Sonnenfels. Young Emperor Joseph II—
24 years old—wrote in his state memoirs: "The first matter for which provisions
must be made in terms of politics, finance, and the military, is the population—
that is to say—the conservation of the state's subjects."

Justi and Sonnenfels were able to combine their thoughts on population with
the theory of society of Christian Wolff (1679–1754), who was a philosopher in
Halle. An understanding of this theory is important for us because Frank adopted
it completely in his *Medical Police*. As Wolff did, he regarded the relationship between
the ruler and his subjects as that of a father to his children. While it is recognized
in modern social medicine that the individual has an inalienable right to enjoy
good health, the people in Wolff's concept were not much more than the object
of governmental care.

The ruler's right of guardianship of his subjects was derived from this patriarchal
attitude which he held. Furthermore, just as the father is obligated to educate his
children (normally using forbidding words and orders), likewise is the monarch
obligated to educate the subjects of his State in matters of health, and the physician
is at his side to help. As one can read in the second volume of *Medical Police,* Frank
was criticized for being a disciple of governmental intervention, since he "out-
rageously limits innate personal rights, which have already been curtailed too much;
violates the rights of fathers, husbands, and parents, and takes away that which
has been authorized them, and gives these rights into the hands of a despotic government." Frank could not, in fact, imagine his task to promote the people's health
and welfare in any other framework than that of the science of police, a branch of
which resulted in his own sanitary program. Having surveyed all these concepts
and theories we can also understand what Frank comprehended under the term
'medical police.'

From the definition of internal security which Frank offers at the beginning of
his introduction to *Medical Police,* we can see how closely connected the work of
Frank is to the ideology of a welfare and police state which has been briefly sketched
here, and to the concept of internal security as used by Sonnenfels: "The internal
security of the State is the aim of the general science of police. A very important
part thereof is the science which will enable us to further the health of human beings
living in society . . . acting in accordance with definite principles; consequently
we must promote the welfare of the population. . . .".

In the same chapter we find a second definition of medical police, which he char-
acterizes as a "'defensive art,' a doctrine whereby human beings and their animal
assistants can be protected against the disadvantageous consequences of crowding
too thickly upon the ground . . ." Striking in this definition is a new word, unusual
for the cameralists and the theoreticians of the doctrine of population. It can be
shown (E. Lesky, 1960, pp. 20 ff) that Frank is delving here into the terminology
of the Genevan citizen and philosopher Jean Jacques Rousseau (1712–1778),

especially in his *Discours sur l'origine et les fondements de l'inégalité parmi les hommes* which appeared in 1754. In this work the spiritual father of the French Revolution surpassed his *Contrat social* (1762) in developing a theory of the origin of culture, that is, society. In this theory, the primitive man who lived in harmony with nature was happy, strong, and healthy. Not until men were thrown together in society did trouble arise, or man-made diseases begin to exist. The moral as well as the physical process of degeneration began. The climax was reached in the cities, those sloughs of vice and luxury. From Rousseau, who is evident in page after page of Frank's introduction to *Medical Police,* Frank learned that degeneration and disease are a necessary attribute of social inequality. Against these disadvantageous consequences stands the social challenge which the physician accepts from the philosopher—to protect human beings.

It is in this light that Frank criticizes the prevailing bad habit of mothers not wanting to nurse their own children. The social reference becomes evident as he accuses the rich "Welche endlich erlernt haben, die meisten ihrer Pflichten in der Fron von anderen tun zu lassen" (2,284).* He criticizes the bourgeois and noble society for letting daughters, who were expected to be the mothers of a strong future race, be coddled in a monastic upbringing with no physical activity. Pampering just increases our needs. While our ancestors made much use of their arms and legs, the trend today is ."deren Funktionen durch Maschinenwerke verrichten zu lassen" (1,26). However, coddling and pampering characterized the upbringing of young people in the age of sentimentality, the overwrought atmosphere of which Frank excellently portrayed. In the postulate of a healthy, natural upbringing in the fresh open air accompanied by much physical activity one can see the influence which Rousseau's great educational novel *Émile* had on Frank.

A past era wanted to view Frank the cosmopolite—who had served Germans, Italians, Austrians, Lithuanians, and Russians regardless of nationality—as the Germanic eugenist par excellence. This is a misrepresentation and must be corrected. Frank advised against marriage between unhealthy partners, and even demanded initiating a statement of nubility. But he makes it perfectly clear that these suggestions are to be understood in the context of Rousseau's thesis concerning the degeneration of the human race, as measures to combat that degeneration. The concept of race which was later to cause so much confusion was far-removed from Frank's ideas.

We also see the influence of Rousseau when Frank takes issue with the clothing fashions of his contemporaries, with their eating and drinking habits and with their sexual adventures which he sees as the main cause for the "decline of the human race." Frank and Rousseau believe that all of this luxury affords the people a pleasant euphoria which allows them to feel happy in an actual state of decay (1,29). As

---

* [References to quotations appearing in this Introduction are to the original German volume and page number.]

Frank stresses the value of moderation and of a simple and natural life, he becomes relevant to our present luxury and consumer society.

FRANK AS A CRITIC OF FEUDALISM

Frank, who stood on the side of enlightened absolutism with his demand of governmental care for the subjects of the state, saw in reality great obstacles to attaining this principle. His oration *The People's Misery—Mother of Diseases* delivered in Pavia in 1790 has gone down in medical history as a classical document depicting this deplorable state of affairs. This speech can be taken as an example of the fruitfulness of the new medical thought which was oriented around Rousseau (E. Lesky, 1960, p. 20 ff). In this oration the physician Frank shows in detail what physicians and philosophers must realize to be socially caused illnesses. These are not only temporary workers' disabilities which can be treated in doctors' offices and the hospitals. He is speaking of a permanent reduction to misery of an entire social class, the farmers of the Lombardy, which was wasting away at every age level from infancy to old age. As professor and high governmental official (*Gubernial-rat*) Frank had the courage to denounce serfdom as the source of this pauperization and the resulting diseases, and he demanded to have it abolished, for an enslaved folk is a cachectic folk.

This speech was delivered on 5 May 1790, and was rightfully received as a classical document of thought in social medicine. The fact that this speech had several pre-liminary steps has been overlooked until now. *Medical Police* began to appear in 1779. We want to seek out these preliminary steps in the first four volumes which appeared up to 1788. It can be shown that Frank's social criticism increased in a continuing crescendo from the first to the fourth volume.

Once again it is typical of the philosophical milieu in which *The People's Misery—Mother of Diseases* has its roots, that the first formulation of its *Leitmotiv* can be found in a footnote to Rousseau's *Discours*. Eleven years before Frank's address in Pavia he wrote in the introduction to *Medical Police* (1,16): "Verschwendung gebiert Armut und Armut Krankheiten." Here he does not discuss the misery of the Lombardian serfs standing knee-deep in water of the rice paddies, but the children of the German farmers who are crippling themselves with the backbreaking labor of the vineyards. The three-page digression moves from the children's misery to the diseases of their laboring parents. Several pages later, another facet of the farmers' misery (1,37) is exposed: because they have been forbidden to gather firewood from the forest, peasant families are freezing to death in the winter's cold together with their cattle. Serfdom has not yet been mentioned. The personal physi-cian of the Prince-Bishop of Speyer merely dared to warn "the Great" that they must revoke this prohibition of wood-gathering. Frank points out to the rulers that another defective situation could have very serious results. For if the healthiest

and strongest of the 16-year-old farmboys are called to military service, a degeneration of the population would follow. It would remain the task of their brothers
and sisters left behind—who are already atrophying due to premature labor, destitu-
tion and misery—to reproduce and replenish the state's population. Not until one
reads Frank's *Medical Police* intently, as historians and sociologists should do,
does the extent of child labor become clear in a frightening and devastating manner.
Not only the farm children suffer. Among the bourgeoisie 10-year-old boys are
forced to work as tailor's apprentices from morning till night until their spines are
so crooked that it is impossible to raise their heads. The degree of Frank's farsighted-
ness is shown by his demanding as early as 1779 a law protecting the young. He
gives us an excellent view into the social structure of the time when he describes
the dangers which threaten children. At harvest time there are entire villages where
farmers' infants lie unattended in their cradles, hungry and screaming because
their mothers must work in the fields. Sometimes, while the parents work, the babies
are attacked by dogs and swine, who gnaw away parts of the children's bodies
(2,226 f). In the twelve years alone in which Frank served as district medical officer
in Baden, five or six such terrible accidents occurred. At that time Frank also became
acquainted with the hard lot of the peasant wives far advanced in pregnancy. They
not only had to haul water and firewood but do hard labor in the fields and at harvest,
since their husbands had to harvest in the landlords' fields (1,483 f). The word
serfdom is used here for the first time. Frank attacks this human state as the actual
cause of all the farmers' misery with this grotesque illustration (2,485): A mare
is freed from servitude for twelve weeks during her pregnancy and after foaling.
A peasant wife, in contrast, since her husband must serve his lord, is destined for
hard labor. Frank, as a doctor experienced in serving his ruler, expresses his criticism
in the form of a question to the rulers of the German principalities: If a horse is
given a twelve week rest during pregnancy, should not a human being be given at
least as much?

By the fourth volume (1788) in which Frank dealt with the Security Institutions
as they affect Public Health, Frank's criticism of feudalism has become much
stronger. In the preface he himself gives the reason. Joseph II, his patron and protector, had even established human rights in Pavia where previously "Nichts als
zähneklappern und winseln an der geweihten Inquisitionskette" had dominated.
With this new feeling of freedom, Frank dared to write "whatever he thought"
(4, Preface).

The hunt was a popular recreational activity of the feudal lords, especially the
hunt *par force*. Beaters were needed to drive the wildlife together. The peasants
were made to do this as one way of serving their master. While often forced to abandon
their own fields for weeks at a time, they were permitted to "Bei Wasser und Brot
dem Vergnügen ihrer Mitmenschen zu frönen" (4,110). Now and again it even
happened that a wild huntsman would shoot down a peasant as if he were a beast.

Frank, who once said, "Die Errettung einzelner Menschen muss eine grössere Tat scheinen, als die Eroberung einer Provinz mit Bürgerblut" was utterly disgusted at the indifference with which such occurrences were received in German court circles. He was also thinking of the families left without means. Frank's philanthropic and social sensitivity moved him to make a passionate appeal to "the Great" in 1788 (4,229 f).

Once more he deals with the entertainment of those men now referred to by Frank as "the most merciful sovereigns of the people." The topic here is again the hunt. Once again the farmers have lined up, but this time not as beaters. Now they hope to protect their fields from the terrible damage which the wildlife causes at harvest time. "The poor little farmer, the deserted man" lies awake throughout the frosty fall night in nothing but his coverall, trying to protect his little bit of grain. These night vigils often last for several weeks. Illness, mutilation, or death caused by animals attacking might be the consequence. Even if the whole portrayal of the situation seems affected in word choice and emphasis—where Frank is normally so sober and even dry in his writing—in the face of this terrible social injustice it results in such a crescendo that can only end in a cry of "My God!"

The revolution in Austria started from above. In February 1789, five months before the French Revolution began, Joseph II, who would always be the immortal Emperor to Frank, issued a generous law calling for the emancipation of the farmers. The law was to go into effect on 1 November 1790. But Joseph II died on 20 February 1790. This background has to be considered to appreciate the fact that Frank's oration in Pavia on 5 May 1790, and his demand to do away with serfdom were not only matters of concern to him as a doctor, but represented the political concern of the Emperor whom he so admired as well.

ENLIGHTENMENT, WITCHCRAFT, AND MAGIC

In the fourth volume of his *Medical Police* which appeared in 1788, Frank dealt with witches, exorcism, and magic. By illuminating these 'dark' realms of human superstition with the light of reason, he considered himself an enlightener in the original meaning of the word and did justice to the task set for him by his century at the beginning (4,461) and end (4,571) of the chapter. As a doctor who came into intimate contact with all social classes—his classification as "nobility, bourgeois, and paupers" (4,485) is sociologically noteworthy—he knew of countless magical practices which had tenaciously survived since pagan times and could be reconfirmed daily at patients' bedsides.

Frank's century was not completely the enlightened one; as late as 1781, seven years before the appearance of the fourth volume of *Medical Police,* a witch was burnt at Glarus in Switzerland. The practice of exorcism had reached new heights, since the minister Johann Gassner (1727–1779) with cross and supplication of the

Lord exorcized the devil from thousands of people in Ellwangen, Swabia, where he reached the peak of his career as exorcist. The pilgrimate sites overflowed with hundreds of votive offerings, wax facsimiles of all body parts of humans and animals. "Ich sah dort," so reports Frank (4,510) from a pilgrimage site in Southwest Germany with the enlightener's mocking superiority: "den Mönchen so viele wächserne Gebärmütter und Weiberbrüste bei jeder Messe auftischen, dass diese guten Väter lange den grössten Ekel vor dergleichen Gegenständen gefasst haben sollten." The success of Cagliostro's conjuring of spirits in Parisian high society was just one more piece of evidence for Frank, "Dass wir noch nicht weit genug im gemeinen Menschenverstand vorgerückt sind, um dass es unnütz sein sollte, von diesen Gegenständen ein Wort zu erinnern" (4,486).

Our selection from Frank's chapter on sorcery, devilry, and magic cures is arranged to give an impression of the comprehensive analysis of witches and magic, which he examines in their many-faceted forms among widely differing people and in different epochs. Everything is laid out, from the priests of the Tartars, the mandrakes and incantations of the Germanic people, the witch trials of the Renaissance, and the slowly gathering resistance to all this by enlightened individuals (Weyer, Spe) up to the miracle cult of baroque, Catholic piety. And with Frank's meticulousness and enormous erudition it is documented in an immaculate literary manner. The psychiatric-historian, the psychologist, sociologist, cultural historian, and folklorist have only recently discovered this almost inexhaustible source, which Frank compiled in his well-known efficient manner. For how many people then have been led astray by crude superstitious practices, who might have otherwise been saved through the intervention of an enlightened physician!

Let us now analyze Frank's attitude, which is also the attitude of the Enlightenment, toward the most important phenomena. First, there is the belief in witches, i.e., the belief that they are capable (as are demons, evil spirits or magicians) of causing (among other evils) diseases, for which reason they were to be hunted, tried, tortured, and executed. The accusation of one person led (by means of torture) to denunciations of many others until all the mothers and daughters of entire villages were exterminated (4,526). Frank regrets that physicians often failed: As the bold Weyer had demonstrated, it ought to have been their task to discover, by using scientific methods, the real cause of the disease instead of resorting to convenient explanations such as "diseases caused by the devil" and thereby hiding their ignorance and pride. And what about the witches themselves? Most of them were victims of their own "twisted imagination." With ointments from hallucinatory spices, for instance hog's-bean, crab apple, or poppy juice, they fooled the "sick soul in such a way that even after awakening he lived on in his dream world." The enlightened and philanthropic attributes in Frank made him refer to witches in most cases as mentally disturbed people.

Frank himself had the opportunity to study the phenomena of exorcism in patients of the most famous exorcist of his time, the minister Johann Gassner (who was born in Klösterle in the province of Vorarlberg) and of his clerical imitators. One must only read the amusing story of an exorcized girl (4,510 ff) who reportedly vomited cat hair and passed pebble stones as feces, and whose mother Frank questioned about the matter, in order to understand the enlightened eagerness with which Frank tried to rationally explain the "Hottentot terms for the causes of diseases."

Exorcism (like celibacy and monastery education) offers Frank another good opportunity to criticize the clergy. He stresses three factors (4,554 f) as driving forces for "our artful exorcists": greed, sanctimoniousness, and craving for admiration. It might be tempting to deduce from these and other remarks to be found in all volumes of *Medical Police* an anticlerical or even antireligious attitude on Frank's part. Frank's criticism of the abuses of exorcism or of the baroque miracle cult originates in the attitude of a person who sympathized with the movement of Reformed Catholicism of his time. It would be a rewarding study to trace Frank's standpoint regarding religion which was only touched on here.

In general, the whole chapter is intended to secularize or naturalize the hitherto supernatural causes of diseases. Frank is convinced that many phenomena that were regarded as supernatural or miraculous could be explained by a more critical study of nature. Above all, this was true regarding the alleged sleep of the tortured (in reality they were unconscious), or the infamous witch-swimming practice to determine whether a woman was a witch or not. In this context, Frank relates (4,532) that he, too, observed hysterical persons swimming "like blown up frogs" on top of the water in the baths of Baden.

In his enlightened zeal to find a natural reason for the supernatural and the occult, Frank and his like-minded colleague Franz Anton Mai (1742–1844) unknowingly touched on the phenomenon of autosuggestion. The exorcist Gassner had once again stimulated the interest. He was capable of stopping the pulse in his arm by invoking Jesus. It is interesting to read (4,543 f) how both doctors, all credit due to the enlightened medicine of their century, tried to stop their own pulses by experimentally pressing their arms to their chests, using a tight undershirt. Mai was successful, but Frank only partially so. At the conclusion of this experiment Frank wrote the words which may be considered the maxim of the Enlightenment in regard to all supernatural and paramedical phenomena (4,557 f): ". . . Ein vernünftiger Mann wird nicht auf übernatürliche Ursachen schliessen, sondern er untersucht zuerst und wenn er den Schlüssel zu dem Geheimnis nicht findet, so gesteht er lieber seine Unwissenheit als dass er zu Erklärungen seine Zuflucht nähme, die der gesunden Vernunft widersprechen."

The Text

The first edition of Frank's *Medical Police* is described according to the accepted rules of bibliography by L. Baumgartner and E. Mapelsden Ramsey in *Ann. Med.*

Hist., n.s. 6, pp. 83–89, 1934. For the present selection the third revised edition of the *System einer vollständigen medicinischen Polizey* was used. The first and second volumes of this edition appeared in Vienna in 1786, the third in 1787, and the fourth in 1790. The other volumes conform with the first edition as described by L. Baumgartner and E. Mapelsden Ramsey.

In selecting excerpts from Frank's complete text of 6262 pages, the editor was fully aware of the difficulties lying before her in presenting a collection which represents the intentions of the author and his era. His work quotes a large number of ordinances, includes descriptions of customs at all phases of human life and of a wide variety of peoples from different epochs and is therefore archaic and subtle while at the same time presenting extensive historical digressions. Frank's erudition and his thoroughness is reflected in the enormous number of footnotes.

The abundance of factual material made it necessary to find some guiding principle to aid in the selection of topics for the English edition. The editor's primary concern was to present Frank's main streams of thought and the problems that moved the 18th century. Another criterion for the selection was to show the philanthropical mood of the period, its thoughts on population which were combined with Rousseau's theories and, finally, the enlightened author's liberal standpoint on social problems.

The division into parts, sections, and paragraphs of the third edition was retained. Omissions are marked by asterisks, thus enabling the reader to compare any passage with the German original. Transition sentences help to maintain the continuity of the text.

The editor is conscious of the fact that such a comprehensive work attains its greatest value for the reader when accompanied by a well-constructed Index of Subjects and Places. In this index we have made an effort not only to present the medical subjects but also to analyse the psychological and sociological procedures portrayed by Frank in the language of the 18th century, and by so doing to make them manifest to the modern reader.

A SYSTEM OF COMPLETE MEDICAL POLICE

Volume One

Human Procreation and Marriage Institutions.
Preservation and Care of Pregnant Women, their
Fetuses, and of Lying-In Women in Each Community

PREFACE

At the beginning of 1776, in a special letter of invitation to scientists,* I explained in detail my intention, and gave my reasons for undertaking such a difficult task as providing a coherent system of Medical Police, for which material is difficult to find and new trails often have to be blazed which sometimes lead further than the individual's range of vision. I may truthfully admit: I imagined all kinds of obstacles beforehand, and in the execution I really encountered them abundantly, but why all this did not deter me from my undertaking, I beg my readers not to demand of me any other account except my mere silence for the future, if I did not in my first attempt give proof that I did not seek to inflict on the world, under the pretense of affected patriotism and philanthropy, my printed thoughts, but that I really put everything I had into this work.

It seems that in my letter I did not express my thoughts sufficiently clearly as some scientists received the impression that I intended to compile a mere collection of medical police ordinances from different empires and provinces and have it printed, for although I recommended to my acquaintances and other philanthropists the communication of such ordinances, this was done only so that I could submit by way of example excerpts of the good that has already been usefully executed, and so that I could find out what has been done in this area in one country which is ahead of another, and what has its own specific traits, and how much preparatory work had already been done on the whole.

To friends and well-wishers who have so far assisted me with contributions from their respective regions, I hereby publicly express my gratitude. Although the number of those who did not confine themselves to mere approbation is small, even approbation provided part of the encouragement which was so necessary to my undertaking.

To come to the point, I wish to explain that in preparing this work I diligently endeavored to eliminate everything that was either impossible or especially difficult to execute. Nevertheless I have no hope, even if I shall live to an active old age, to live

---

* "Epistola invitatoria ad Eruditos, de communicandis, quae ad Politiam medicam spectant Principum ac Legislatorum Decretis," Mannhemii, apud Schwan. 1776. 8.

to see half of my proposals fulfilled. Bad enough, I thought—with the inner conviction that the matter would be possible and useful despite all—bad enough that this is usually the expectation of all those who propose laws:

> Importunis frustra laboras rebus,
> Araneorum telis similes sunt leges,
> Parva quidem & debilia volentes cohibere.
> A potentioribus autem rumpuntur facile.

Could this vexing thought make me reverse my decision? . . . No! . . . For I would think too little of our descendants if I did not consider that they will do better with what my contemporaries and I leave to them, and from that good, I seek my reward. For I myself thought that a work such as the present one is either completely insignificant or else of importance forever to all mankind. I imagined that the interest of states changes from one country to the next, according to the different conditions of their neighbors and the changing times, but what is based on the healthy state and longevity of the citizens, on the way they spend the years of their lives, and on their healthy procreation is never subject to change and that truths had to be recorded which applied as much in the remotest ages as in our own days. Therefore, I was proud enough to think that the broad field which I opened to myself was one in which the influence of medical science on the well-being of the states would attain a new splendor if my diligence were blessed and that physicians would cease to be regarded as men who are only more or less successful in making others healthy in the republic.

To those who consider that all improvements are superfluous because to them things seem to go well enough, I have nothing to say. One must have a certain amount of warmth and love of mankind otherwise one finds fault with or sees something ridiculous in many arrangements, if they are aimed only at saving a few persons or children per year and what occurs in some district or other seems of little consequence. But in large states, where the people's need makes improvements valuable, they have their undoubted usefulness. I ask, therefore, expressly that my ideas and the possibility of their implementation not be judged from the standpoint of small districts, for it is not feasible for a dwarf to wear with seemliness the coat of a well-built man without many changes which can be easily effected since enough cloth is available.

On all occasions I enquired about the habits and customs of people in different countries, and I have attempted to report them here with an accuracy that may seem objectionable to some; for I believed that it is not amiss to give hints of this or that kind when things are being discussed which deserve to be abolished or imitated, or which prove that somewhere, a long or a short time ago, something was considered useful or detrimental to the community which elsewhere was not deemed worthy of attention at all. Perhaps, I said, thereby I shall give some philanthropist an impetus to new and useful thoughts for the benefit of the people; and then I will again have attained my purpose.

The frequent quotations here are not made to show my erudition, but because I believed that I should not disown any source from which I drew, and that I should facilitate consultations of books on such an important subject. Those police ordinances that seem to merit special attention I shall quote, if they are, or will be, known to me, in full or give a faithful excerpt. However, since in different places enactments concerning the same subject have been made, I shall give only individual examples, if there is no important difference, and add my thoughts.

Since this work deals with the most varied subject matters, I expect leniency if the reader does not find the same wealth of material everywhere. For although some of these subjects have already been treated by other writers more or less successfully, there still remains a considerable number of such concerning which deep silence has been observed so far, although it will become clear that these subjects are worthy of all our attention. As regards other subjects, it is still worth the effort to have them corrected by a physician or treated from a point of view closely related to the police.

Forensic medicine, even by its nature, is distinguished from the Medical Police: the former deals only with the thorough solution of juridical questions concerning natural occurrences, the detailed determination of which is the physician's task. The latter has as its subject the general health, care and appropriate order in it. Thus there is sufficient cause why I treat Medical Police separately, quite independently of forensic medicine. Moreover, in spite of all its imperfections, forensic medicine lacks less in elaboration and systematic order than the Medical Police which in many regions does not consist of more than what can be read about it in the introduction to an ordinary pharmacopoeia.

I do not know if it requires an apology that some matters in this book are treated at some length. It seemed necessary to me that in a work such as the present one, the task is not to present new discoveries and inventions, but to acquaint persons in authority in human society with the necessities of the nature of their subjects and with the causes of their physical ills, not to leave out anything that may have a bearing on the detailed knowledge of important subjects. Besides, since least of all I write for physicians, I had to make myself understood by everybody. This could not be done without occasionally explaining things that are not completely unknown. Henceforth, I shall express myself more briefly, and subjects will also come up for consideration about which so far nothing important has been said at all, or concerning which I shall be able to give eminent outside examples of measures that have already been taken. I have no doubt that the important considerations expressed in the second and third parts belong to those about which so far nothing has been said, at least by physicians, which might have made my endeavor seem superfluous.

Nowadays, endeavors are made to make various useful improvements in economic and other matters. But they concern only the wealth of a country and of its rulers. Even assuming that someone succeeded so well, which does not seem likely, that in one province there would be abundance: would it therefore be right to say that one single region was made happy? . . . Certainly not! . . . A golden waistcoat does not make a sick body happy, and a silver bier does not make up for a good citizen who was carried off in his bloom.—What is there above health? all people ask, and experience shows that nothing is treated more wastefully than health. And yet, in most countries, very few measures have been taken, although they could be expected to be among the duties of the authorities. One hardly sees anybody other than physicians take care of the noble jewel of public health, until suddenly a deadly epidemic raises its head: then everybody who wants to seem somebody shouts about the tardiness of the police. On the other hand, the police then expends more vain efforts and spends more money in one week in order to provide relief than would have been necessary to prevent the disease by prudent regulations. Health measures are almost like the fire-engines which have to be mended and put in order when a village is on fire; the fire dies of its own accord before they arrive, but the village is left lying in ashes. I thought long about the inactivity of some excellent men, men who stay awake many a night for the sake of their country, and it pained me that I had to accuse them of careless negligence. I said to myself that they are too busy to pick up the complaints of physicians from afar and to learn from other people's experience. Certainly, the physicians complain to each other in their books about the miserable state of public health care, but the medical title of a book results in only physicians reading it, and physicians cannot stop bad habits, or if they can, very few.

It was natural, therefore, to believe that a work of the given title would arouse the interest of various persons in authority, that these, although their time is very dear to them, would gladly listen patiently to the voice of a philanthropic physician discoursing on the general misery and ways of remedying it as far as possible, and that the detailed development of many subjects, some of which may seem minor, would never lose its value in their eyes if they were to be able to promote the general well-being of people.

Since the married state is the foundation of human procreation, I devoted special reflections to it, and I did not omit anything that seemed important to me in judging such an important matter. Therefore, I called things by their own names and described nature without a veil, as it were. Although I had great doubts finally whether or not to publish this first chapter, a special cause finally decided me. For I saw that in the Roman Catholic Church, which I also profess, and where abstinence is imposed for life on the spiritual members already on their receipt of subdeaconry, there are many young persons who, frequently without any consideration or testing of their nature, temperament and moral strength, and even without much chance to weigh them for lack of timely consideration, hurry posthaste into a profession which they can leave only very rarely. In most Catholic provinces which I know, I saw such a large number of members of the clergy of both sexes who, by their obvious regret, proved that they had deceived themselves in the choice of their profession, that I made up my mind out of pity for such a considerable number of annual sacrifices of a rash youthful zeal who are torn away from society without fulfilling the good intentions of the Church and without doing it honor, to describe with complete openness all the difficulties and obstacles that may be in the way of fulfilling a great vow. And to do it in such a way as to facilitate for every candidate of the priesthood the judgment of his physical predisposition for observation [of the vows] and to enable prelates and church authorities to proceed in the choice and acceptance of candidates with special caution and with some distrust based on experience of human nature, on the transitoriness of hasty, though pious, intentions and promises of young and inexperienced persons. Thus a good part of my first investigations is written more for my co-religionists than for others. The rest concerns only secular celibacy which, although much has been said in various places against it, increases daily, according to the greater moral debauchery, and must have a strong influence on the good condition of the world's citizens.

If, in such investigations, without my knowledge, I should utter an expression or thought that is against the general opinion of the Church to which I belong, I hereby withdraw it in advance, and I submit publicly to the authority of this Church.

There are many subjects which have a considerable bearing on public well-being but they are not to be treated by police laws, they are matters of mere good advice, and these I endeavored to avoid here because I would have had to digress. Others, which some of my readers may deem to belong to the same class, I considered worthy of the attention of the authorities. I believe that often nothing more is needed than the realization that a remedy may possibly be useful, in order that one may rise above the general prejudices and introduce an order, even if the majority of people laugh derisively, for precisely this largest part of mankind is almost always the most insignificant one where correct judgment is involved.

The general health of a state has its incidents and certain stubborn diseases, like the body of an individual citizen. Heroic means are then required to remedy the ill, and it would be a great loss of time if one went to work timidly and gave too great heed to the melancholic premonitions of faint-hearted physicians.

I found an example of such courageous efforts, which in certain German provinces perhaps would never escape criticism, in the police regulations of Paris. For several centuries the judicious care of the police authorities of this immense city has been concerned with the minutest details, and beneficial order confirms the value of most police regulations which originated there. I have profited so greatly from these that I hope I shall do my compatriots a service by acquainting them more closely, and at the appropriate place, with such regulations. And I do not doubt that the worthy authors of these regulations will not take it amiss if one believes that they are capable of greater perfection. By comparison and closer examination of these and similar laws which I shall quote successively, I shall endeavor to fill to the best of my ability the large gaps which, despite the obvious care taken hitherto, still exist on the whole in the Medical Police, to the obvious detriment of human society.

And if the unexpected lethargy of the scientists from many regions, whom I exhorted to cooperate, had not hindered it, I would have been able to provide, in addition to my own thoughts, the history of the medical institutions of most neighboring provinces and states simultaneously, and to the certain benefit of mankind, and the blessing of the founders of beneficial regulations. If in view of the lack of cooperation, I am deemed worthy of elaborating this subject further, the loss can be made up to a certain extent. This was also the reason why I decided not to publish my work at once but by and by, and thus in every conceivable way to prevent shortcomings that generally are unavoidable in my first attempt of a general Medical Police. Very few of the subjects that appear in this first volume have had many or important regulations issued about them as far as I know. Therefore, further philanthropic contributions by state governments, health counsellors, or individual well-wishers of this work will find their appropriate place. And although I already possess an ample stock of beneficial edicts on the health system, I do not doubt the usefulness of an extensive correspondence with philanthropists in whose support I shall not see any obstacles, not even of common passion that in such undertakings is easily foreseeable and of which it is said:

> Sick of a strange disease, his neighbor's health:
> Best then he lives, when any better dies.
> Is never poor bot in another's Wealth;
> On best mens harms and griefs he feeds its fill.
> Else his own maw doth eat with spiteful will,
> Ill must the temper be, where diet is so ill.*

According to my first plan, this work will consist of several volumes but I cannot determine their number more accurately; I only believe that I shall be able to conclude with the fifth volume. Nor can I stipulate the time which will elapse between the publication of each volume, for the judgment of the public about this first attempt will serve as encouragement for me or otherwise, about the decision whether to continue with my work or cease.—Since in the present volume I treated everything that was to be said about human procreation, and endeavored to put all subjects of Medical Police up to the instant of the birth of a new citizen into a bright light, it was left to me only to treat of extramarital procreation, and of abortion of the fetus. Since there is so much of importance to say on this subject, however, which might have caused this volume to become too thick, I had to leave it for the subsequent volume. All the more so since I have to speak there in another context simultaneously of the abandonment and murder of children by unmarried mothers. —If it is a valid excuse for a writer, who himself recognizes unequal quality in his utterances, faults in style, and other shortcomings, to say that he was often distracted, I am entitled to expect every indulgence from my readers, for I have very few moments

---

* Fletcher's "Purple Islands."

as free as I could have wished in my zeal for elaborating such important subjects. I leave it to the judgment of the public whether my confidence in their patience is wrong therefore.

Written at Bruchsal in the Bishopric of Speyer 1778.

PREFACE TO THE SECOND EDITION

Since the first printing of this volume of Medical Police, according to my publisher's reminder, is out of print and a new edition is necessary, I endeavored to enrich and improve it as much as my position permitted me. But to prevent the owners of the first edition thus being deprived, I saw to it that the additions and changes in the new edition would be supplementarily supplied by the publisher in an appendix at the end of this work at a low price. The third volume of Medical Police already represents half of my plan; the remaining half will be published by and by, as my other occupations permit. Whoever bears in mind how much space the appended foreign regulations and examples require, will not be surprised at the size of the planned extent of the work. I wanted to elaborate Medical Police in detail, and not publish a mere excerpt of a teaching which before me nobody supplied coherently (as has been generally admitted to me). I had to convince the public with pertinent reasons of the necessity and the utility of this science. I could not have achieved this with a compendium, which I could have written more easily.

Will the increased field of the police (as has been feared since the first publication of this work) thus immensely limit the natural freedom of man, which is being more and more curtailed anyway, abuse the rights of the family fathers, husbands, parents, and will that which is thus wrongly taken from them be put into the despotic hands of the authorities?—After what I said in the introductions to the first, and especially to the third volume, I shall gladly leave the decision to every philosophical observer of human nature. I only believe that I must add the following.

It is incomprehensible to me how anyone can hope to retain natural freedom in social life without curbs, and it seems to me this is philosophizing a la Rousseau. Can one not raise equally valid objections to all laws? . . . And will the time ever come then when we shall return to our half brothers, the other animals, into the woods?

I understand the objections well; people want fewer laws, and with the few laws they want to retain their complete freedom.—But is this not a clear contradiction? . . . I must not rob, must not take revenge, must not abuse, beat, murder anybody; I must not, like the ancient Romans did, abandon my newly born children, execute my children, tyrannize my servants or have them flogged and strangled . . . my natural freedom suffers from that; but is it not better for me, for all members of the state, to know that in those matters and a thousand others, our hands are bound because of the care of the authorities? Yes, but Medical Police! . . .

Well, it will make every father of a family responsible for the behavior of his family as regards public safety. It will force a husband to fulfill his most important duties toward his healthy and his ill, pregnant wife, his wife just giving birth or lying in childbed. It will, if necessary, take to task the parents concerning the life, the physical education, punishment, and employment of their children. It will place difficulties in the way of a marriage between a lascivious old woman and a greedy flourishing young man, between a declared consumptive and a healthy hopeful maiden. It will prevent the citizen from driving his cattle, suffering from infectious diseases, among the healthy communal herd; prevent him or his family, if suffering from an infectious epidemic or the plague, from walking about the open market and infecting the whole town; prevent him from engaging in trading with goods which even in the present century threatened not only Marseilles and Toulon, but the whole of France with destruction; see that in populous cities he does not direct his latrine toward the public road and dig a deep dung pit in frequented roads; or that he does not carry on a murderous trade with Aqua tofana, Poudres de Succession, and with abortifacients, etc.

In all this and other tasks of Medical Police, there is nothing that could possibly violate freedom in a community, or make the sensible citizen a slave of the law-giving authorities. They only take care of him and, so-to-say, take away from their children the knife with which they could injure themselves gravely.

It is remarkable that Medical Police is charged with too much curtailment of civic freedom and with aiding legislative despotic power, and that the wrongly understood word freedom is used as a weapon, while on the other hand it is not realized that by attempting to defend mankind against some unwarranted attacks by ill-advised laws and detrimental, albeit sanctified, customs, I may have exposed myself to the danger of being considered in various places a preacher of excessive freedom! . . . What can one do to avoid both reproaches?—However, by such a complaint, by replying to the objections of a single man, or at the most two skillful men, who judged my work very favorably, I put myself into the danger of seeming ungrateful to the German public which received my system of Medical Police with such flattering and loud approbation! . . . Therefore, only one more remark:

Although in such a work mere classification is not all that important, if only the exposition of the matter is orderly, I nevertheless cannot see how the separation of Medical Police from forensic medicine can be subject to the slightest doubt. The former is as much different from the latter as any state government is different in its actions from any high court of justice; I think the comparison fits perfectly.

Bruchsal, St. Lawrence Day, 1783.

INTRODUCTION TO MEDICAL POLICE

Of Medical Police, of the population in general, and of the present state of public health among civilized nations

The internal security of the state is the subject of general police science.* A very considerable part of this science is to apply certain principles for the health care of people living in society, and of those animals which they need for their work and their sustenance. Thereby the conditions under which the population** live are improved so that the people can enjoy with pleasure and for a long time the advantages which social life really offers them, without suffering too much from the risks and the degeneration to which such a life had to debase them once they had made up their minds to tame nature in its wildness, and to renounce for ever certain advantages which in no province were as predominant as in the rough and iron-like state of the still unaffected humans.

Medical Police, like all police science, is an art of defense, a model of protection of people and their animal helpers against the deleterious consequences of dwelling together in large numbers, but especially of promoting their physical well-being so that people will succumb as late as possible to their eventual fate from the many physical illnesses to which they are subject. It is strange only that this science, so indispensable to our race, has been kept to such a trifling amount down to our times, and is treated only piecemeal here and there, and as far as I know, has not been treated

---

* Von Sonnenfels, "Principles of the Police, Commercial and Financial Science," Part I, §29.
** By population, I do not mean to say that it is more advantageous to plant people everywhere more densely; it is known that this is not the way to go about it if one wants to obtain abundant harvests. I only believe that where they are too thinly planted, it must be made up, but where they grow only like suffocated plants in order to fill a place without any use whatsoever, measures should be taken to replant that place with more useful, albeit fewer, citizens. The task of the Medical Police is to make liberal use of the possibilities of nature and its energy in such a way that from every given couple of persons of both sexes, and under the supervision of good laws, the best, healthiest and most durable fruits will be obtained. After Europe, to its misfortune, sent many of its citizens to the newly discovered America, and after the recent bloody troubles in Germany, it seems to me we should welcome this opportune lesson.

systematically by anybody.* Perhaps this is because people started late to calculate the value of a person and the advantages of the population, and because these calculations gave an impetus only to philanthropic considerations of the causes of a decrease in population about which there have been complaints in some regions?

It is not so long ago that the Medical Police in almost all countries did not deal with anything except complaints and made impotent intercessions against quacks and charlatans. At the most, in times of plague certain precautions were contemplated and certain measures and prescriptions were made known to the public in print, and physicians and gravediggers were allocated their place and tasks. In healthy times, meaning times when no special epidemics were rampant, there was hardly any worry about general health, as if only those diseases which depopulated the provinces really mattered. As if the country's loss was not the same when its citizens died by the thousands because of various specific diseases and bad conditions, and when they were lost due to a single epidemic. The numerous accidents to which people in every community are exposed either due to their own carelessness or the incautious behavior of their fellow citizens, through the nature of their ordinary actions or through violent physical causes, were nowhere subject to the supervision by the authorities, or if they were it was in only a few places where providence entrusted life and well-being of a society to an active philanthropist. Resuscitation of citizens in such unforeseen misfortunes was not even taken into consideration: it was even a crime to alter the position of someone who was found choked in the water or in an open field, or for unknown reasons hanged before a formal court investigation had been held. Such investigation lasted so long that what little life may still have been in the person found, was completely lost. In our times, we have a new procedure: thus several hundred of such apparently dead persons, on whom successful remedies were used, have been wakened from the sleep of death by the philanthropist's hand, and were returned to society and to their relatives. Fifty years ago with what killing indifference in otherwise civilized countries and unfortunately even nowadays in some provinces, were pregnant women and women giving birth left to the mercy of the most contemptible crowd of superstitious women who, upon their appointment, were at the most instructed by the priest about the required rules of baptism. And have we not in our time, when religion preaches true humanitarianism in such a noble manner and says so much about our obligations toward our fellow man, permitted a most abominable law to remain from heathen times—and which even they disregarded—that no pregnant woman should be buried before giving birth. It is true, our forebears founded many hospitals in a most generous manner, and built shelters for the hungry and the miserable, which must immortalize

---

* A short time ago, Professor Baumer in Giessen had printed: "Fundamenta Politiae medicae, cum annexo catalogo commodae Pharmacopoliorum visitationi inserviente," Frfrt. & Lipsiae 1777 in 8vo. 200 pages thick. But this is a handbook intended for his own lectures, which must be complemented by spoken discourse, and it has little in common with my plan.

the glory of their good intentions. But, since most of these foundations lacked prudent arrangement to serve suffering mankind as well as was possible, and their design and equipment reflected more the founder's good will than accurate knowledge of the best way of remedying the worst misery, it cannot be denied that many a hospital is more a source of mortality than of the sought salvation, for lack of good Medical Police, as I shall demonstrate later on. For how long did an incomprehensible prejudice regarding pernicious cattle diseases make physicians completely useless to the state, only because the treatment of sick animals was considered contemptible, and because of lack of knowledge, the state's treasure was calmly left to mechanical treatment by ignorant blacksmiths, shepherds, and other such persons. And well-intentioned physicians, who were ready to disregard the prevalent prejudice, were prevented from making investigations and accumulating practical knowledge.

Eventually, but not much earlier than the beginning of the present century, people began to realize the advantages of having a better order in the public health system. Here and there societies were founded which took over the care for public health, and these, these Collegia sanitatis, or health councils, began to appoint properly qualified physicians and surgeons in the provinces. Botanical gardens were founded in order that the science of herbs might be propagated and to teach how the useful plants could be distinguished from the poisonous ones in every region. It is now known how greatly agriculture and cattle breeding gained by that. Under this supervision, public schools of midwifery undertook instruction of future midwives. Unfortunate mothers, who otherwise would have become infanticides, were looked after in special houses until they gave birth. There, newly instructed midwives and young accoucheurs received practical training; churchyards which exhaled nothing but a smell of death were removed from towns here and there; funerals were banned from churches and temples in which entire congregations formerly had been infected by deadly poison. Care was taken that hospitals were built on better sites, and that their design and construction were better, that the air in the rooms was improved—whereas in former times, more patients suffocated than died of the diseases with which they had entered the hospital. In addition to these improved hospitals, buildings were erected for the dissection of human corpses where practical physicians had an opportunity to discover hidden faults of the body, correct the mistakes they had committed, by thereafter treating unknown diseases more knowledgeably and defeating them. The beginner was able to become better acquainted daily with the constitution of the human body, and now even in small towns, they have an opportunity which previously had to be sought at great cost only at universities. Now provincial physicians had to give an account of the measures they had taken against native and foreign diseases, and the health council used its joint forces against all public ills, infectious epidemics, diseases, and physical attacks. Inventors of famous remedies were rewarded, substantial prizes were granted for the saving of accident victims, and experienced physicians were called upon to communicate their instructive experiences. Public veterinary schools were founded in which the animals that had died of the most nauseous diseases were dissected, regardless of all prejudices, and the cause of death assessed, and thus for the benefit of mankind, a foundation was laid for a better future, curative method, etc.

How greatly useful are such measures, and can the honor of the developing sciences be defended in a better way than by making mention of such philanthropic arrangements beneficial to the community, and which are due only to greater enlightenment and better insight into the general good of societies? With all this, it must be admitted that we are still very backward in the art of defending our health for the longest time, and in utilizing the forces of nature to our advantage as far as the particular constitution of our republic permits; examples of good are less attractive, and notwithstanding the excellent arrangements for the public health at one place, entire provinces abandon themselves to the stream of physical incidents either out of ignorance or out of a certain sleepiness, with no other defense than that of any other dumb animal which does little more than sigh under the power of the pains in its illness, and when the illness does not improve on its own, dies.

Several philanthropists,* therefore, have also mentioned how important a work is which would treat coherently all the important subjects connected with Medical Police, and lecture in good order on the remedies that are already in use, as well as on those which are offered for the promotion of public health and need thorough consideration. Therefore, I shall not go into detail now concerning the subjects which will be treated later, beyond what I have said in my announcement; I want only to point out that all the phenomena, the present constitution of most persons, and the decrease in the number of inhabitants, which is deplored on many sides, are new and certainly important causes for wishing to put the best rules for improving the health system in most countries before everybody and to see them implemented by clear-thinking supervisors.

Are these complaints about man's deterioration justified? As it is, population is a relative matter with numerous relationships to a country's internal budget, its cultivation, and nutritional benefits, which make a natural increase in inhabitants practical and preferable to artificial increase. Thus, even if we knew the number of the former inhabitants of our continent (and it is really unknown to us) we would still undoubtedly lack much knowledge which would be needed to compare the former with the present population. Germany certainly was never so populous as it is in its present state, and in all probability there were only few countries so populous, in spite of the immense armies which were reputed to have taken the field in

---

* Wolfgang Thom. Rauen, "Thoughts about the Usefulness and the Necessity of a Medical Police Order in a State." Ulm, 1764. 8. 2nd edition—Rickmann, "Of the Influence of Medical Science on the State," Jena, 1771. 8.—S.A.H. Reiser, "Of Health and its Influence on the Happiness of Men," Giessen, 1776. 8, etc.

the past.*   But things look quite different when one questions whether the present population is in the same relation to substantial improvements in agriculture in Europe, and to other improvements as [the population] was in the past when our wandering forefathers did not profit from good breeding. Even if this were so, the people's increase in annual expenditures, caused by increasing luxury, a certain change of the earth's surface, new—or at least more widespread—diseases, greater induced effeminacy, even the increased interest in sciences and a tendency toward an idle way of life, senseless customs, and many other motives, would prove more than sufficiently the small advantage of our increased population over that of former times, so long as it is not proved that the fertility of our marriages has increased greatly over that of our forebears. I for my part am rather inclined, for most comprehensible reasons, to believe that the opposite is true. The fact that our lists of deaths year after year show fewer persons who have left this world than were born is, in our times, not too convincing a proof. For it is known, and the English admit it, that not all lists are incontrovertibly correct; many a foreigner is recorded twice or more times in the same list of the living, whereas the citizen who perishes on his travels on the water or in some other way, remains unconsidered, and finally, because roving creatures cannot be counted like trees.

    To compare accurately the present population with that of past times with the

---

* There are provinces wherein depopulation seems certain if one compares the number of their present inhabitants, not with that of ancient times, but with their flourishing state, after agriculture and various arts had already been introduced. Spain lies mostly fallow since the diligent Moors no longer have to till the soil there. It is also known how much foreign acquisitions in America cost this empire and others in Europe in terms of human losses, after the unbelieving innocents had been massacred most cruelly. Italy, although very populous in some of its fortunate provinces, nevertheless suffers a lack of people in other parts, especially in the Roman region (J. Bapt. "Donius De re restituenda salubritate agri Romani"). It is known that France lost a large number of diligent citizens upon revoking the Edict of Nantes, and Prussia's gain and that of other Protestant countries derived from the population increase through those expelled, is France's loss. It is certain that many affluent families were disrupted and reduced their reproduction for rather a long time. Without indulging in detailed calculations, we know that the taste for marriage decreased surprisingly, and the number of illegitimate children increased greatly in all large towns of this Empire; hence, it can be concluded that France did not have the population increase it could have had because of its favorable situation.—The depopulation in Switzerland and its causes were pointed out by Tissot, and recent reports in the "Ephemerides of Mankind" for the year 1777 confirm that in the last forty years in Basle the number of marriages has dropped to one half or less; moreover in the country, too, and in the last ten years in all cantons marriages, and consequently the population, also declined. Sweden, too, has fewer people than before, as proved by Royal Physician-in-Ordinary Bäck in the Proceedings of the Royal Swedish Academy 1764.—Poland at present has barely a third of her possible inhabitants, even if one disregards what the last Turkish war and the many uprisings cost in terms of human lives, and Hungary seems to be open to the same reproach.—But it is not my intention to indulge here in political calculations. Suffice it for me to name means to ensure that the living people and their descendants enjoy enduring health and consequent happiness. A physician looks after the lives and health of the citizens; let the state see to it how to feed them and use them to its greatest advantage.

aid of birth and death lists is a very uncertain procedure, where one must expect inaccuracies of several thousand. Whereas, in the past such lists did not exist at all, one cannot take for a fact the figures given by gullible historians who obviously exaggerated everything, and which defy reason and probability. On the other hand, so instructive are the calculations of these far-fetched relationships, owing to the way of thinking, that the present population accepts them. This contribution indicates that we make up for the losses [of population] by increased food and development of the arts.

The consequences of luxury, if we are to follow just one point, may be considered from so many viewpoints that perhaps both sides are partly right, those who vie in praising and those who jeer at luxury. As it is viewed by the sceptical, luxury on the one hand increases particularly the livelihood [of farmers and peasants] and work for the needy thereby circulating the treasures of the rich, and apparently doubling the possibilities of marriage. On the other hand, increasing luxury destroys this advantage, and the refinement of social life again costs our race dearly! "An unbiased comparison should be made," says Rousseau, "between the state of the citizen and that of the savage. One should search, if possible, what different paths the former, without including his evil inclinations and requirements, paved for themselves to pain and death. If one contemplates the gnawing commotions of the mind, the tearing and exhausting passions, the more than irksome labors suffocating the poor*

---

* Extravagance gives rise to poverty, and poverty gives rise to illness. The more miserable a country is, the more infirm and sick subjects it has to feed. Lack of the necessary foodstuffs emaciates entire families and causes them throughout their lives to haunt their environment like skeletons. It is precisely this lack which forces people to seek the most indigestible means of stilling their hunger, and in recent expensive times moldy bread has been a treat for entire households. The bloodiest war only begins to have its real effect on human entrails when its consequence is starvation; then people drop as they do during the plague, and illness caused by exhaustion soon empties entire empires. Like gnawing worry, the coarse and raw foodstuffs gradually spoil all the body's juices and the children of such miserable persons are weak and vapid creatures, with swollen bellies and constipated entrails, and their mortality is very great. Already at the tenderest age, they must help earning their scanty livelihood by the heaviest labor, and thus sweat out the forces which should support their bodies' growth. Therefore, in most villages, especially in wine country where most of the dung has to be carried on human backs to the high mountains, and the earth constantly scraped in a crawling position (work which formerly was less necessary in Germany), one sees most young people there deformed and stunted, for beauty is incompatible with extreme poverty and with suffocating labor. If one looks at the draft animals which are forced into heavy labor before their maturity, one sees the image of youth forced into all kinds of work before their time. Tallness and strength are lost under the burden of misery, and the most perfect animal degenerates under it. No joy (the most essential vital balm) refreshes the oppressed peasant anymore, and everyone sighs under the yoke of extravagance which raises the price of all foodstuffs, and sucks the blood of the poor to the last drop. In all epidemics, it is the poor who are attacked first. The number of [state] appointed physicians in every region is not sufficient to look after the mass of poor patients in an epidemic, and where there is a shortage of bread, the most essential means for restoring health are certainly lacking. Either for this reason, or because the despairing do not wish to live, the physician is hardly ever called: they know that the physician will come . . . but

and the even more dangerous effeminacy to which the rich abandons himself, by which both die, the former due to want, the latter due to abundance.* If one sees the immense mixing of foodstuffs, their detrimental preparation, their spoilage, the adulterated spices, the cheating by vendors, the mistakes in preparation, the poison which the food extracts from the vessels in which it is prepared; if one contemplates the epidemics which spring from air that is filled with too many people; if one calculates the diseases which we owe to our effeminacy, the consequences of the sojourn in closed rooms from which we again move into the free air, the illnesses due to rash changes of clothing, the extraordinary lasciviousness which has become second nature to us and from which we cannot be easily rid, one realizes immediately how dearly nature makes us pay for scorning its lessons.—One would not be less shocked

---

they also know that his arrival will make them feel their misery even more deeply, as the poverty does not permit of their obtaining the prescribed remedy. This is an important reason why the average person prefers the quack who himself advertises his medicines and offers them more cheaply, although in reality they are not cheap. Thus one sees that the peasant and the needy citizen out of their feelings of impotence fight their dangerous illnesses and carry on their work or day-labor for a long time while half dead and thus spread an infectious disease. Once he remains in bed, the whole house becomes sick, for there the sick and the healthy lie side by side. Under such circumstances if the poor had some attention and the necessary moderate nutrition, nature alone would often help; however, all too often even this is lacking, which makes poverty really terrifying.

However, one should not think that here the object of my description is only the beggar. Misery among the lower classes is almost general, and a silk overcoat often may cover the worst bareness only because the laws of exaggerated luxury demand it. The priest and the physician know how bad the poverty is in some houses the exteriors of which indicate affluence; quiet tears here express the misery better than does the moaning of the poor in the street who, without blushing, may admit their real misery and call loudly for help.

Poverty following upon affluence seeks to hide as long as possible, and even the habit of living extravagantly causes people to resist their fate. This is the moment when morals are in the gravest danger, and all means are tried to maintain the former way of life. A young wife, a well-formed daughter now must be made to jump into the breach, or in order to continue their lavish expenditure on clothing, do it on their own. As physician I would not have to say anything to this, were it not certain that all debauchery is punished by physical penalties, and that in this way almost always an abhorrent disease is fated for households which, without the madness of pretending to be so noble, would never have been made to resort to such desperate means of keeping up the style of life appropriate to their rank.

* All abundance induces gluttony and gourmanderie and it is known that by weakening the mental and physical strength of people these have destroyed the greatest empires: Rome itself has been overwhelming proof of this. It must be admitted that nowadays in Germany people in general eat too much, just as in the past they used to drink too much. In the past, drinking killed many thousand people and was the reason that half the city dwellers in the evening were barely any better than their domestic animals as far as reason is concerned. Nowadays this vice has largely lessened, at least in southern regions. On the other hand, instead of ten large wine bottles, the rich now put twenty more platters filled with unhealthy food, from which the fair sex as well as tender youth help themselves as much as the strong man, and fill themselves with hotter things than the wine which was consumed by only the master of the house and his male guests. Just look in the best houses in the morning to see to what our Haut Goût and the facetious cooks have reduced people, how everybody complains of indigestion, aching

about the number of those whom the sea devours every year* or who perish at sea of hunger, scurvy, by the hands of pirates, or through fire. To these should be added the large number of unhealthy crafts which shorten life or at least damage good body constitution. I have in mind work in mines, the various processes of ore dressing, especially lead, copper, mercury, cobalt, arsenic fumes from foundries, realgar, and other extremely dangerous machinations of the roofers, joiners, bricklayers, and stone-masons which daily cost many persons their lives;** if one puts all these subjects together, one will soon realize that the cause of the decrease of our race,

---

stomachs, and limbs, which we physicians politely call nervous diseases, of which no house in large cities is free and of which droves of persons die every year. Would it not have been more advisable perhaps to correct the old mistake rather than bring about such a sad change? It is true that excessive drinking at least does not have the evil effect on our health that too much and too hot foodstuffs have on us. Our times, beyond a shadow of doubt, have chosen the worst, if one bears in mind that whereas formerly only the best wine was offered in the form as yielded by nature, now all the wines that are brought to table are foreign, and their composition is a secret known only to the spice merchant and poisoning wine merchants. In almost all countries, especially in the north, frequent drinking of brandy has become very common, and this contributes not a little to the deterioration of most nations, as I shall show in more detail later on.

* The East Indian Trading Company, which was founded in 1602 in Holland, reckons that the number of ships which returned to the company back from India up to 1740 is 2000. On the other hand, up to that time, more than 230 ships were lost due to storms and other causes, and did not return (Bösching, "New Description of the Earth," Part 4, Introduction). Between 1734 and 1740 on 73 ships which sailed to and from the Cape of Good Hope and were manned by 15,889 persons, 1,733 died, i.e., eleven out of a hundred. On eleven ships, which returned from Batavia to Holland and which were manned by 1,203 persons, 34 died before reaching the Cape, and 46 died between the Cape and Holland, i.e., a total of 80, thus one out of fifteen (Süsmilch, l.c. Part I, Ch. 24). If one considers the ships sent to sea by other nations, more than before the wars fought at immense distances with formerly unknown nations, the incomprehensible participation of Germany in such foreign quarrels, and the unfeeling sacrifice of German blood in trading persons for a few thousand pounds sterling, which moreover rarely benefits the country but only the princely merchant, and if one adds the ordinary taxes to the expenses which an excessively courageous undertaking causes because of exaggerated confidence in improved knowledge, no matter how much the danger is reduced, owing to improved navigation; if one considers how little the sailors do for the population nowadays, because of their audacious and almost incessant travels at sea, and if one calculates the damage which persons of this class do because of their almost general immorality one can conclude the rest from these chapters alone.

** It suffices to think of the many hundreds of thousands of Negroes and slaves whom European greed buys, to the shame of religion, and puts into the gold mines of Peru and Mexico for the rest of their lives and lets them rot there; of the many persons who must sweat blood in unhealthy plantations so that we can have our sweet tea and coffee, and while talking of unhealthy crafts, just look at the innumerable wigmakers most of whom become consumptive from the large amount of dust with which they must daily powder empty heads, the lace factories in which thousands of young and old people eternally sit and have to become crippled in order to supply us with finely spun yarn with which the women ruin their husbands, the powder mills which cost so many persons their lives, and an even larger number of new towns which boundlessly increase our mortality—of this I shall treat more in the course of this work.

which has been noted by more than one philosopher, lies in the origin and perfection of the way human beings dwell together."*

Just as our increasing love of comfort and pampering increases our requirements and raises them to lusts the fulfillment of which is fraught with manifold dangers, so is it proven also that our perfection in the art of satisfying our sensuality in every conceivable way, and to do as if by machines everything to which our fathers needed only arms and hands,**etc., are the main cause of our deterioration. And no matter what one says in favor of luxury, it is always open to the reproach that for the hundred paths which it opens up to the population it opens up as many abysses to the lives of the citizens, and every state can calculate with horror its loss from these, incurred in exchange for the simpler and much healthier way of life of previous times for the sake of some present comfort. It is the worst feature of luxury that it covers the most deleterious objects with a dazzling gloss, and makes people believe, by a kind of pleasant intoxication, that they are very happy, while in reality they are in the midst of perdition. Later on I shall have an opportunity of going further into this subject, where it will then become clear that the strongest proofs against luxury must be sought in its effect on our physical constitution and on the general health and well-being of people, and that even if a large part of our incomes should be lost by reducing luxury, human society would still gain very much by it.

The history of the artificial changes of the surface of the earth cannot compete in numbers and magnitude with the pictures which Nature itself has left us frequently enough of its own regular revolutions in and on the globe. But it is an indication of the influence which these changes have exerted on the health and well-being of empires, and on the character of their inhabitants, and these are of much greater importance to the inquiring friend of the human race. Social life and the sciences have turned immense cleared woods into populous provinces, and extensive swamps into fertile plains.

* * *

There follow examples from history.

Whether this is a gain or a loss, after what I have said before, will become clear elsewhere; but this can be stated with some confidence already now: assuming that our forefathers had a special way of life, and that through constant change of their residence they were hardened against the effect of the changed atmosphere on their less sensitive bodies, a moist and swampy region was not to them what it is to their coddled grandchildren. Human nature in its original strength becomes used both

---

* J. J. Rousseau, "Discours sur l'origine et les fondements de l'inégalité parmi les hommes," p. 139. N. 7.

** In all of Italy, there is no greater disgrace for persons of the least nobility than to walk on foot, and even foreigners who know better, must acquiesce in using a carriage for distances as short as 20 paces, if they want to be received in society and not to be looked upon with disdain.

to the greatest heat and cold, as well as to considerable dryness or humidity of the surrounding air; it is sensitive only to the excessively abrupt changes in these, and sometimes they are deleterious. Against this a country is well protected if it has large and well placed forests which cut off various winds and thus prevent the communication of some terrible ills and keep at bay the effect of burning summer heat, which is such a widespread cause of illness and death in the country during the harvest.—By the clearing of forests to gain land for other use, our climate undoubtedly became milder, just as Italy enjoys a milder climate than in Augustus' time since the neighboring empires Hungary, Poland, and Germany itself are to a larger extent under cultivation and therefore warmer than before. Even the inclement climate of Sweden, according to Gaddi's remarks, has become milder since so many forests have been cleared there.—But it is just by this increased warmth that people became weaker and more coddled, and today's young German man with his light silken dress would be like a woman, compared to his manly forebear clothed in deerskin; moreover, stagnant waters, swamps, and lakes have become more deleterious to us since they evaporate infinitely more rapidly under the continuous sunrays, and begin to decay sooner than they did in the past. Also, for good reasons, southern countries have the advantage over northern ones with respect to health due to the large amounts of snow and ice water in northern regions, these giving rise to many swamps which become dangerous in summer because of their great evaporation. The inhabitants of Jamaica and the island of Barbados have been robbed of needed shade by the rash clearing of most of their forests, and now they suffer more from diseases than ever before due to the great heat to which they are exposed. The great usefulness of trees on earth, and especially in hot countries is, according to some experiments, that the exhalations of plants greatly improve the air which is putrified by the constant exhalations of animals and other causes. As mentioned before, the usefulness of the many trees in diverting certain winds is not inconsiderable, and forests lying to the south may, according to certain experiences, be considered especially good dams against many diseases, but here the importance lies in which regions the winds usually blow over, as what they easily receive, they also communicate to others on their journey. The Romans, therefore, did not permit large forests to the west to be cleared because these were a natural protective wall against putrid and poisonous exhalations and against the terrible Sirocco, or southeast wind.

* * *

Further examples from history follow.

It is true that if forests are too plentiful and too dense, they prevent the soil from drying up and choke off almost all the salutary movement of air from refreshing winds. They must, therefore, be almost as harmful [as too little forests], but this is a shortcoming that can be remedied within a short time and by little skill. I believe that our fathers saw to it that our forests afforded some ventilation, for they crisscrossed them day and night when pursuing their ordinary food, namely game, and with their tame cattle, and in so doing they had to clear or burn out the valleys to convert them into meadows and pastures. But they did this without shaving the entire surface of the earth, as we do, thus exposing their bodies to the violent power of storms and winds and sharing the putrid atmosphere with their unfortunate neighbors in a dry region.

If, in addition to that, it is borne in mind that the taste for large towns is getting the upper hand everywhere and that, after large swamps have been dried out, people have been led into artificial but much more dangerous swamps and have been lured to live in them permanently, that almost everywhere there is a shortage of wood* and entire nations have to use the stinking pit coal for cooking and heating and thus fill the air with unhealthy exhalations, if one bears in mind that the ease of hostile attack in dry plains forced these people to take recourse to the old advantages by which nature protected nations mutually from each other, and to lower themselves into fortresses, between artificially created morasses and moats full of stinking puddles, and to poison themselves in order to save their lives, if, in order to live in constant idleness, one has to scrape the soil all year round and have a class of people, who are devoted only to work, cover entire fields around human abodes closely with putrid filth and manure at certain seasons and have the air filled with exhalations which would force the most insensitive passerby to hold his nose, if all this is borne in mind it is easy to see whether the former aspect of the surface of the earth or the present spectacle is more conducive to health, and whether the change attained, which is often only dazzling gain on a small scale, is not really very deleterious to the public health of entire empires and the good state of the human body altogether.

* * *

Subsequently, Frank blames the appearance of new diseases for the increased mortality, and deals with the history of these diseases (smallpox, leprosy, syphilis, German measles, typhus). He sees other causes in the pampering of the female sex and the bad state of the public health service, and he arrives at the following conclusions:

---

* Shortage of wood, especially in countries that have neither pit coal nor peat to burn, is a very important cause of illnesses among the poor who often lack clothing and blankets. Parents, grownup and under-age children sit stiffly next to each other and seem to be awaiting their death when the greatest cold has already caused several of their animals in their stables to freeze.—Previously, things were different; the poor man collected the wood he required without the inhuman cries of the forester, and in view of the general abundance, did not have to carry it far because he was at home in the forest. In good time I shall mention the necessity of eliminating this injustice which we commit against the poor, and of establishing in every village one or several rooms where near-frozen wretches can recover.—Hail to those great ones who, in view of the inevitability of such a prohibition, think of the misery of the poor, and by their compassion and by frequent gifts of wood in winter, make the blood that curdled because of the cold, flow again in their honor.

With such a state and situation of public health in most regions, philanthropy requires all authorities and heads of republics to consider most carefully and examine thoroughly how to prevent further deterioration of the human species, how to diminish mortality by all available means, as far as it depends on people, and thus to return the human race gradually to its previous strength and dignity. . . . . For there is still hope that through wholesome efforts the growth of our race and its former esteem can be enhanced. For why should we be less successful in experiments with the animal-like man than in experiments with other animals whose races we have learned to improve sometimes in a whole country by diligence and art? . . .

One should only take in hand with the same diligence a much more important matter than this; one should not be deterred at the first contemplation of the frequently occurring difficulties. One should first seek with a certain doggedness all the causes of our ruin and the slow poison in the nation's veins, in order to develop then, if I may express it as a physician, the status morbi under which mankind groans. One should become as well acquainted with the small loss in people which a state suffers annually for some reason or other as with the annual increase in the number of citizens, and should thus learn ever better to know the true value of a person. Philanthropic physicians should investigate the nature, situation and condition of the smallest village, its diseases and their causes, the ratio of the sexes, of the different classes of men, calculate the ratio of births and deaths, and thus produce a kind of geography of each district. This geography would indicate the boundaries of life and death, the width and length of the dangerous lakes, and the safest routes between the reefs on which many thousands founder because of mere ignorance. The saving of individual persons must be viewed as a greater deed than the conquering of a province at the price of citizens' blood. All obstacles, especially those that violate public well-being, must be removed in every possible way, and public safety thereby actively restored, even for the as yet unborn citizen who is locked in his mother's womb. It does not suffice that a certain class of people is calmly left to look after the public health; wise laws must provide for order and advantage from such activities, only the worthier workers must be charged with the task. And, in regard to painstaking obedience to the necessary rules, which concern the maintenance and improvement of general health, those workers must take such measures as are of undisputed quality and feasibility in execution.

Of all these and many other useful subjects does Medical Police have to treat, and I shall consider it my duty not to omit the smallest matter that has any bearing on general health.—Subsequently the subject matter will be richer, and by the nature of the subject with which I deal, I shall enjoy more freedom; its lack often makes the exposition mournful, and the expressions seem labored.

PART ONE

Section One

Of human procreative urges in general, in respect to public health

§1

If it is said that the first concern of prudent statesmen should be that the population is commensurate to the nature, the food situation, and other circumstances of the country, this means only inhabitants who jointly carry the burden of social obligations and who can buy the fruits of social cohabitation by making alleviating contributions.—Society must view the addition of miserable and sickly bodies as a bunch of idle boarders whose maintenance must double the efforts of the working class. Thus, the means of increasing the number of inhabitants of a country is a drawback to the state, if it may be anticipated that the number of the infirm will increase.

§2

If the increase in the number of people were left to the free play of the instincts of the sexes, we would soon attain a number that would cause mankind to suffocate itself. Quarrels, want, and increasing misery would be the general fate, and thereby, masses of superfluous persons would be soon destroyed by the stronger. The same happens in the mother's womb when it has to nourish several children simultaneously: one child usually consumes the available juices and grows to the detriment of the others.

§3

All this was remedied by religion and our present constitution, apparently much later in one country than in another, where most people previously lived as the ancient Greeks had lived:

> Graecorum prius mulieres per Graeciam,
> Non quemadmodum nunc, conjugebantur legitimis viri;
> Sed instar jumentorum miscebantur omnibus volentibus,
> Erant igitur unius tunc naturae filii,
> Solas agnoscentes Matres, non patres.*

* "Tzezez historicus chiliad." Lib. V. cap. XVII.

24

§ 4

By means of such changes, which in cultured countries have finally become general, it has been made possible to forecast fairly accurately the size of the future population from the number of marriages concluded and, according to these calculations, it is in the nature of things that the number of persons in an otherwise well administered country may double within fifty or even fewer years unless this is prevented by plague or long drawn-out wars.

§ 5

Few countries are in as fortunate a position as their nature could permit. In most of them there are obstacles to human procreation the complete treatment of which cannot be expected of me since a large part of it is outside my field.—I select only those subjects that deserve examination by a physician either because they seem somewhat at odds with nature or because, due to physical causes, they reduce very much the fertility of married couples.—But before I communicate my thoughts on this subject, I consider it necessary to say something about the power of human procreation as part of our animal nature. This is not for physicians . . . For the Creator hid the secret of procreation so well from us that there is nothing I could tell them that would be outside the boundaries of known discoveries.

§ 6

When our nature was endowed with the ability of procreation, this was incorporated in the mechanical structure of certain parts which, since their functions necessarily depend on the circulation of our juices from the heart to them, are forced to carry out this function constantly, just as happens with the secretion of gall and saliva.—Nature has taken care that nobody, if of sound body, the maintenance of which is a duty, can completely suppress the constant effect of the natural forces fashioning the seed of posterity, if he cannot first stop the coursing of the juices in the genitals from which the excretion of semen depends.

Moreover, the Creator added to the procreative ability of animals a burning lust to appear active, so that it does not always depend on the free choice of the creatures, who do not always think or act in accordance with their intentions, on their comfort, or other seeming advantages and who might sacrifice posterity. This is the same as the urge to eat originates from a certain rubbing together of the inner surface of the sensitive stomach skin and on the stomach juice excreted there. This [procreative] lust likewise is produced by a sensitivity inherent in the structure of these implements and is produced by the semen excreted here. I do not know of any means that is able to withstand this mechanism with constant certainty in the physical sense; whoever (for no matter how noble a motive) resists while waking, is shamed in his sleep. So powerful are the mainsprings which nature instituted for the procreation of posterity . . . and the intention was worthy of the arrangement.

* * *

Subsequently, Frank deals with the anatomy and physiology of the male and female genitalia, using examples from the animal kingdom, also. He is particularly preoccupied with the consequences which in his opinion are due to the accumulation of semen.

* * *

§17

It has often been remarked that those who observe strict abstinence against their physical inclination and without being aided by nature with nocturnal or unintentional pollution, are fairly frequently the weariest of human society and are immersed in themselves. For often the disposition of a person suffers as much from complete retention of the otherwise so invigorating semen as from the opposite, namely its squandering. Therefore, it is said that it has been observed in England that out of twenty persons who have been torn away from society by taedium vitae, more than half are citizens who had been living alone.

* * *

There follow several examples.

Indeed, nothing has such a terrible power over our souls as the accumulation of semen. The difference between castrated and whole people is obvious to every observer, even if he is not very attentive. Compared with the whole bull, the draft ox seems to belong to a different species; likewise cows, sows, and some fishes whose ovaries had been removed, live free of all inclination to the act of procreation.

* * *

There follow several examples.

Thus two or three drams of a juice stored between the bladder and the rectum make us commit acts of foolishness which we would not commit for anything in the world when we are rid of that juice! . . .

* * *

PART ONE

Section Two

Of clerical celibacy

* * *

In the following paragraphs, Frank describes the various causes of ecclesiastical celibacy observed by various nations, and then he states:

§ 5

The generality of clerical celibacy in many religions

Yet it is a strange thing that so different nations have similar notions and accordingly almost universally hit upon the idea of forbidding their clerics any intercourse with women, either completely or at least for as long as they are engaged in the service of the deity; and that almost everywhere the opinion is held that one pleases the deity more easily by sacrificing certain desires.

* * *

There follow examples of different forms of ecclesiastical celibacy observed by different nations. Very courageously, Frank warns against making too early a decision on this matter.

§ 12

Danger of vows of chastity made too early by many persons

According to the frequent aforementioned experiences of physicians, it is certain that continence is a rare gift of nature which requires, in addition, special attention in itself, as well as to the external objects that cannot be easily avoided, so as to gradually dry up, if possible, an excretion, the continuance of which would cause worry because of future inappropriate and not easily explained evacuations. It is incomprehensible, therefore, how rashly the inexperienced young man, still ignorant of himself and of nature in general, and either out of religious fervor or because of persuasion by his relatives, or from longing for a rank which combines veneration with the certainty of an easy livelihood, or for other reasons, can decide as early as in his 18th or 20th year* to enter a profession whose proper observance requires so much.—How is it possible that such a man waives so early and forever all the rights the nature and relationship of which to his own physical constitution may be as unknown to him as the future development of his mentality—which in more mature years well may change greatly and those circumstances which so often determine our moral character . . . Surprised by cunning education, disguised examples, and artful pursuit, the inexperienced maiden, often brought to a state of taedium vitae by disappointed love, wraps herself in the wretched veil, and, after a few years, waters it daily with tears of desperation. Then time and changed circumstances demand that desires are to be denied which cannot be so easily dismissed by mutilating tender limbs and by enfeebling the body, which thereby is made just so much more suscep- tible. The Church does not approve of ways that are unknown to it, but as experience leads us to conclude, are now and again trodden, and it is against obtaining consent from the gullible weakness of youth, against which all nature rebels in more mature years. One forgives youth many moral lapses, which are often committed at a point of the human life which, compared with more mature age, deserves to be called a continuous enchantment, and are committed out of lack of reflection and experi- ence; . . . and at just this age, twenty-two or twenty-three years, sometimes even much earlier in the weak sex, the rash person makes a vow that presupposes so much experience and strength of character, because for one or two years of probation they made a very uncertain test of their moral strength against physical enticement;— should these be less worthy of the compassion of the Church and the superiors of the persons in whose power it is to provide aid?

§ 13

In various Catholic empires and countries the secular arm already a few years ago put a certain restraint on the so-called vows in monasteries by stipulating a more mature age, and thus curbing the rash zeal of youth. In the Austrian hereditary countries the twenty-fourth year for men and the twentieth for women were stipu- lated, in France the twenty-first for the former, and the twenty-eighth for the latter, and before this age no ecclesiastical vow will be accepted as valid.

Nevertheless, as long as there is no strict supervision of this, and as long as the

---

* In the oldest times not only seven-year olds, and after the Council of Trullos ten-year olds, but even children in their cradles were consecrated by their parents to monastic life, whereby the parents at the same time assured their donation in writing and promised God in the name of the minor all that was necessary. They also took all possible measures to prevent the entry of their children into the world, which might be possible in time. Eventually St. Bernard declared publicly that he was against this, nor did he even shrink from calling the consecration of children a human sacrifice. And at the end of the twelfth century, Clement III also forbade all Christians to make such dispositions in regard to their children at such a tender age. "Too Much Is Too Much, or Capitulation of the King of France with His Monastic Clergy," p. 194 ff.

ecclesiastical authorities do not help, and while public and ceremonial vows in monasteries and convents will have to be deferred up to the stipulated time, the binding force of vows made quietly will seem no less to the zealous candidate to the order, and the effect of the resolution will be no less certain, for resistance will only inflame it all the more.

§ 14

I do not want to assert that the usual age of 24 years, which is required of those who devote themselves to the priesthood, is insufficient for arriving at mature judgment of the inner relations or the mental strength against the impending wars of the natural desires. Nevertheless, as a physician I tremble for the full-blooded with very sensitive nerves, for I am afraid that the volatility of his temperament sometimes constitutes the most important part of both his good and his ambiguous decisions. I admit that I often believe such persons are less indifferent at that age than the decision of the question seems to require, a question which is to decide almost irrevocably the fate of an entire future life.

§ 15

Whether everyone may be permitted to make such early vows

Because of the character of persons who enter the service of the Church, it is to be feared that perhaps the largest number of young persons of both sexes who desire to enter the Church are liable to be rash. Lacking knowledge of themselves and being completely inexperienced, they make the mistake of not knowing how time and matters occurring in the world can change both the human heart and the human mentality. Thus, they choose a vocation in which an inner turmoil can arise so that either their vow or their health will be exposed to great danger. That being so, I leave it to the consideration and judgment of the ecclesiastical authorities to resolve the difficulties of a long delay of the vows, and to compare them with the advantages to be derived by a class of people in whom the foresight of various physical effects may make the moral decisions seem very ambiguous. In view of the great respect which I have for their excellent judgment into the matter, I forgo examining further whether it would not be better for the inner calm of the human conscience, for the good of the community, for the good of the Church itself, and for the sake of maintaining many thousand persons in good health:

Firstly, that the choice of suitable subjects for the clerical profession be made with much consideration to their maturity and physical predisposition.

Secondly, that never should a vow be accepted from either males or from females before the 28th year of the human age.

At that age, a more reasonable decision about whether he is suitable for fulfilling the law of abstinence can be reached by a person, on the basis of his having had more experience, and a better knowledge of himself. Thus, the now dissolved order of the Jesuits used to proceed carefully with its candidates who were admitted very young to the novitiate and to appointments of public teachers, but not readily to the profession of priest before their 28th or 30th year. Therefore, even past the age at which members of other orders have already been priests for several years, one saw several young men return from their [Jesuit] colleges to worldly life without hindrance, and therein, these young men did honor in the world to the good education which was typical of the order. At a riper age, they were better able than others to judge themselves and to save the order from the embarrassment of having to ascribe to youthful rashness the presence of an unhappy member who had fallen victim to his self-deception.

On the other hand, already in their twenty-second year, upon their request, other aspirants are usually granted the subdiaconate and the diaconate, or the first two great ordinations, and even if consecration to the priesthood is deferred until the usual time, the vow of abstinence is no less firm, and the future of their entire life is determined by a deed performed in early youth. It seems useful, therefore, even if the above proposals do not find the hoped for approval, that:

Thirdly, those young men who, having once decided to devote themselves to the priesthood, seem unable to await the stipulated time, or when they are refused, constantly entreat the ordinary and write petitions for the required age to be dispensed, and offer all kinds of pretexts, should be emphatically exhorted to have their suitability for this vocation thoroughly examined. This is most important in every respect.

Fourthly, as the priesthood is considered in several Catholic countries to be merely an opportunity for the younger sons of good families to be provided for, especially in France where the third son is always supposed to consider himself a born Abbé whether he has the necessary inclination and willpower for this profession or not, I leave it to higher judgment to take to heart the consequences that society must expect from this custom which is not in agreement with the spirit of the Church. It does not matter whether or not the frequent victims of their families submit to the vows that often clash completely with their nature.—Sometimes there may be very important reasons for not delaying the vows beyond a certain early age; nevertheless, it seems that here, more than with other candidates of the clerical profession, it is desirable that the vow is put off until a more mature age is reached, and that perhaps the noble young man is given time to do honor to his birth in some other way. If there is more freedom from the parents' coercion, or now and again some fortunate change in his family affairs, dispensation from the vows is usually demanded anyway, and sometimes given by Rome, thus making a free choice more easily possible.

Fifthly, that it should not be easily permitted to exaggerate the recruitment in convents by excessively attractive means and praise and thus, according to the saying of a popular writer, some human fields are laid fallow in convents. It is known that there are many young women who now regret having rashly chosen their monastic state, that it was the many tendernesses and exhortations of others who were either very satisfied with their profession or, in the opposite case, sought at least a friend with whom they could share their misfortune, which made them miss their true vocation and be placed in their present misery. It is not enough that the weak sex seems to require a more mature age to be exposed to such adult decisions, it also seems to be required that a maiden not be admitted easily to take the vows unless she has spent at least two years outside the convent before her novitiate or has gone through a novitiate lasting two years. This should be so that she learn to know herself during that time and be better able to judge everything the knowledge of which will be so closely related to her future fate and to her future peace of mind. It seems a kind of injustice to make use of the person's lack of instruction and experience to persuade a gullible and innocent person to take a step which may in time drive her to desperation if an unexpected chance event or awakening nature cause to be felt the error committed in the choice of profession. Thus, since 1778 convents in Tuscany are forbidden to accept young maidens for board and lodging before their tenth year, and these are not permitted to choose the ecclesiastical profession before their twentieth year and an absence of six months from the convent.

§16

Of invalidating holy vows

My insight into the internal constitution of church discipline is insufficient for examining the question of whether the above considerations can bestow a greater semblance of justice upon the desire of an unknown person. Of course, if the return into the world from the ecclesiastical profession were permitted, it would be the greatest contribution to the prevention of all kinds of bad physical consequences of abstinence, but I must confess that from my point of view, I consider the complete reversal of the hitherto existing mode of life of our male clergy and a general abrogation of abstinence a very ticklish matter. Although I have no doubt that both the Church and the state would gain immensely by a better choice and more thorough self-examination of the candidates to priesthood, for it is impossible that persons, who in more mature years would be made to waive their decision to devote themselves to the priesthood by a mere natural instinct, would not bring with them a fruitful set of virtues whose procreation would be all the more advantageous to increase a class of righteous descendants; thus procreation would become more than it is now the business of well educated and mature persons, who have not yet contributed their best juices to disorder; thereby the recovery of the human race, which has visibly deteriorated in its quality, could be substantially promoted.

PART ONE
Section Three

On secular celibacy

§ 1

Unmarried life for healthy adult persons who are not constrained by pious vows protected by the Church, nor by lack of food to support a family, nor by the nature of their civil employment, cannot be a matter of indifference to a state in which there is still a lack of inhabitants; therefore, among almost all nations whose religious system permitted it, the taste for such a way of life is considered extremely deleterious, and bachelors are considered members who are obviously detrimental to the state.

* * *

There follow examples of regulations issued by different nations against secular celibacy.

§ 4

The longer I view the unmarried state of laymen from this aspect, the more I find that its influence on the healthy state of the citizens is usually not judged with sufficient accuracy. What, indeed, can society expect of a class of people who, without being able to provide a sufficient reason for their chosen way of life, are of insouciant demeanor, and roam about in a continuous search of desired opportunities and, where they seize them, would like to provide themselves against possible future shortage?—It is known that a frequent change in love provides the body with certain strength enabling it to rush more quickly toward its exhaustion. This is so because new objects renew the stimulation which sucks out the last reserves of vital spirits and ends the debauchery early.—Moreover, it often happens that the desire to get rid of an unwanted stimulation does not occur opportunely, and under such circumstances a painstaking choice by the bachelor is not to be expected.—The spread of venereal poison among the street whores, who are then sought [by the foregoing], indicates vividly all the misfortune which springs from such disorder. But then, in an unfortunate hour, after having laid a thousand traps, the incontinent one gains the favor of a married woman and, regardless of any other consequences of the wicked intercourse, the infectious disease also spreads in an innocent family, a disease which should really punish only the disturber of the general order in his guilty parts. What increases the misfortune so much is the following: the physician who is called in has to cure diseases in the most innocent children and in fathers who are free of any suspicion, and every effort is made to conceal their origin from him. Close questioning gives rise to suspicion which might destroy the well-being of the family in one fell stroke. This, because the guiltless husband believes that the physician, who expresses some doubts, despises his family, and he then seeks uncertain help. Or else he hits upon thoughts which, no matter how justified, are no less damaging to the family than the ill itself, yet without making its recognition as certain for the physician as would be required in the interest of curing it.—I speak from experience which many practical physicians share with me.

§ 5

How important is help against such ills

There are the physical reasons by which the disadvantage of the unmarried state among laymen who have no particular inclination to it must be judged, and the further development of which could rightly be expected of me here. In as much as this state has begun to become so general, for several years, I leave the investigation of the causes of our deteriorating morals to others. I have no doubt that even according to the reasons given, unmarried men who could maintain a family and who despite that evade the married state without reason, seem worthy of the same treatment which they would have meted out to them under the same circumstances in Rome.

But freedom? . . .

Well, this is a chimera if it is to be based on the detriment of all society.—I know: "According to the teaching of our Church, abstinence is better than the married state"; but one should beware and not waste this precious title on such a widespread class of people who use it only in order to mock the world and to give free play to the passions under a piously painted blanket under which virtue and posterity are suffocated.—But whoever nevertheless is of the opinion that the reintroduction of the law that promotes more marriage is against the Christian freedom should consider this: whether it would not be good, in the case of such freedom, as Süsmilch already advised, if an affluent bachelor contributed annually to a special fund from which the marriages of impecunious and diligent couples could be facilitated and supported, and that, according to the saying by a popular writer, "the bachelors would have strange children conferred on them, like a hen receives strange eggs for hatching."

According to Roman Law and customs introduced in Germany, it was fairly common for the estate of dead bachelors to go to the exchequer, and the so-called bachelor law is still in force in Brunswick, Württemberg, the Palatinate, and other lands.—Thus one can see that the state does not receive any compensation for the loss it suffers; what is there to prevent a man, who during his lifetime in the midst of society enjoyed all the advantages of that society without helping to make good the loss which society suffers daily in citizens, unless he can prove his special vocation to the unmarried state by blameless behavior, [what is to prevent him] either to get married or at least to compensate the state by an appropriate contribution to the dowry and marriage fund; thereby he would enable others to provide the fruits of which he robbed the state by his stubbornness.

* * *

There follow examples of such regulations.

§ 6

How such measures against bachelors should be taken

Whoever has ended his thirtieth year in a community, should be made to give an account of his way of life and his circumstances to a certain authority. It would help if every town and village compiled special tables of unmarried men and maidens, the former over twenty-five, the latter over twenty years old, listing name, age, health (whether they are blind, crippled, badly or well built), nutrition, skill.—The principals of police would annually compile these circumstances in order to make the bachelor pay a stipulated sum of money (unless he had to provide for old parents, or a widowed mother, small siblings, or he could plead a special vocation to unmarried life and prove his endeavor to fulfill this punctiliously), upon whose correct annual payment he would be free to continue his otherwise doubly disadvantageous way of life.

§ 7

However, the female sex, which is not free to enter into marriage at will, should receive in all earnestness as much assistance as possible. It is incomprehensible how little is done for this useful class of members of society. A large number of the healthiest and most fertile young women in almost every village are forced without any guilt on their part to languish at their worried parents' place, and to resist the advances of dangerous bachelors, without anybody giving it a thought how such parents could be relieved and how their daughters could be employed as useful mothers in the state. Yet, especially among the peasantry are the most maidens who are able to help the population and be useful in increasing it. Therefore, Süsmilch counted among the causes of lesser fertility in the country that the women there marry almost too late, often not before the thirtieth year and sometimes even later.— What a disadvantage must it be, therefore, in every small village if so many maidens die unmarried, since it is certain that only lack of help and of a small contribution prevented them from becoming worthy mothers!

Poor unmarried women, especially young fecund widows, to whom even the Apostles (partly overlooked by today's apostles) recommended remarriage for several reasons, and altogether maidens of healthy and promising body, if well-behaved, would receive certain sums from the dowry fund, and affluent young men, who would take them in marriage, would receive certain advantages, such as relief from taxes for several years, etc. The taxes imposed on bachelors would have to be in proportion to their affluence, so that effective contributions for poor married couples could be raised. Therefore it would be especially meritorious toward mankind if their legacies in regions where bachelor law is still in force anyway, would be diverted by magnanimous regents, to the aforementioned dowry fund, instead of to the exchequer, so that at least from the ashes of bachelors, children would be produced of whom he robbed his country in his lifetime.

§8

Bachelors should be punished more strictly for incontinence

In case a bachelor forgot himself and deflowered a maiden, he should be punished incomparably more harshly than a young man of less than twenty-five years of age, and he should be made to pay a special contribution to the marriage fund, unless he decided to marry the deflowered maiden, or, where this is not feasible, another woman.

To deprive unmarried life even more of its attractions (unless it be bound up with an eminently virtuous life), and to weaken the taste for debauchery more and more, in case of equal deserts, the married man should be given preference before all others, and also younger men should receive a flattering distinction before others of their rank who are neither married nor have produced children if married.—Thus in most imperial cities only married citizens are eligible for posts at the magistrate, and in deeds set by Mühlhausen to the law faculty of Helmstadt, the following is said of such applicants: "because married men are entitled to this, and the unmarried ones are not half-masters but only quarter-masters." Likewise in Switzerland, bachelors are excluded variously from public positions, and it seems natural, especially in free republics, that such posts also are entrusted least to those who do not want to tie themselves to the country by any closer bond, or are by their reproachable manners inappropriate to such a special virtue.

* * *

PART TWO
Section One

Of too early marriages

> Est in juvencis, est in equis patrum Virtus.
> Horat.

§1

General stipulation of time for marrying

The determination of the proper age for marrying has always been an important subject for the legislator, and there is no cultured nation which did not stipulate a certain age under which people were not permitted to attend to the business of procreation. It is only a pity that the health and well-being of the citizens was not always the prime consideration of the regulation, and that in drawing it up, economic, and also moral reasons, were taken into consideration.

* * *

In the subsequent paragraphs, Frank gives various examples of regulations and laws for late and early marriages, and he develops his own point of view concerning the correct age for marriage as follows:

§6

Important influence of procreation on our state

Procreation is a subject on which the more or less good state of animals depends completely, and it presupposes certain conditions which only the complete maturity of the parents can fulfill.—Most functions in the human body occur either early, or at least in the first years after birth, and all nature works daily with visible success on the tools necessary for this. Only in man does the procreative power remain undeveloped, and here nature seems to sleep for many years, in order to deal exclusively with the growth of the rest of the body.

Finally, after the person has attained a certain size, there are phenomena, made known in girls around the twelfth to fifteenth year and in boys from the fourteenth to the sixteenth or eighteenth year, which indicate that nature now has wakened from its slumber, and also begins to work energetically on the tools of procreation.

Yet, just as all tools of animal functions during their first employment show a marked weakness, there is an even greater immaturity in the first development of procreative power. This distinctly teaches that there are even more important requirements of the animal economy, and that the daily growth of the entire body forbids a freer discharge which seems to be intended only to create our posterity from the overabundance of our vital spirits.

Nature certainly is not at cross purposes with itself; it does not hurry with the discharge which costs the still incomplete body so dearly;—and thus we often see a well brought up young man, eighteen to twenty years old, well guarded against depravity, with daily signs of budding virility, yet living quietly, without great stimulation to lasciviousness, which otherwise occurs mechanically due to discharge of semen. His body wins the great advantages of his late employment of his procreative powers, whereas the lascivious at that same age is a bogy of nature and lives only in order to be a walking proof that he has wilfully forced nature to work toward its own destruction, and to use all nourishing matter for the discharge of an ingenious juice which will be so greatly needed for the complete development of the rest of the body.—Even in animals, one can notice that a male colt that has been used for breeding too soon never regains its strength. And it is one of the more important aspects concerning the breeding by immature colts, that wild horses do not easily grow as large as tame ones where this mistake is prevented. This is really detrimental even to the mare which is brought to foal before her fifth year.

Yet, in regard to the female sex, things are quite different from the male sex; its formation is rarely incomplete once the usual signs of its maturity occur in the proper order. Every month there is a discharge of superfluous juices which nature does not require for its further perfection.—Besides, the fair sex also suffers less fatigue from matrimonial work, and nature carefully saves the monthly excess for nourishing the fetus in case of pregnancy; thus the fetus is less demanding of the mother's body which has already attained maturity.—Giving birth, as is known, is less hard on young mothers; and everything indicates that nature, which makes the male sex attain maturity later, but also makes more lasting claims on the business of procreation, quite deliberately endows the female body with earlier maturity, in the 16th year, whereas male maturity is attained around the 25th year. Thus, the male can await in uninterrupted propensity for procreation the time when nature also begins to command the man to provide more for his own daily uncertain maintenance rather than for the production of others.

For if one places the limit of female maturity in the sixteenth year, and its fading in about the fiftieth year, but concedes the male sex the ability to produce children from the twenty-fifth up to the sixtieth year without danger to well-being, I do not see any contradiction in the interval of procreative ability of both sexes;* on the

* How else could one find a probable explanation for the fact that the female sex ceases being able to

contrary, I find that the Creator clearly stipulated, also according to general experience, the time before which it is doubtful and often dangerous to the detriment of one's health to engage in the procreation of posterity which will inherit all the symptoms of the paternal immaturity and will continuously lower the quality of the human species.

* * *

Frank describes the consequences of immature marriages and subsequently deals with the difference in the age of sexual maturity in different nations, whereupon he returns to European circumstances:

§12

How things should be handled in our region

If a law were to be passed stipulating the safe time at which marriage should be permitted as an advantageous union for the common good for the inhabitants of our temperate regions in Europe, in such an important matter I would suggest that because of the aforenamed reasons the age for females should be lower than for males. Nevertheless, only very rarely should marriage be permitted before the eighteenth year. Young men in the country should not be easily permitted to marry before their twenty-fifth year, but in towns, because of the earlier mentioned danger of exhaustion and loose life, it should be somewhat earlier, but not before the twenty-second year, especially since procreation depends mainly on male maturity. Without such provision such married couples are lost for the population even in their best years, for the fertile husband, once he has reached his fortieth year, lies next to his already infertile partner, and all the wife's efforts only amount to a *mutuum adjutorium*, in which the state cannot be greatly interested since it wishes to extract the greatest possible effect from all its members.

Therefore, Müller has already advised the authorities to restrain those young who hurry too soon into marriage;* and Heister wished that such marriages simply should not be permitted in society.** However, the Supreme Consistory in Dresden had some objections, because in some cases a much greater misfortune had to be feared when marriages were refused even at an immature age.†

This may be correct in some respect; yet, I wish that in such cases the disadvantages to the general health of the people to be expected of immature marriages were

---

procreate just at the time when the man is in his best years? And that, therefore, between marriage partners of equal age all cohabitation for almost twenty years usually fails to achieve nature's purpose? . . . Is it not reasonable to draw the conclusion from this inequality of the sexes that polygamy is based on the specific propensity of the man to desire procreation for a much longer time.

* Pet. Müller, "Dissert. jurid. de calore juvenili," Jenae 1680, Sect. V, thes. III.

** Laur. Heister, "De principum cura circa sanitatem subditorum."

† Müller, l.c.

always thoroughly considered, and we should be induced to make exceptions only in rare cases in view of some advantages which cost the human race so dearly. And I believe that every time such an exception is made, it is only just to demand a contribution to the marriage fund, and thus the damage is made good to a certain extent by promoting a fruitful marriage between more mature persons.

* * *

There follow examples of various regulations aimed at preventing early marriages.

PART TWO

Section Two

Of marriages that are too late and unequal

§1

Of marriages of elderly people

The mother of Dionysius the Tyrant demanded of her son that he should give her in marriage to a handsome man in her old age; and Dionysius replied that although he had despotically suspended the laws of the land, he had not got so far as to dare to mistreat the laws of nature also. For the first purpose of marriage is the procreation of children, and it does not require more than sound reason to realize that people who marry at an age at which it is foolish to hope for children, cannot possibly have this in mind.

§2

Spartan laws for old men who had young wives

For this reason the oldest laws forbade marriages of such persons with younger ones, and the Spartan legislator introduced in his republic [the law] that an old and impotent husband who had married a woman and thus gained her entire fortune, had to permit her to produce children with one of her closest relatives, and thereby to compensate the state. Therewith but one standard was established among the marriage laws which ordered that the matrimonial duty to such a woman had to be performed at least three times a month.

* * *

Further examples of regulations against late marriage follow.

§5

No matter how the ancient legislators strove to prevent marriages between old and young persons or at least to make them useful for society by extraneous contributions, nevertheless, both secular laws and orders of the Church declared marriages between old and young people valid, for the consolation of human frailty, as it was put, and only ancient habit of various nations testifies to the former disdain toward old persons who married young ones. The young people often congregated in front of the dwelling of the unequal couple, made a dissonant noise with various instruments (charivari) and jeered; the police chief and the Church usually punished this.

I leave it to the reader to reflect whether this very old custom does not teach the opposite of what is somewhere stated: "that the ancient Germans never denied marriage to those of their men who were more than 60 years old," although I do not deny that our forefathers seem to have maintained their procreative power longer.

§6

Doubts concerning such marriages

If one considers thoroughly how much store a state in need of people sets by the fertility of marriages not being weakened by anything, one must admit that such changes deserve deep thought; partly because the calculation of the children from a given number of concluded marriages is thus subject to important doubts; partly because health and morals are often endangered in such married companies; partly because the children begot thus usually do not have the good quality which matters so greatly to the country and the individual citizens. Not to mention the fact that such parents rarely live to see their children provided for, and thus the number of widows and orphans increases. This ill is rarely remedied by getting married again: for there is reason to believe that if children are brought up by stepparents, their mortality increases in various ways.

§7

No matter how the fertility of marriages is calculated, it is always correct to say that in marriages between very unequal persons, one partner ceases to be able to procreate, and must be considered *pro civiliter mortuo*, while the other partner is still in full strength. Therefore in such marriages only half the number of children, or even less, are produced than is otherwise the case. The inequality of temperament and natural impulses, which depend on the age of people, may even bring about complete relative barrenness; for how often can one see that young women spend many years with old men, and though these cannot be considered impotent because of their age, they nevertheless do not have any children. On the other hand, the same women, when remarried, immediately become pregnant from their active husbands.

§8

A man who is otherwise in good health cannot be declared impotent at any age, for many examples (though some of them ambiguous) have been recorded of the oldest men, some even a hundred years old, having given proof of their potency in procreating. However, I believe that these still rare observations do not sufficiently justify the complete rejection of the most ancient marriage laws, because such laws do not have in mind only the mutual well-being of the married couple, but also the expectations of the country. The Roman censors saw to it that the fields were culti-vated, and they punished those who left their fields untilled or who tilled them badly, although it seems to be only the affair of individual households whether they look after themselves, and to blame only themselves if something is lacking because of their own negligence. How could they calmly acquiesce that those of their daughters who were capable and affluent enough to get married and bear children, wasted away in the arms of cold, old men, without real hope of bearing children, and thus disturb the natural order in the necessary replacement of good citizens?—Or is it probable that perhaps it was unknown to the great legislators of those times that even an old man can sometimes still become a father?—Certainly not; for the pro-hibition shows that then, too, old men sometimes procreated children; therefore, they had to have similar experiences to ours: and since these did not prevent the prohibition in its execution, it can be easily seen that the spirit of the law was not based, wrongly, on the supposed inability of old men but, on tenets which are found to be true also in our days: individual persons and most of all their offspring suffer too much by such unequal marriages for the civil dignitaries of the country to remain unperturbed.

It is known that changes occur in the human body at a certain age. Nothing is more equal than age with its infirmities and frailties:

> Plurima sunt juvenum discrimina; pulcrior ille
> Hoc, atque ille alio multum hic robustior illo;
> Una senum facies, cum voce trementia membra
> Et jam laeve caput, madidique infantia nasi.*

However, among all the [body] parts those deteriorate first which are intended for the procreation of the race and for the first nourishment. Regard in her fiftieth year the gem of creation, the body of a beautiful woman who was alluring in her youth, and see what has remained of all that nature endowed this sex with in order to subjugate our sex at some time and make it commit acts that would be completely repellent if it were not for the mutual feeling of both sexes, and if our sensitive fibers were of coarser structure. For, "how small," says Langhans, "would be the number of patriots who would produce children only for the sake of the general well-being of the world, so that it be everywhere well populated and cultivated, if the business of procreation did not entail such a strong attraction and pleasure?"**

Shriveled, blackish brown skin now takes the place of the alluring hemispheres which give one half of the human race their desires, and the whole human race its first and most necessary nourishment. And this wonderful source is now so decrepit that it is very rare, as is sometimes told of some old mothers, that in their sixtieth

---

* Juvenal, ("Sat.") Lib. IV, Sat. X.
** Of vices which take vengeance on the health of people; §20.

year they still gave of their miraculous fruit. Well behaved maidens also may sometimes suckle infants: for their breasts, too, sometimes swell up, filled with a kind of milk. Just as nature itself in time deliberately lets this important part dry up, it also stops the bleeding which distinguishes the fecund from the barren women. From a certain age onward, all differences disappear, and no woman menstruates any more without this being due to ill health or a natural disorder.—The changes in the inner sex organs are no less considerable: the vessels of the uterus coalesce and mostly close themselves; this entire organ shrivels and becomes cartilaginous; and the vagina and the other parts lose the fine discriminating feeling with which nature endowed them for the act of procreation.

In men no part of the body undergoes as great a change as the penis which gradually shrivels into itself and disappears. Like lasciviousness itself, the scrotum becomes limp and flabby, the vessels for the outflow gradually disappear, and there are only a few drops of an ambiguous moisture in the receptacles for semen. Therefore, erection and ejaculation require lengthy stimulation; and it is here that nature, to its disadvantage, is robbed of the little necessary balm, where, however, the continuing tension of the body and of the imagination contribute most to the convulsive evacuation of this small amount of fluid.

For this, and for even stronger reasons, the old man, who as though he had become a boy again, is now forced to avoid such waste, which is against nature, and for lack of the stimulating semen, and the former sensitivity of his genitals altogether, nature comes to his aid by endowing him with a quiet calm freedom from violent passions:
—Minimus gelido jam in corpore sanguis
Febre calet sola.*

The night is not to him what it is to the young man in his prime with honest intention. An unintentional dream leads him into much worse company than the one which he was taught to flee while awake because this dream causes him often tiring pollutions which at his age are deleterious. The old man, thanks to nature which is engaged in maintaining him, does not feel any of this after long years, and it is daily proved to him more and more that the necessity of such evacuation has passed for him. He also feels the effects of mutual behavior fully after forced cohabitation: the body, which is already sick anyway, feels a general lassitude, whereby the special feebleness of various parts, of which a person at that age is rarely free, apparently increases; the digestive forces are suppressed, and thereby are laid the foundations of strokes, palsies, and lingering consumption, which could be avoided for a long time yet if his way of life were more appropriate to nature. Rightly one may say with Young:

O how disor'd our Machine
When contractions mix!

* Juvenal, ("Sat.") Lib. IV. Sat. X.

When Nature riakes no less than twelve,
And folly points at six?*

* * *

§9

Yet there is a difference which must be mentioned here, whether it is an old man who marries a young maiden or a young man who marries an old woman. For from the latter marriage one cannot practically expect any fruit whereas from the former, perhaps a few fruits can be expected: for it is certain that for every woman who really bears a child after her fiftieth year, at least thirty men above sixty can be found who still have certain abilities for begetting children; nevertheless, they will only rarely be in the mood to fulfill the requested or tacit requested obligations, and in this they will be unequal to a young wife. Therefore, when the legislator called the fruits of such old mothers a miraculous birth, it was the mildest name that could be given to such a game of nature.

§10

From this follows that all the foregoing objections must apply doubly to marriages of young men who are greedy for money and therefore famous men considered them totally unnatural, and consequently extremely sinful.**

If one trusts that nature at least acts according to the intentions of its Creator, one has to be convinced that as it deprives the fair sex of all attraction at a certain time, when the male sex only appears in its true maturity, and as nature terminates the ability of women to procreate, in which they differ markedly from men, it stands to reason that such a woman has little claim to the caresses of a young man. On the contrary, such lusts excited at the wrong time must cause a really deleterious exhaustion, which also entails the most pronounced loss for it.—In fifty-year old women, the uterus must be considered an atrophied part of the body, and any influx induced by ingenuity or nature is, as mentioned before, either the cause or the effect of an unnatural constitution. Although the female sex suffers less from the consequences of caresses, the strength nevertheless begins to suffer more from untimely exhaustion than before, and continuing bleeding, sharp effusions, drying up of the juices are consequences that can only be expected from the natural order of things.

Fortunately the bribed young man is of little help here: nature denies him the fire of imagination of which nature otherwise makes such good use in order to awaken the sleepy. Soon the dead object of his caresses becomes to him a horror, and under

---

* Young's "Resignation," pars. II.

** See: Joh. Fr. Eisenhart, "Thoughts on the Marriage of a Young Man and an Old Woman," Leipzig, 1757.—Süsmilch l.c., Part I, c. V. §90.—Henr. Bodinus, "Diff. jurid. de conjugio illicito," Hal. Magd. 1704.—L.B. a Wollzogen & Neuhaus, "Diss. juridico-politica, de connubiis infantum," Jen., 1734, c.I. §VII, p. 13.

constant endeavors to deceive himself he must use up his youth in enforced fulfillment of his obligations, and cultivate a field which, without a miracle, cannot reasonably be expected to yield the slightest harvest.

In the meantime jealousy gnaws because of the certain loss, either of posterity, or of the young man so bought. If it is well founded, it entails disorders; otherwise, it requires from the man proof which, when he supplies it, entails resentment and much greater enfeeblement of the male body than double that employment between persons of equal age and with a better relationship would cause.

Such tasteless consummation, bought at such a high price, incites all the more to buy at least a happier hour for the unhappy night, to be paid for with the shamefully gained money and to be spent in the arms of a sinful love which, however, is less of an abuse to the laws of procreation. Who can fail to see that the direct cause of this ordinary occurrence is the constitution which permits "that a woman whom nature has excluded from procreation, to her own shame and to the loss of offspring, can possess herself of a fertile young man, against charming and hopeful maidens, and who teaches him base thinking by dangling shimmering gold before him, induces him to eternal dissimulation, and kills *civiliter* for the population. Or does this practice perhaps contradict nature less than the legally prohibited marriage of a castrated man with a young woman?"

* * *

§12

In my opinion it would not be wrong, in view of the earlier procreative ability of women, if this time difference were taken into account and men were permitted to marry younger women, with the provision that a woman of 48 years would not be permitted *ad mutuum adjutorium* to marry a man less than 60 years old; conversely, a man even 50 years old should be permitted to choose a person of 28 years or older, who up to the higher and feebler age of her husband, would have paid her debt to the state and to nature and would not have great claims left. On the other hand, a 60-year old suitor would not be permitted to marry a person less than 38 or 40 years old.

* * *

§14

It goes without saying that the above-named reasons do not apply to marriages where both partners are equal in procreative power and the marriage is not merely friendly company of elderly people who have abandoned procreation. But the police must watch that a couple, unlike in age, does not pretend to seek merely friendly society, and so that by stealth and pretense, a healthy and fertile member of society, the best property of the state, does not get into dead hands.

PART TWO
Section Three

On unhealthy marriages

§1

At first sight it may seem harsh to try by law to deprive someone of his natural right to procreation and the fulfillment of his instincts, as long as this business is taken as what it is to most married couples: "an act for their mutual pleasure, and since it usually leads to the production of their like", which every right minded person still considers important enough to gladly see the race maintained. However, if one considers that marriages in the eyes of the state are something of much more consequence, the statement loses much of its roughness: "that one cannot indiscriminately let people take part in a matter on which, in reality, the fate of society and of all mankind most intimately depend: first, because marriage under certain circumstances may be for the partner himself a disadvantageous, or even a lethal, matter; second, because in such unhealthy marriages almost no children are born, or only such children who are only a burden to the community and who do not last long; third, because this sustains even more the transmission of hereditary diseases."

§2

It hardly needs proof that sexual intercourse is an act that requires most natural powers, and where it is indulged in excessively, these forces are squandered. Therefore semen is not discharged until the time of body growth is almost past, and again, it ceases completely as soon as [the human species] is weakened by age. As regards this effect, semen was compared to the so-called vital spirits, and this comparison is borne out by nature: for one single untimely ejaculation of semen weakens, as Galenus already remarked, more than the strongest bloodletting; its effect extends as far as the soul, and according to an old saying, all animals become sad after sexual intercourse. The convulsive shocks which attend cohabitation testify to the strongest motion of the invigorating fire in our veins and nerves, and the terrifying phenomena observed in those who wantonly waste this juice teach sufficiently what a weak creature may expect who condescends to such evacuation.

§3

Let us now recapitulate all the lengthy and chronic accidents the nature of which forbids such weakening. It can then be seen how little is the general freedom of contracting marriage at will compatible with the true advantages of individual citizens and with the common wealth. Therefore, a person suffering greatly from a chronic disease can be seen rapidly approaching his destination soon after having contracted a marriage, for the inner fever (the worst companion of lengthy illnesses) obviously increases, consumes his last strength, expedites death.

§4

Thus it is with the sick part itself, but how much reason has the healthy, who is joined so closely with the other, to detest such a marriage! Without mentioning the infection to which he exposes himself by close intercourse with the sick partner, there is no hope for him of pleasure or inner peace. Is it the lofty final aim to produce children, which induced him to get married?—There is little hope that a part which hardly exists itself could be instrumental in helping fulfill such intentions. . . . If it is the soothing of the passions—what satisfaction can be expected of a person who due to his sad circumstances is before God and the world more than excused from it? And how can people be mutually bound by a contract, when they know beforehand that its fulfillment will be prevented on the one side by danger, on the other by eternal apologies?

Yet there is no lack of mutual allurement: the senses are inflamed and only very rarely soothed; the necessity of satisfaction increases with the feeling of mutual deficiency, and causes a certain illness of the soul and of the body which becomes the source of many physical, as well as moral, disorders in society.

* * *

After the statement that diseases of the parents can be transmitted to their children hereditarily, Frank arrives at the conclusion:

§6

It can be confidently expected that very sickly parents will usually produce not only weak children, but children who suffer from the same illnesses or who have at least the special ability to contract them at the first opportunity. The diaries of physicians are full of such persons, and it would be a grave injustice to charge the physicians with ignorance and lack of skill in healing.

It is fortunate for society that many marriages between sick couples remain without heirs, or if there are any, their life is rarely durable. Nevertheless, it sometimes happens that such a hapless victim of an ill-advised union of sick libertines reaches a ripe age, and in his turn contributes to the perpetuation of the family failing. This human misery is then propagated carefully from generation to generation.

§7

If one considers the matter more in detail and bears in mind the danger of infection to which the healthy partner is exposed through close contact, be it cohabitation itself,* sleeping together, or other intimacy, it must seem to the moral judge, as well as to every good citizen, that it is highly irresponsible if a woman, created for [a member of] the healthy population, gives her hand in marriage to an emaciated consumptive, or a man afflicted with a contagious disease, and thus publicly declares her willingness to make not only her offspring, but her herself unhappy. I could fill many pages with such examples, but there are everywhere so many such cases that I do not want to lose time over them. I only want to point out that the habit among poor and lowly people of letting their children sleep with them up to a certain age, who in view of their inherited predisposition for the diseases of their parents are prepared anyway, that this can only speed up their early infection, and therefore in this respect we must view marriages between sick and healthy people as another cause of a constant spread of human infirmity.

§8

It is, therefore, clearly the duty of the leaders of the community not to let those of their subjects who suffer from particularly grave and deleterious ills get married without thorough examination.** It is understood that, although the male sex seems to have the greatest influence on the formation of the fetus, nevertheless the female sex must be subject to the same compulsion because of the closest relationship between mother and child.† Of course, in view of the great variety of human incidents it is impossible to be too strict in this matter and always to lurk in wait for even the slightest physical shortcoming of the citizens. On the contrary, as I mentioned several times before, it is correct to say that the mutual constitution can be improved in the offspring by a certain mixing, even if there are some visible defects. However, matters are entirely different if there are grave defects, especially in the juices of the human body. Their diseased state is so important in some illnesses, and of such a quality that there is simply no possibility of rapid change through favorable mixing, and the venereal [diseased] father even infects his still healthy wife, his children, and grandchildren in the same way as the comsumptive transmits his weak chest and other illnesses down perhaps to the fifth generation. There is, therefore, nothing

---

* This kind of contagion of different diseases has been correctly demonstrated in "The Philosophical Physician," Part 4, p. 73.

** According to Indian law those born deaf and blind, among many others, or noticeably crippled in body or mind or enfeebled, are not even permitted to inherit. See Gött, gel. Anz. Supplement 1778, p. 246.

† "One recognizes very often in the young stock, not only in some, but in each and every descendant of the mare, the distinguishing stature and the character of the mother, even if they do not have her color and have been sired by different males. I could name many such mares from the Württemberg stud farms." Hartmann, "Horse and Mule Breeding," p. 136.

more natural than not to be indifferent to the situation of the persons who are preparing to marry. Such illnesses should really be a cause of prohibition of marriage
if it can be said of them with great probability that they will increase the class of
miserable and ailing people, promote the mortality and spread of the most dangerous
diseases, and further the gradual deterioration of the human race. I will, therefore,
endeavor to determine as accurately as seems necessary for my purpose the conditions that are important enough to prohibit marriage in any well-regulated community, until they are completely eliminated.

* * *

*In the subsequent paragraphs, epilepsy, various wasting diseases (Phthisis pulmonalis,
tabes), and faulty pelvis formation are cited as obstacles to marriage. In §13, Frank
thereupon expresses the wish:*

§13

How desirable would it be if some of the care that is given to the breeding of good
animal strains, to the painstaking distinction of those which are to be used for breeding, while inferior, sickly, unclean fathers or mothers are not used, would also be
applied to human beings, in every community, and the marriage of completely degenerated, dwarfish, very crippled, and disfigured persons never permitted.* Care
should be taken that beautiful persons with well-built and healthy bodies, even if
they have no means, be supported in concluding marriages with partners equally
healthy and physically perfect, and in bringing up a large family of similar children.
Thus, the number of strong and well-built citizens be gradually increased. At least
there would be a very good opportunity for arranging this if, for some time, the great
princes would marry a certain number of poor couples and provide their dowry. In
this way the state would obtain its own children for whose good behavior and health
it would take better care, and from time to time the state would transfer the surplus
into those regions where human perfection seems to have suffered most. Similarly,
there is now hardly any town which does not have its own tree nursery through which
its citizens obtain ever more abundant and better kinds of fruit, since it has been
realized that in the place where a crippled tree stood and bore badly tasting fruit, a
noble trunk now has room and can help increase internal wealth.

I again express my regret that the [social] class of soldiers causes a constant and
irreplaceable loss of the most beautiful male youth, and that the business of procreation in the country is left to only a small and badly built race of persons whose
growth has been stunted either by starting work too soon or by want and misery. As
soon as one finds a somewhat well-built boy among his depressed peers, one who

---

* Waldschmid, "Dissert. de Sororibus Gemellis," pag. 25, fqq. cit.—Frid. Lud. Curds, "Dissert. de
jure monstrorum," Gissae 1712, §XI.

excels by his better growth, a colored ribbon is tied to his hat when he is in his sixteenth year, and he is ordered to hurry to the nearest garrison where he is incorporated into a group who are dead so far as the marital procreation of our race is concerned. It is as if only those who seem to be created to fulfill the business of procreation in the community were fit to be exposed to the enemy's fury, as if the peasant's son, even if only five and a half feet tall, could not equally well fire his own firearm. I ask every philanthropist to take into account this origin of human degeneration among the peasantry, and to judge how much the now general system of having large armies constantly ready must deprive general health of our days in view of the mania of inducting into the army only selected young men, the nucleus of the population. One should consider the imperfections of the married men who are not fit to be soldiers, or the way of life of those whose better physical condition gave them cause to be incorporated in a class where the forces of future legal employment for the population of the fatherland are little spared or not at all spared, even if the limbs and lives of these warriors were spared by fate.

All these considerations apply primarily to small states, of which a large part of Germany is composed, for here every regent uses the right according to which the sons of his subjects are obliged to serve him, often for a long time. These usually return with the worst morals (and therefore exhausted by debauchery) to the country. Their smaller siblings, who in the meantime had to look after the fields together with the parents, and who have been prematurely weakened by excessive work and prevented from growing are therefore almost the only ones of whom the country may expect most of the population. Thus, the good race in a small country is gradually extinguished, especially if foreign male blood freshens it only rarely, and thus reduces the disadvantage which must occur due to the inclination for a disproportionate military class. It is just as if the mares of a country were fertilized for many years by the most miserable sires, and the best stallions were admitted only after the mares had run the posts for a long time.

In large towns it is moral decay which mostly degrades the respect for, and the beauty of the human race. A maiden of the middle class, of beautiful form, needs rare courage to resist the thousandfold pursuits of the lascivious youth, the soldiers, and the bachelors. And since for this sex, a beautiful body is the surest pledge of the advantages to be derived from the incontinence of the men, it seems to them often to be easier to devote themselves to a free way of life than to wait without good prospects for serious suitors. But it is known how much such debauchery degrades the perfection of offspring, and how little the state can count on the fruits procreated by fornication under present circumstances.

It must thus be admitted that a law is important which would forever prohibit the marriage of all crippled, maimed, very stunted, dwarfish persons, and leave the work of procreation to a healthier class of citizens. A law which would endeavor to conserve and maintain in every community the number of those who were endowed by nature with excellent form. And it is very desirable that measures be taken so that these persons do not deliberately squander the advantages of their bodies, or to the disadvantage of posterity lose them in an ambiguous bachelor life.

* * *

After treating of various infectious diseases and mental diseases, Frank arrives at the conviction:

§17

In the case of all the diseases mentioned above, marriage is a wrong that is done to mankind, an attack on one's own life and on the life of posterity. There is therefore no better comparison than to say with Unzer that, people, with all this who want to produce children, are like spiders which devour their own young. I am convinced that no means would be as effective in promoting strength and health in our race, and that consequently a state could not be made more to bloom, than by putting procreation on a better footing by eliminating all those who sow only bad seed into the field of the community, and that the class of sickly and miserable people were deprived of the power of sacrificing half of posterity to their impulses.

Whoever in our country wants to get married, has to produce his certificate of baptism in order to prove that by being baptized he acquired the right to belong to a Christian community. Who could say that it would be unjust if the community in the midst of which the young couple intends to join each other in order to fulfill the intentions of marriage according to the intentions of nature and of the country, made them promise, as if by oath, in the presence of secular representatives, "that they, as far as they could and had to know, do not suffer from any grave, infectious, or hereditary disease, whereby the intentions of the married state would be frustrated and the country cheated in its expectations, and only miserable and sickly fruits be produced. Also, if they should have been so diseased knowingly or unknowingly, insofar as their future cohabitation should be deleterious for one or the other, or for the country, they solemnly now undertook to waive the right which their present act gave them to each other, to submit to the laws of the Church and to its commands, and to endeavor altogether to raise such children as providence might provide them from their marriage, not only as Christians, but for the good of the country, also healthily." But those who were afflicted in the past with known grave diseases, or still seem to be afflicted, should be charged to give proof "that their former ill has disappeared already several years ago, by itself or through good remedies, or that it has been removed, and that their health did not suffer any of the bad consequences for them or for their family of which there was mention above."

Thus the first and very necessary step would be made toward the physical improvement of the human race, on which moral character certainly depends to a considerable extent also. The children, thus born to healthy parents, will have a durable life, and their mortality, which so far has been incomprehensible and in some regions greatly increasing, will be reduced. They will also get over otherwise unavoidable illnesses such as teething and smallpox much more easily, and they will be less susceptible to many other diseases. Dropsy, consumption, etc., are becoming rarer in every community, but matrimonial fecundity will enrich the country with young citizens who have the greatest skill for all social activities and a natural gift for the most difficult undertakings. The person who is insensitive to such gain and would calmly forgo its attainment, a difficult remedy, merely because of sleepy contentment with the arrangement of things as it was until now, must have been born to a father whose sickly mental state must have exceeded by far all the physical illnesses the presence of which makes the procreation of his race seem like punishment from heaven.

PART TWO
Section Four

Of matrimonial fecundity and some of its physical obstacles

> La stérilité en tout genre est ou un vice de la nature,
> ou un attentat contre la nature.
>
> Quest. sur l'Encyclopédie

§1

The procreation of one's equal, by intimate intercourse with the opposite sex as the noblest intention of a married couple, requires a certain disposition of both partners, on the strength of which the tools of procreation must be in natural and healthy condition. Moreover, between man and woman there must also be a special relationship, which is still partly incomprehensible to us, without which nature seems to deny its assistance to and greatly reduces the initial dignity of the act of procreation. This ability to create with the opposite sex a like being is called fecundity; however, it is usual to call fruitful only such a marriage which has proved this ability in practice by actual procreation. Fecundity is either complete, if a person is so fecund that he can produce children with any other healthy partner of the opposite sex, under natural favors as to age and certain circumstances;—or it is incomplete and relative if he can procreate only with certain persons and under a more restricted relation. Nothing, not even the climate, prevents a perfectly healthy couple from bringing this creative gift of nature to blessed fulfillment, and the courageous European fertilizes equally reliably his white, blond woman, the chestnut-colored woman from Ava, and the gleeming black beauty from Ethiopia.

§2

Of course, the natural fertility of the man can never be determined accurately, but it can be least judged where the natural freedom is curtailed by law. Not even a palace brimful with women can provide a sufficient idea of the possible fertility of its owner, as long as the palace is filled only with bought or forced female slaves. For freedom invigorates everything, and the procreative power in particular. Polygamy is far from being able to determine the true fertility of the sexes, and there is reason to believe that if one man has many women, and in view of the fairly proven equality of the sexes, polygamy must be a hindrance to fertility, although in individual cases it may serve as proof of what can in case of necessity be expected of the forces of healthy citizens.* If the thing which the more metaphysical European calls love is also known in wild regions, then love of the same beauty among free men must hinder proof of the procreative power, for its effect must be, with its tender steadiness, at the later signs of pregnancy and in view of the urges of the opposite sex, which do not cease simultaneously and for long, but without effect, to cultivate an already sown field and leave many another good field fallow. It is possible that a healthy man, from the time of his maturity up to his fifty-fifth year, is disposed to indulge in more than a hundred cohabitations annually if he is not disturbed by anything, and at least one fifth of these will be fertile, if change of the females is sought and if they do not apply all their ingenuity to prevent conception. There are sufficient examples that one man has produced a large number of children, either with many or with few women, although, as mentioned before, even polygamy does not remove the many obstacles to natural fertility. But from one single marriage there are everywhere examples known of fathers who produced 16, 20, or up to 28 or 30** children, and I myself know of cases of 24 and 25 children.†

§3

Although such fertility is rare, it is usually the woman to whom the cessation of further procreation is due, and it is unusual if a woman bears sixteen to twenty children, unless several of them are twins, if she takes over all the mother's duties and also nurses the children with her own breasts. It must be put to the account of the female sex, therefore, that matrimonial fertility on the whole does not easily exceed four children in one family. It was usual with all nations, therefore, but especially with the Jews, that in case of childless marriages, only the woman was exposed to reproach of barrenness, and that the life of these unfortunate ones was made difficult by a chance the prevention of which was very rarely within her powers.

* * *

* It is not my task here to determine whether polygamy is appropriate to human nature or offensive to it, and more than mere physical reasons are needed in order to speak of the suitability of its introduction as something satisfactory, or to say something more on the subject than has already been said on many occasions. As for myself, according to merely natural principles, I believe that polygamy, even disregarding the evil of venereal disease, recently brought to Europe, is prone to more objections than is the community of women, proposed by Plato, and kept in order by good laws, where the children of these women would be educated according to their abilities in a certain profession at public expense and according to a well thought out plan.

** v. Haller. Elem. VIII. p. 460. Twenty-four children from one mother is nothing rare in Switzerland.

† Otherwise it is usual to calculate two years for each child, including pregnancy and nursing. As the time for which females may procreate is about 25 years, 12 children can be expected naturally in marriage, if health remains unimpaired. Süsmilch, l.c. [Div. Ord.], §82, p. 108.

*After treating of female sterility and male impotence, Frank attempts, in §7, to arrive
at statistics of sterility in marriage:*

§7

It cannot be determined with any degree of certainty how a great a number of marriages do not have any other proof of their reciprocal barrenness than the time of
their childless cohabitation. It seems to me, however, that this much is correct: the
assumption that out of 1000 marriages there are only about ten childless marriages
does not seem to tally at all with experience. Thus the Swedish priest Hedin found
in his country-parish Kracklinge, in Nerike, which has about 800 people, that
every ninth woman was barren.* Whoever is not satisfied with this one observation,
let him take his own region and examine it. He will find that in most places, where
there are only three or four hundred married couples, at least six or seven out of a
hundred, if not more, are without heirs and always were, without there being any
stronger proof of barrenness from their external condition and abilities. Also, if
one calculates the number of good families and great houses which die out in each
century because of barrenness of the marriages, and which represent a small proportion compared with the class of burghers, one will see more clearly whether natural
barrenness is such a rare occurrence in each state. It is true that debauchery and
youthful intemperance often cause barrenness of the marriages in rich and noble
families; this happens much more rarely to persons who lead a moderate life. Therefore, the class of the noble and rich citizens must not be taken as the basis for such
general calculations. However, it is an unfortunate fact that the middle class in large
cities is beginning to imitate the unnatural way of life of the nobility, so that gradually
the mistake in this calculation will be put right. If one assumes that among each
hundred marriages there are only five childless or barren couples, and that one
marriage has four children on the average, although in the ordinary calculations all
marriages are included without exceptions, this amounts to a loss to the state of 20
children because of this lack of fulfillment of matrimonial intentions.

To this must be also taken into account that the procreation of children, at least
for females living a married life, is not only beneficial to health but almost indispensable. At least, one sees that most women living in barren marriage are ailing
until they have given birth several times, whereupon most of their illnesses seem to
be cured. Apparently they are to be viewed as cause or as effects of barrenness. The
women themselves are so familiar with this observation that when they consult a
physician about their state, they immediately reveal and put to him for consideration
that they had never yet borne children, and that they only hoped for better health

* Joh. Andr. Murray, "Medical-Practical Library," Vol. III, Part I, from the 37th volume of the Proceedings of the Royal Academy of Sciences.

when they would become mothers; in this they are rarely wrong. Van Swieten often heard women in Austria, where they are usually very prolific, complain that they had only borne 6 to 8 children, being firmly convinced that after every birth something left their bodies, which, if retained in the body, they feared would cause an illness.* If one takes into account also those women who lack this beneficial revolution and who, in spite of constant stimulation, remain barren and gradually waste away, one sees that the damage of barren marriages has a very extensive influence on the number and the good quality of the people, not to mention the disadvantage to, and the fate of dying out of the most respected families, and consequently to the political well-being of the states.

* * *

In §8, Frank deals in detail with various causes of sterility, and he wants to eliminate it by the following proposals:

§9
Necessity of provisions against the causes of sterility

The considerations contained in paras. 7 and 8 and concerning an institution that has been found to be good, do not intend to attain an important change that cannot be easily expected or to eliminate at once all kinds of causes of sterility in society. Nevertheless, the persons in authority should be better acquainted with the nature of this shortcoming, they should be shown the obstacles which prevent the intentions of nature, namely to make a country happy according to its disposition, and finally, according to my best knowledge, I want to state the best means for eliminating it in the easiest possible way.

1. A general improvement of the nation's morals will necessarily have the greatest influence on the increase in human fertility because the squandering of the forces is thereby prevented, and health is best preserved. Nevertheless, it is worth the effort to make an accurate list from time to time of all sterile marriages according to years; this helps to throw into relief the ratio of the loss caused by them to the gain that the country enjoys from fertile marriages in each region. The list should note as far as possible: whether sterility was due to certain obvious diseases of the married partners, and if so, which, or whether it was due to obvious continuous discord of the minds, to debauchery, or even to provable impotence. Furthermore, it should be examined whether in some region or other, under equal circumstances, procreation proceeds better or is more on the decline . . . And what, with some reason, should be considered the most probable cause of it? Because mankind, although it makes out better in all

---

* "Commentar." Tom. IV. §1354.

regions of the globe than all other animals, seems to develop better in different situations and to have less difficulties in its procreation or multiplication.

And because it is certain at the same time that because a large number of children is viewed as a burden in the household, a vice has taken root in some regions (§8) which was a horror to our German forebears;* as mentioned before, the time between two births, as well as inadequately low fertility in individual places should be scrupulously noted (so that after prudent assessment of the possible causes, if they are only of physical origin, wholesome measures can be taken to prevent more general evil. Or if there is perhaps suspicion of immorality of citizens living in married life and detesting a larger number of children, that this terrible enemy of human procreation can be fought with the aid of the clergy and with religious arguments). The sensual inclinations of every nation have to be examined with the greatest care by the persons in authority so that if they should tend toward an aspect incompatible with the laws of nature, they can be controlled. When in lascivious Rome, marriage began to be looked upon with almost general loathing, boys were sold shamelessly on public markets for the most horrible abuses, and they were kept in hundreds by nobles in special palaces, Augustus endeavored to control this terrible evil by indefatigable promotion of marriages and by inescapable punishment for bachelor life. Constantine believed that he could attain this purpose with more certainty by imposing the death sentence for this offense; each legislator has his special way of effectively controlling public ills. The best of them is the one that bases itself on the best knowledge of the nature of the nation which is to be improved.

So that the minds of persons living in marriage are less inflamed against each other, and procreation be prevented less often by continuous quarrels in individual households, the police must see to it strictly that parents never transgress the boundaries of their power over their children in regard to the choice of a spouse, and give their children reasonable freedom. It will also protect the inner calm of families, and consequently married harmony, and forcefully castigate all public, voluntary or arbitrary separations of marriage because of quarrels, and not permit that husband and wife choose separate abodes and remain separated for good without reason, each tormenting himself by suspicion against the other, and not infrequently giving cause to it. Therefore, information on such occurrences must be obtained in time, and endeavors should be made by all possible means, by clerical and secular exhortation, to reunite the minds. If necessary, recalcitrant persons should be made to toe the line by force of authority. The police should punish harsh treatment of peasant women by their coarse and ill-bred husbands. This harsh treatment embitters the minds more and more every day, and intercourse (at least between married couples) often does not take place for years. The peasant altogether holds his wife in too low esteem; and in his eyes she hardly takes precedence over the cattle. This is the reason

* "Numerum liberorum finire, apud eos flagitium est." Tacitus, de morib. germ.

why few of them think of seeking remedies for their wives should any of them fall ill. I know of many instances when such negligence caused the death or permanent loss of health of the women, and nothing is more affected by this than fertility. Since every husband has certain duties, imposed by civil law, to aid his ill wife, and if his wife dies because he did not call an approved or experienced physician, he loses his claim to her dowry, it is only required to enforce more than has been done hitherto in many regions the fulfillment of such a natural duty, and that the police aid the weak sex.

Also agreed indifference of married couples and their mutual debaucheries should not escape the police authorities; even if the two contracting parties believe they can absolve each other of the given promise, this is not the case when the country may lose by it as much as in this case, and where religion and the political system make marriage an insoluble bond. Likewise, concubinage of married people should be prosecuted because the damage that is done to marital fertility cannot be made good by the procreation of illegitimate children, for their survival as well as their future good education are much less certain than where fatherly love and unhindered tenderness protect them.

2a. Expecting that those countries which to their eternal shame still carry on trade with eunuchs will soon abolish this atrocity and learn to sanctify the rights of nature, endeavors should be made in our country to bind the hands of those who under the pretext of healing abdominal injuries or hernias, often enough still castrate. An example should be a well-thinking and great prince who saved many miserable people by banning castration in his country by a special decree.

* * *

There follow various regulations according to which operations on hernia have to be carried out without castration.

Therefore all foreign vagabonds and hernia cutters, who by their smooth chatter are too easily able to talk the afflicted peasant into taking such daring steps, should be forbidden immediately upon their entry to rove about in the villages, and all mayors should receive the most emphatic order not to permit any of these persons to make a surgical operation, especially cutting hernias. In case an operation takes place, however, they should be made to compensate for the operation as well as for the damage ensuing from it. The clergymen, who are usually consulted by their parishioners before such operations and are asked for spiritual aid, could render mankind a service here, too, by explaining to the patient, as well as to his relatives, the consequences of such an undertaking. Or, if all this does not help, to report this to the proper authorities, so that assistance could be rendered by them.

* * *

After dealing with the proper treatment and prevention of hernia, Frank stipulates the conditions under which a sterile marriage should be dissolved:

§10

Finally, and so that at least the damage caused to the general well-being of the citizens by matrimonial sterility not be irremediable in cases in which neither ecclesiastical nor secular laws prevent this, it should be ensured that the parties who can prove the inability of the spouse to procreate or have some other valid cause for separation, be enabled according to the practice of their Church to obtain such separation without objection, that they are not beggared thereby, or are not deliberately deprived of the time and ability for another marriage due to the lengthy process of investigation. It should be permitted, therefore, to take a married couple to task and question them if the marriage is sterile after ten years, to what cause they believe this unnatural state is due, for thereby some women, who are unhappy and out of excessive shyness avoid all explanations of this kind, though healthy and able to bear children, could be helped and informed of the freedom permitted them by the Church. However, if the cause can be removed, they could be instructed to use the means provided by the Creator against an ill that is deleterious to the state and even to general health. Against this ill only the richest or nobler citizens are used to seek help so far, although the middle-class and working-class is precisely the one whose healthy multiplication matters most to the persons in authority and to regents.

According to a circular from Berlin, dated 27 September 1751, "spouses among whom there prevail *inimicitiae capitales & notoriae*, and from whose marriage nothing but trouble and calamity for one spouse or the other can be expected, if they seek divorce, this should not be made difficult for them; on the contrary, if such hostility is properly proven, the bond of marriage should be immediately dissolved, without previously deciding on separation from table and bed."

However, "according to the rescript of 29 December 1751 the punishment for divorce also shall decide that whichever spouse is guilty has to pay the innocent one."*

According to public information, the above rescript has been somewhat restricted because there was frequent abuse of the petitions for divorce. However, although these restrictions may be necessary, the impossibility of just divorce would weigh heavily upon the innocent spouse, if theological difficulties rather more than the law of natural justice should prevent the dissolubility of a bond which may gain in esteem through the dignity of a sacrament, but which had to degenerate in every community into a chain of calamity to which virtue and uprightness often find themselves shackled, without there being any cause why in a state from which the public and private well-being depend so much, the mere whim of a base person should be the

---

* Collection of Edicts for the Years 1751–55.

reason that the innocent spouse, though not prevented from separation from table and bed, yet for the rest of his or her life be unable to find solace in the company of a worthy subject. About 16 years ago, a middle-class wife gave her diligent and living husband a good dose of fly poison, whereupon he was close to death. The woman poisoner escaped for years; the man who had been saved was unable to remarry, although nature and domestic circumstances pressed him hard to do so . . . Was it his fault that he had been deserted and poisoned? However, these are things that are beyond the comprehension of a physician, and I leave them entirely to the judgment of those who know how to apply reasons of a higher kind in order to solve such otherwise insoluble difficulties.

PART TWO
Section Five

Of the damage done to the healthy population through obstructing free choice in the selection of a spouse

§1

Love is the spice of the married state, and nature, which wants people not to await the act of procreation with an indifferent expression, has used this spice to advantage so that tasty fruits, and not only yawning children are born. Whenever I see some sluggish and sullen temper, I am tempted to think that the mother enjoyed herself at the wrong time, and the father, still half asleep, thanked her. Children who were begot more from duty than from natural emotion, always look as if they were not really serious about playing their assigned role in the world, and they only serve for filling the stage where human life runs its course. Just look at the fruits of most marriages which were concluded in accordance with rank and according to some clever arithmetic, without reciprocal liking having lit the marriage torch. It proves that to beget persons who lack neither liveliness nor activity, a certain degree of warmth is required, as is required for every eminent deed, without which one in every republic is only a left-over. The children of love, most of whom are unfortunately illegitimate, have always been distinguished by lively looks and a natural efficiency which is almost unknown to the dutiful heirs, and every friend of human society must certainly desire that the act of procreation between spouses does not become a merely mechanical act.

§2

The persons in authority in the police, therefore, must ensure that nobody in the community abuses his paternal powers by forcing his marriageable children into unions against which the heart rebels, and to which the imagination refuses its necessary assistance.* Not that intractable youth should be permitted complete

* According to the former customs of the Romans, dependent children and daughters of marriageable age were often married by dint of paternal power, as can be seen particularly from one place in Gellius, "De Sponsalibus," lib. IV. Vid. L.B. a Wollzogen, "Diss. de Connubiis Infantum," c.I. p. 17.

freedom to sacrifice the well-being of the family to an unfortunate or ill-advised infatuation. But it should not happen that obstinacy, greed, or irresponsible intentions prevent marriages between courageous couples who have the necessary fire in their veins for begetting, and thereby could promote the work of procreation in accordance with the intentions of nature and the country. In France, there is a law which permits marriageable maidens to give their yes and their person to any honorable man who offers them his hand in marriage, unless there are well-founded objections against him. If the father of such a maiden refuses his consent out of obstinacy, the daughter repeats three times in proper form and with due deference the exhortation (sommations respectueuses), whereupon she is entitled to proceed with the marriage, even without such consent. On the other hand, how often does one find elsewhere that an ambitious father, or a father who has been left with the maternal inheritance for the maintenance of his daughter, fights against any sensible union of his daughter until his child either takes recourse to dissoluteness or becomes part of the class of hopeless virgins, without properly claiming her natural right to being lawfully provided for and to holding a position which by dint of honor and nature is her vocation.*

§3

One would think that nowhere is there a freer choice of a wife than among the peasant class, where unintentional friendship should join the hearts and enable everybody to attain his aim without much hindrance. But this is not so. A large number of healthy maidens in the country remain for ever unprovided for because they do not find a suitor in their own village, and outsiders cannot court them without danger to their lives. As soon as the young men in a village notice that a suitor from another village is after one of their maidens, in most places there is no persecution that he would not have to suffer from them. It is not rare that several killings are the consequences of these senseless customs. There is indeed something strange in the rancor which entire communities harbor because of their unmarried women, without anybody ever thinking of deriving lawful benefit from it.

§4

On the contrary, in some places there is the custom that does not permit a young man to marry outside his village, and to fetch a strange maiden as his wife if he is unable or unwilling to buy himself off by a certain sum of money,** and this is often

---

* According to an old custom (coutume), in the provinces of Anjou and le Maine, a maiden past her twenty-fifth year may let herself be deflowered (déflorer) without her father being entitled to disinherit her because of that. "Encyclopédie," Tome X, art défloration.

** Or the maiden herself must leave part of the fortune behind because of the reigning so-called bondage; this led to the suppression of many thousands of marriages. Perhaps this also explains the influence of this old custom on the general welfare.

accompanied by bloody brawls. Expectation of this deters many a young man who cannot find a suitable wife in his village from marrying altogether, or at least for a long enough time.

* * *

After Frank has dealt with the consequences of inbreeding by animals and human beings, he proposes to prevent them by encouraging free communication between neighboring communities:

§7

Why should not thought be also given to devising means of enhancing unity among neighboring communities? Certain joint celebrations, where both sexes of different communities, under the eyes of their superiors and fathers, could meet several times a year in peace and love and become acquainted with each other through friendly intercourse, would perhaps be the best means of countering the hitherto existing hatred between communities. Freedom of persons to talk to each other without having to fear somebody's jealousy would have to be upheld by good laws, and troublemakers would have to be ejected at the first move, and strictly punished. Many opportunities would thus arise for concluding alliances favorable to the state, which at present occur only rarely in view of the prevailing wild manner, i.e., mixing like untamed animals only after bloody wars.—Our forefathers gathered their youth in the shade of broad oaks to tender dances, where many a marriage was concluded, just as in our times at parish fairs and wedding dances in the country many a young man sincerely grasps the hand of the red-cheeked maiden. This is a reason why such public festivities and congregations of young people can be abolished only to the real detriment of those concerned, merely because of some easily prevented disorders. It seems that by excessive strictness the laws could easily do more harm than good, the legislators' forgiving insight should therefore moderate it.—The Jews (a people which understands the advantages of procreating, regardless of all unjust oppression, better than any other extinct nation, who have seen this mostly during their beginnings and survived their end) still keep up the custom of assembling their youth on holidays, and thus, arm in arm, to run joyously through the wide streets, whereby the point is always emphasized that the unmarried lacks five things: "The blessings of heaven, a true life, pleasure, succor, and all the best."*

---

* M. Just. Fridr. Zachariae, "Dissert. philolog. felicem matrum curam, educandis liberis adhibendam, proponens." Kiliae 1732.

PART TWO
Section Six

Of public physical education of grown-up daughters as future mothers in the community

"Par l'extrème mollesse des femmes, commence celle des hommes. Les femmes ne doivent pas être robustes comme eux; mais pour eux, pour que les hommes qui naîtront d'elles, le soient aussi."

J. J. Rousseau, "De l'éducation"

§1

Nature itself molds every physical human being into what he is to be in time, and if nature is permitted to do its work unhindered, it produces masterpieces almost exclusively, and leaves to us the great art of raising trees and human children as dwarfs. Most persons, who are contemptuously called savages, are of the most magnificent physical build, the maidens slim and ready for all the functions of their sex, especially for giving birth, which with them is much easier and auspicious than with us, so much so that according to Graunt's observations in America, out of a thousand women giving birth not one dies.

§2

Things are entirely different where, as with us, the usual manner of education is that any female who is only slightly above the peasant or lower middle class, or supposed to be, is almost paralyzed from the time she has attained her tenth year, up to her adulthood, so that eventually we achieve the weak and pampered sex that we want. A woman brought up according to what is called good taste is a really miserable and pitiful creature compared with what nature raises without us. At the slightest continuous motion, she feels all the sensations of a sick person, palpitation of the heart, shortness of breath, trembling and lassitude. Eternal sitting and the noninterrupted leisure of their motor muscles are the reason that circulation takes place only in those vessels to which the strength of the feeble heart is sufficient by itself to convey the juices. But there is no trace of internal motion of the blood in such parts where this strength alone is not sufficient, and whose smallest veins can be filled only by the combined forces of the circulation. The genteel deathly color and the bloated appearance of city beauties are the consequences of half-strangled circulation; on the other hand, the healthy blood of the merry peasant lass tends toward the firm cheeks and proclaims the fortunate abundance of the soothing juices from which the future vigorous citizens will be produced.

§3

The influence of such an education on the general state of health is the worst, as is obvious from mere observation. It is here that the key to the disheartening observation made everywhere must be sought: that the mortality among noble children is so much greater than among the country folk. The vital strength of the pampered mother does not suffice to convey with sufficient emphasis to the fetus the required nutrition which is essential for its best development and the greatest possible perfection of all its parts.—How can watery blood, heated only by an artificial fire, convey to the creature who grows so fast out of nothing more than a merely light spongy nature, provide it with substance suitable to provide the human body with the durability required by all its functions, and convey external impressions to the soul with a certain agility and elasticity?—Look at the fate of such mothers; look how the woman, product of the current method of upbringing and with some advantages of a superficial education, soon collapses after having given birth to one or two children, and how extraordinarily this natural function exhausts her. On the other hand the quick peasant woman who is not overburdened with work, briskly goes back to work in the field soon after having given birth and, without change in her good condition, is soon ready for further pregnancy. The city woman receives more help than the peasant woman, for as already mentioned earlier, the midwives in cities are usually more skilled and, together with the physicians, they help remedy many bad situations during birth, which would mean death to a lone peasant woman. Nevertheless, the danger to women after birth is only slightly greater in the country than in cities. It is true that many a village woman causes her own death by excessive vigor, by getting up too soon after birth and going out, and also by all sorts of carelessness, of which the city woman giving birth in comfort knows nothing. Yet, in giving birth, the latter must do the same work as the former; in relation to her strength she must become more heated and strain her nerves more than the hardened peasant woman; therefore, frail women after birth are exactly like persons who have overworked, they sink into a consuming lassitude, or are prey to inflammations and childbed fever, due to excreted juices or juices coagulated in fine vessels which in the very first days after birth become gangrenous and septic, or leave obstructions in the internal genital organs which may cause future complete sterility.

§4

Everybody must judge whether things should be left as they are and whether indifference to this is in place: that every citizen lets himself be dictated to by the current vogue, locks up his daughter in good Turkish fashion, and thus fashions instead of a worthy mother of future citizens, a creature whose natural predisposition it is to produce only useless weaklings.

§5

Of the influence of convent education on the health of future world citizens

In our country, it is a generally accepted custom among all from the middle class to the higher nobility, that maidens, as soon as they have reached their twelfth or fourteenth year, are sent to convents in order to refine their education there and to train them partly in the French language, or in other work (which, however, also cannot make a man very happy). In the past, when opportunities for education outside convents were rare, this custom may have been very useful; at present, however, I do not see how one can look on with indifference at the continuation of this custom, without achieving a great physical improvement in such educational institutions which, however, can hardly be expected. As regards religion and notions of virtue, certainly the necessary concepts of religion can be taught to all classes; as for virtue, it is not important to fill the heads of young maidens as is partly done with strange ideas that all worldly persons are adventurers, and thus induce in their hearts a certain distaste for their peers, so that when these good lasses rejoin the world, they have learned to look at everything askance. It is seen that most young women bring back from such homes a certain prejudice against all worldly society, for each of them was treated as a recruit of the order, and endeavors are often made to induce in them a distaste for their future destination in the world, in order to persuade them to take up a profession to which only the fewest have a natural calling before their 25th year.

It is not only the state that loses when the most affluent women, although often without any predisposition whatsoever, get stuck in such homes; I have noted that the education of most women in convents may be deleterious for the health of future female citizens, and consequently also for their future procreativity. How detrimental must it be for a future worldly person to be locked up between four walls for several years, where a maiden rarely has her own room to sleep in, where so many, in an often less than spacious room, have to sit on their chairs for hours on end every day as if nailed down, and to work; whence they do not get out anywhere but to the church of the house, to the table, and rarely to a garden that is surrounded by a high wall and robbed of all air? Food and drink are placed before them exactly on a certain hour; it may be good for those who can always have it so, but not for persons who may have to conform to others in time. The same applies to sleeping and waking.

Most women, who spent most of their youth in convents, cannot bear change of air without greater danger than those who have been brought up outside convents. Their bodies, used to the closed-in air, are as sensitive as their souls seem to be, and they often bring back into the world the impressions, and the special mental faults of their frequently dissatisfied and sullen companions. In short, if the many physical shortcomings of convent education are remedied, I do not see what there is to approve in the custom of hurrying our daughters so much to the convents, and I would suggest an entirely different style of life. Its aim would be to base the quality of our descendants on the health of the parents, and to produce children who will come to enjoy their existence.

* * *

There follow examples of forms of educating the female sex in use by different nations; then, he states in principle:

Necessity of physical exercises of future mothers

The movement of the body in fresh air is equally necessary for both sexes; it maintains the circulation of the juices and the animating fire of the nerves, without which only half-live children are born. A state which is indifferent to the mode of education of the future mothers, waives at the expense of posterity all the advantages of health and strength which our forefathers, leading a completely different life, maintained so long and so carefully. What good are embroidered pictures and shoes, the shapeless laces and cuffs, and all the dallying at a time when the female body should be hardened for its future destination and for all the functions of social life, and a solid foundation be laid for future durable health? As regards the state of their bodies, is not the fate of common peasant wenches so much better, the more their busy life differs from the sleepy pampering of city beauties?

Therefore every worthy person in authority must consider how he could, by prudence and good example, inhibit the natural yearning of city women for comfortable indolence, and how he could correct the fault which has penetrated all the education of noble and middle-class young females everywhere, but especially in convents, where persons live in such a way as if all the faculties of the soul had to be bought by immobility of the body, at the price of the loss of one's health.

* * *

§8

Better arrangements regarding dances

Though all the recommendations are intended to enhance movement of the women, this nevertheless should not be exaggerated. Various dances are an important cause of many illnesses of unmarried women, who often have an incomprehensible passion for such pleasures, and consider it an honor if they have danced several partners to exhaustion. Almost in every medium-sized town there will be several examples of such dance heroines, who soon after the carnival entertainments have lost their lives because of fever or inflammation. This happens more so if one drinks while still hot, or if the company at night goes home while full of sweat. Even some kinds of dance, where the motions are very violent and protracted, or very disorderly, cause the blood to seethe, which is difficult to subdue and may be dangerous. Now if a female, while in the midst of the monthly purification, commits such a fault, and this happens frequently, it happens rarely that she escapes without some obstruction and all sorts of detrimental effects on the internal genital organs.

The authorities, therefore, are rightfully entitled to determine the duration of balls. Also because of the health of the participants, it would be very desirable if certain excessively violent dances, the so-called waltzing, etc., were forbidden.

The police will forbid parents and relatives to let their daughters to attend such violent amusements without supervision, or at uncertain times. And the police must forbid dancers to disperse before half an hour of quiet has passed since the dance came to an end. Everybody, but especially young girls, should be acquainted with the consequences of infringing these arrangements.

According to public reports, the Basle Municipal Council meanwhile has forbidden waltzing at all dances in the city and in the country. Contravention of this is to be punished, regardless of the standing of the person concerned, by a fine of 50 pounds. The decree of 17 December 1719, enacted by the Canton Solothurn, and which has to be read again on 14 December 1780 before Shrovetide, deserves to be quoted here.

"His Grace finds himself obliged, for very important reasons, to forbid in town and country waltzing, which is very detrimental to health and contrary to propriety, and to punish contravention, regardless of the standing of the person concerned, by an irrevocable fine of 50 pounds; this is to be publicly announced at all places."

§9

Disadvantages of certain pieces of clothing to future mothers

The police must furthermore make provisions that no fashions in clothing which inhibit the natural growth of young maidens and harm their health are introduced and tolerated by parents. On this subject I shall say more elsewhere. But here I must at least recall that for the love of mankind the usual corsets should be struck from the number of permitted garments. They prevent the natural formation and expansion of the abdominal cavity in which in future pregnancies the uterus must expand in order to obtain sufficient space for the daily growth of the fetus. Through the constant pressure of the corset, the abdominal muscles become either too stiff and do not yield to expansion, which often leads to premature births or miscarriages, or else these parts are in a certain way paralyzed and are too weak during the timely birth of a child to afford sufficient assistance. Equal attention is due to the fact that the rash lacing of these fish-bone suits of armor prevent the growth of the breasts, and especially the natural protrusion of the nipples. This usually makes women unable to nurse their children. It suffices to see how badly off most mothers are who in their youth were laced in too much, when they want to nurse their children themselves: most of them have nipples that protrude too little, some have nipples that do not protrude at all from their breasts, the children cannot hold them with their lips, and they and their mothers are thereby exposed to all the consequences of neglected breastfeeding.

One should altogether take care to make the clothing of future mothers light and comfortable. Corsets and excessively tight-fitting clothes are detrimental to health and procreation, for they force the juices from the surface to the inner parts; this causes full-bloodedness in the vessels of the internal genital organs which promotes future excessively violent bleedings, miscarriages, and hemorrhoids.

* * *

The subsequent sections contain advice on behavior during menstruation, and demand clarification of the mutual duties of marriage partners.

PART THREE

Section One

Of pregnancy in general, its rights and advantages in the community; of the necessary care for maintaining pregnant women and their embryos

§1

Natural dignity of the pregnant

The female sex deserves veneration and all possible consideration in a condition through which the whole is maintained by the daily replenishment of new world citizens, the development of all states promoted, and individual families perpetuated. A good police, thus, must be watchful for the sake of this most necessary class of persons, maintain them in their good state, and respect, and protect them. The police must use all possibilities to see that all matters, evident and even unobtrusive, are vigorously removed through which the great work of procreating our posterity, and thus our population, may be weakened or even smothered. Therefore, the police must use real paternal care to avert the dangers which threaten mother or child, or both together, so that every woman in her blessed state may attain her aim joyfully and in comforting security.

§2

All civilized nations believed to have found in this condition something so venerable that they gave it the most respectful names; however, most of them are due to the oldest legislators, and subsequent times have done little to add; on the contrary, gradually almost everywhere, many of their prerogatives have been lost, and in many regions this most worthy condition is mixed with the large mass, almost without distinction.

The Athenians venerated their women citizens, who were blessed with pregnancy, so much so that they even spared murderers who fled to a pregnant woman and reached her in their flight. Every pregnant woman received a double gold coin as a gift from the ancient kings of Persia. The Jews who, as is well known, always observe their laws so strictly, permitted those of their pregnant women who could not resist, to violate the prohibition and eat pork if they so wanted. Whereas in Rome, everybody who encountered a person of the magistrate was made to step aside and make

70

room by the vehement calls of the lictors, a married woman and even her husband, if sitting next to her, were permitted to drive past unhindered "so that she not suffer damage through compulsion or a blow."

* * *

More examples follow:

The freedom of pregnant women has an even greater range: the greatest nations on earth either seem to have once observed the law, or to still observe it "not to have marital intercourse with a pregnant woman"; and this circumstance is probably one of the most important causes of polygamy which is permitted among many of these nations.

* * *

The subsequent sections contain examples and further advice concerning the behavior of pregnant women.

§5

First of all it must be ensured that pregnant women in every country and class are held in respect by everybody. Youth must be educated in time in this sense and even the slightest fault in the due respect, the smallest insult to a woman who is with child, must always be punished twice as severely, just as greater crimes against pregnant women are subject to more stringent punishment anyway.

§6

It is not enough that pregnant women enjoy all the prerogatives of their irksome state; endeavors should be made to increase their advantages by ordering that on public occasions pregnant women should take precedence over nonpregnant women of equal rank, once they are more than halfway through pregnancy and their motherhood is certain. Though this may not have much substance, one knows people too well not to realize how infinitely flattering it is to every pregnant woman when she sees that a better rank has been allotted to her in the republic.

* * *

Further rules for the treatment of pregnant women.

§10

Nobody should dare tell a pregnant woman tales and accounts of sudden misfortunes, especially accounts of births with unfortunate outcome and of women who died in childbed, and thus scare them. Midwives and attendants are to be given special orders not to brag in front of their pregnant women, in order to gain their respect and display their indispensability, telling of their heroic feats which they accomplished with this or that woman in difficulties by turning the child, etc. ; I know of cases where women had been entertained with such tales during their pregnancy, and then, when labor set in and not everything went immediately as desired, suffered the greatest fear and anguish, which even embarrassed and alarmed the garrulous midwives.

§11

On the contrary, in order to lessen fear, the danger of giving birth should be represented as less serious at every opportunity, and since the death of a single woman giving birth immediately frightens the entire community, the women should be taught that some such case or other does not mean anything, that it is impossible, since human beings of every rank and in every situation are still mortal, for pregnant women alone to be a complete exception. But, according to experience, women during pregnancy die incomparably more rarely than at any other time, and according to credible calculations the conviction is justified that of all women giving birth only one out of sixty, seventy, or as in Sweden, out of eighty, two or three dies. Of course, the surest means of preventing such fear is to provide every community with efficient midwives on whom the pregnant women can rely.

* * *

In §12 it is stated that—and Semmelweis later forcibly pointed this out—even the tolling of the passing bell may frighten a pregnant woman.

§13

Imagination of pregnant women

As regards the imagination of pregnant women, there are important reasons to doubt its effect on the formation of the fetus. Of course, there are always reasons which may be suspected of having caused the malformation of the fetus, without imputing to the mother's mental images any metamorphosing power. However, without examining the matter more closely, it must be admitted that a pregnant woman in general shows a more high-pitched imagination, and that in this respect, there is always some danger for the fetus, for every violent passion of the mother, but especially fright, brings the circulation of the juices into disorder, which is detrimental to the tender build of the fetus, and daily experience has confirmed that this causes some children to be miscarried before their time.

* * *

There follow examples of the imagination (fancies) of pregnant women.

What can the police do here? . . . Of course, it cannot remove from human dwellings everything that could induce a sudden fright or loathing in sensitive pregnant women. But the police can first see to it that on various occasions women in general are informed of the ineffectiveness of the imagination. Second, it can insert into the general educational system of the daughters, better acquaintance with objects inducing abhorrence and fright, without seeming to do so, and thus enhance intrepidity. And finally, the police can endeavor to remove at least some of the most prominent frightening images, and prevent all preventable surprises to excitable pregnant women, and thus, so-to-say, cut off the nourishment of their imagination which is out to seek adventures.

Thus it will be useful if a good police will see to it, as far as possible, that all such objects be banned from streets, highways, gardens, avenues and public places where there might be pregnant mothers.

* * *

Various recommendations are made in §§14–17 for preventing pregnant women from being frightened (establishment of homes for cripples, prohibition of lying in state in churches).

§18
Necessary cessation of heavy work of pregnant women

Townspeople and peasants often burden their pregnant women, long after they have entered the second half of pregnancy, with much and difficult work. While the otherwise diligent peasant lies idle behind the stove in winter, his wife in advanced pregnancy, in the greatest cold and sometimes on dangerously iced paths,* fetches water (in our country carrying it on the head, whereby the pail has to be lifted by the raised arms), brings firewood into the kitchen, and lights the stove. This, because these classes view and treat their wives as their first servant. It would be useful if it were borne in mind that it is punishable to make pregnant women in the last two months of pregnancy perform excessively heavy work, especially threshing, which is still very common in the country, although it is very detrimental for women in advanced pregnancy;** moreover, though distress has no law, and the poor day

---

* Only because of pregnant women, should sand, sawdust, cut straw, etc., be spread in front of every house as soon as there is ice. It is terrible to see how many persons fall on the slippery ground in every street and suffer injuries for lack of such precaution. See public safety.
** Van Swieten saw a woman miscarry because she wanted quickly to raise a two-year old child who had fallen. L.c. [Comment.] T. IV, §1299. How detrimental must it be when women in advanced pregnancy in the country are forced in a stooping position for days on end to hoe the soil, mow grass, etc.

laborer with 5 or 8 children, of whom half cannot walk yet, has his hands full enough with outside work without being able to help at will his pregnant wife in the household, it should be ensured that malice, greed, or laziness do not contribute, as sometimes happens, to force such women to carry out heavy work. In a nearby village, I once lost a pregnant woman and her child who had come in the eighth month of pregnancy when, instead of her husband, she had stood for hours up to her calves in the mud to clean the creek; the mayor, who was present, did not send the poor woman away. She started bleeding violently, and the midwife, who was called too late, could not prevent it. This was fatal to mother and child. In the countries of Baden, a mare in the last six weeks of pregnancy and six weeks after foaling is exempt from compulsory labor or her owner is not obliged to compulsory labor on her account. Why is the peasant not exempt when his wife is near giving birth? Especially at a time when he has to work outside all day for others and she alone bears the entire burden of the household. Therefore should not the husband of every pregnant woman be completely exempt from all personal compulsory labor at least during the last six weeks, so that he could help his wife more? If this were too difficult for communities, the compulsory labor could be made up after this time has elapsed, and could be distributed over the entire year. Of course, most peasants would not be glad of that because it cannot ever be brought home to them that a pregnant woman during her blessed state is entitled to twice as much consideration and kindness.

But to make even more certain that no citizen will force his wife to perform excessively hard work without dire need, everyone should be held responsible for the consequences of every kind of unjust coercion, and the neglecting of such clear duties should be strictly punished.*

* * *

Further prohibitions for pregnant women (dancing, sledging, wearing constraining clothes).

§21
Nobody should beat a pregnant woman

Among the coarser classes of people, especially the peasants, the right of men to chastise their wives by beating should be completely rescinded during pregnancy. Those who infringe this should be strictly punished, for the fetus is always maltreated thereby, and the pregnant woman is not only the wife of an individual citizen, but also the hope of the state whose protection she now has to enjoy. Since, however,

---

* Most of our peasants are similar to the Hottentots who pile onto their wives who carry small children an additional 15 or 16 skins, which the women carry on their heads, while the men with their rifles calmly walk next to their 'beasts of burden.' "Allgem. Histor. all. Reis.," III, Vol. III, Book 6, p. 152.

cases may occur where the wantonness or inflexibility of a woman may overcome the patience of a Socrates, at least for an instant, and where complete freedom from punishment might cause much greater disorder, it must be seen to that chastisement is a lighter correction which will not damage the fetus.

§23

Among poor couples, one pregnancy often follows immediately after the other; perhaps because intercourse is rarer and occurs only after the complete maturation of the seed, and fertilization of the woman, just achieved, is not immediately undone by new dissipations and a hundred other causes. Also there are cases in every community where the extreme poverty of the pregnant women prevents them from obtaining the necessary support and even the simplest food. As a poor woman she has a just claim to the charity of her fellow citizens, but it is known how slowly and sleepily things move in such a case, and what grief the pregnant woman must overcome while the fetus sucks the enfeebled blood from her veins and makes immediate succor imperative.

In France a special "Arrêt"* stipulates that when a poor person, especially a destitute maidservant, declares herself pregnant, the man whom she names as the father (or if she names two, the one who seems more likely for the time being and until more information is obtained) has to provide her with the required food and also the necessary support during her confinement, because anything might happen if such a wretched woman were neglected.

Why should not every community apply the law likewise that every married woman in advanced pregnancy be permitted not only to appeal to the compassion of others, whose hardheartedness and refusal must be so depressing to her, but directly to the highest authority of the community, and demand as a right the double portion of a citizen who cannot earn her bread either by work or by begging, and yet is employed in furthering the well-being of the state.

* * *

Still further prohibitions for pregnant women (corsets, high heels, excessive drinking of wine and coffee, bloodletting, praematuri concubitus).

§30

Proposal to have an accurate list of all pregnancies in the community which have completed their first half

As nothing of what has been said about this subject hitherto can be observed, and the rights of the pregnant women cannot be safeguarded, nor the proper care be

* Of 18 February 1679. In several other countries the same has now been stipulated.

taken of them, if the persons in authority are not informed in time which women are entitled to these privileges, I therefore submit to the judgment of those who are not prejudiced against a matter only because it is new or unusual, whether it would be useful to keep everywhere an accurate list of the women who are in the second half of pregnancy, a time at which there are certain symptoms.—That way, not only the number of citizens actually living in each state would be recorded, as has been done hitherto, but the tender trunks in the human tree nursery that are the budding objects of the hopeful country, would also be noticed and recorded. I shall explain myself in more detail.

These lists of pregnancies would contain the rank, name, age, time of marriage, and the number of children already begot according to their sex. The report would be recorded from approximately the last half of the new conception, and next to it the time of birth, whether it was too early (and if so, in what month, especially because of which presumable, probable, or certain unavoidable or punishable causes) or at the right time, dead or alive, well formed or unnaturally deformed, the sex of the child, whether the mother escaped with her life or whether she died because of a special (and which) cause before, during, or after birth, whether she intends to nurse the child herself, or intends to employ a wet-nurse, feed it on animal milk, or other food, or already does so.

Such reports would be heard and recorded immediately by certain discreet persons and every father of a family would be free to choose whether to make the report himself in writing or through his relatives. Or, as regards the circumstances of the birth, the midwives of each town and village could be instructed to report everything that should be known, and that they found in the course of their duties. It seems to me that this arrangement would be very useful and important.

Few persons who know something of the inner management of a state deny that it is an important advantage if the marriages and their fertility, as well as the ratio of births to deaths is accurately known. So far, according to fairly complete lists, it has been found that in general in most countries, the number of births exceeds the number of deaths. An accurate list of those human beings who between the instant they were conceived and the ordinary time of birth, die in the mother's body, are miscarried, or aborted, could apparently contribute to obtaining more details. During the first half of pregnancies it is not advisable to concern oneself with recording them (for until then their knowledge is fairly uncertain), although perhaps most human embryos die or are lost at that stage. But what is there after this period to prevent us from informing the persons in authority of the women's blessed state by a fairly clear announcement that will not be a burden to anybody? Are there not very important causes to justify such an arrangement? Is it not important that the secret ways of nature are thus more and more discovered, and that one learns thereby that even in its squanderings it observes that divine order in the procreation and maintenance of our race which Süsmilch and others found and proved to exist from birth until death? How useful is it if the state is acquainted with the annual loss of hoped-for citizens, and thus has its attention drawn more to the causes which in some region or other increase this loss every year, and are the reason why only a few children are born in time out of a certain number of pregnancies, whereas others are aborted before their time, because of lack of consideration for pregnancy, because of bad supervision and enforcement of the duties of the pregnant women, even out of wantonness or deliberate use of force.

In the cases of unmarried pregnant women, it is necessary that pregnancy be reported immediately its first half is complete, so that better supervision can be ensured, and all misfortune thus be prevented. Yet experience shows us that in many places many a fetus is aborted in the most punishable way even by married mothers; one would think that it is superfluous to care for the safety of the not yet born posterity, and to give this class a guardian who could safeguard the right of such human beings and give them our most tender protection, and put a limit to the wantonness and malice of presumptuous and irresponsible mothers.

* * *

Various advantages of the suggested list of pregnant women are discussed subsequently (i.e., establishing the age of aborted embryos for one).

Before I end this article, I must mention another advantage of this arrangement. An accurate list of pregnancies and births supervised by the secular authorities can be used in every community with greater confidence as proof of origin, time of birth, rank, and names of both parents. Until now, only the certificate of baptism has been used; in most regions it is issued exclusively by the clergy, and since their records were not made in duplicate, an unfortunate occurrence has caused complete loss of the books of baptisms, with important consequences. This [loss] would not have occurred so easily if the secular authorities had recorded their new citizens as conscientiously as the clerical authorities had.

* * *

Now if this is done according to the described proposal, simultaneously at the secular authority, or possibly when the child has not come to be baptized, or should have had a public funeral, all the advantages which I mentioned above are obtained and it will be possible to judge according to certain criteria the fertility, as well as the diligence and care of each woman citizen for her embryo, and thus do away with disorder.

* * *

After Frank dealt in the greatest detail, in Part 3, Section 2 with the dissection of

cadavers of pregnant women who died before giving birth, and the saving of their em-
bryos, he turns in the last part of this book to the care of women giving birth and in
childbed.

PART THREE
Section Three

Of the necessary care in every community for pregnant women and women in confinement

§1

The state of a pregnant woman approaching confinement naturally imbues every sensitive heart with a quiet veneration which causes everybody to feel considerable sympathy for her fate and leaves us in a kind of disquietude up to its auspicious end. During that period, the pregnant woman has a certain undemanded right to our tenderness which the Creator makes express itself in favor of the human race, even among barbarians, when all other feelings are silent. I do not know whether it is the much lowered respect for the married state that has in recent times played such a large part in the indifference which many people exhibit toward the child-bearing sex in its most dignified function. But this much can be said confidently: the most ancient nations displayed their respect for women giving birth and in childbed (except for what has been said in the last fifty years about the business of giving birth) much more solemnly than certain centuries did.

* * *

In the subsequent paragraphs, Frank demands sensible consideration for women in childbed, and then he analyzes the magic notions of popular opinion, that she is unclean.

§6

After a brief mention of all those customs and rules of behavior which have been considered beneficial in various times and regions in regard to women giving birth and in childbed, it must be admitted that after so many examples attention must be given to such an important matter in the community. A state without which all of us would not exist certainly deserves our respect, and one would have not been born by a woman if one would not help promote all kinds of good measures to improve the fate of the child-bearing group. No animal creature so greatly needs someone else's help in giving birth as does the human female. The cases where unattended women gave birth with good results are as nothing compared with the ease with which most animals bring forth their young. This, for good reason, has been ascribed to the great size of the human head. It is very probable that the greater sensitivity of the human form also contributes much to this, for we see that, other conditions being equal, in general, the least tender mothers provided with coarser fibers await birth with less worry and suffer less during birth than the sensitive city woman who lacks almost all vigor for this great labor, and so often perishes either because of excessive strain, excessive sensitivity of the nervous system, or because of complete lack of strength and labor failing to take place because of some kind of paralysis.

* * *

§7

In order to be born without mishap, members of the human race generally need assistance by other human beings. And it depends on the skill of this assistance and on the timing of its correct application that the danger of birth is greatly reduced. Among the oldest nations, as among the Americans now, it was the men who assisted their wives in labor and received their children from them. Even among us, fathers of families now and again render this service, or they at least keep the woman giving birth on their lap, instead of letting their child be brought into the world in a labor chair and with the assistance of the first female neighbor who is available.

§8

But for reasons which I will state in more detail later, when treating the subject of appointing midwives in a country,* it is very irresponsible to calmly leave the fate of women giving birth in such inexperienced hands, and to look on indifferently while a number of fertile women citizens and upright mothers are killed in the most repulsive manner, and every year a number of innocent children are killed even before they are born. The persons in authority are responsible for this loss, and they cause the lack of the most important thing if they do not make efficient arrangements to provide every community with well-trained midwives, and every moderately large district with an efficient and experienced accoucheur. How can a pregnant woman retain her courage when such bad arrangements have been made for her safety during birth? And how else but with trepidation could she approach the time, when in obvious danger, she will see herself delivered over to the hands of ignorance for life and death? I have already mentioned how dangerously the prospect of such an uncertain fate must affect the mind of the pregnant woman and the embryo. And one should also consider how much cause one gives to a woman to protect herself against becoming pregnant by all kinds of ways, or even to be glad of a miscarriage, since so

---

* I had to postpone the treatment of this subject to the time when I should reveal my thoughts about the best way of arranging in an orderly manner the medical system in the state altogether.

little has been done for the safety of such a serious act on which, after all, the welfare of the state depends.

§9

But it does not suffice that efficient midwives be appointed everywhere and thus care is taken of unnatural and difficult births. It must also be ensured "that every pregnant woman immediately sends for the midwife as soon as labor pains begin." It happens all too often that they wait until an emergency is here and the child is about to emerge. Many women even brag that in this way they often bore their children before the midwife arrived, and I know some who almost always chanced it.

* * *

There follow examples in which emphasis is placed on the deleterious consequences of calling in the midwife too late.

But in order that such negligence be hindered, every midwife must be obligated, for her own safety and as a warning to negligent mothers, to make a proper report as to whether or not she has been present at the birth at all or whether she had been called too late to provide proper assistance, or that the woman in labor, out of misplaced or irresponsible shyness, did not suffer a timely examination to be carried out on her. For it would be the greatest wrong to leave a free hand to a heedless and audacious mother to sacrifice herself and her child to her obstinacy, without any punishment being meted out by those whose first duty it is to ensure public safety.

* * *

In §10, Frank puts forward the demand that only sworn midwives or accoucheurs should be called in.

§11

Necessity of good accoucheurs in every region

There are not rarely such childbirth cases that tax the skill of the most experienced man, and consequently are far beyond the ordinary science of an otherwise efficient midwife. Therefore, as mentioned before, several accoucheurs are required in every country so that midwives can turn to them for assistance in times of need. At some other time I shall examine the question as to whether it is useful to leave the business of midwifery completely in male hands as was done in the larger French towns in the past. But this much is certain: we shall never reach the point where country midwives will learn all the science needed to enable them to cope with every case that may occur, and there are strong reasons why they were long ago forbidden to use most of the tools. Therefore, since sworn midwives must be advised to ask for an accoucheur in case of extraordinary births, it must be ensured that the intention of this instruction not be thwarted by the stubbornness of the woman giving birth, or her relatives. In most cases, the accoucheur is called far too late, either because the midwife relied too much on her own resources, or because her expostulations concerning the necessity of calling an accoucheur were disregarded. This last happens either out of shyness, stubbornness, or fear of the costs.

Safe measures must be taken for meeting all these cases: time and limits must be stipulated for the midwives' attempts to deal with difficult births. One must endeavor to eradicate the prejudice against male accoucheurs in difficult births by reasonable representation, to which clergymen are most suited, but also by legislation. For the accoucheurs themselves certain modest fees must be stipulated, the refutation of which can be easily prevented by a few measures. And finally, every community must be empowered to demand for poor women giving birth immediate gratuitous assistance by an accoucheur who is paid [by the community] for this purpose.

* * *

There follow expositions concerning the use of delivery chairs and obstetric instruments.

§15

On the state of women after birth

I now come to the state of women in childbed. Either the birth went well and the woman feels as well as circumstances permit; or she suffered damage during the birth and is really ill. Here I do not take into account the necessary care for the newborn child, for in this first volume I do not yet deal with newborn children; this I leave for the next volume. On the other hand, the state of the woman who has just given birth deserves all my attention, and I ask every one of my readers not to ignore the least detail of what I have to say and advise concerning the safety of a class of persons which is so widespread and so in need and deserving of our compassion.

If a woman giving birth has been very much exhausted and damaged through the bad position of the fetus, or through delay of the birth, through various accidents or some fault, her state deserves the quickest assistance, the husband and the relatives have a double duty to do their utmost to have her health restored by suitable means. Since in such cases one relies mostly on the midwives' statement, these must be well acquainted with the most usual symptoms of an incipient or impending worsening of their women in childbed, and they must be admonished in their instructions to reveal her bad or serious state without loss of time to her relatives, and to remind them of their duty. But to prevent the relatives from blaming everything on the omission of this warning, the midwife in such cases must in good time make a report to the clergyman, and if this does not help, also to the secular authority: that this or that woman in childbed is sick and requires rapid assistance. This should be heeded by those concerned, as was mentioned earlier in §9.

Neither the midwife nor anyone other than an authorized physician or accoucheur should be permitted to prescribe medicines in such a case. For even with other conditions being equal, cases connected with childbirth are usually difficult to treat and cure; consequently, if the life of this ill woman is not to be exposed to the most obvious danger, no time should be lost and the last hope of saving her should not be squandered through unskilled treatment.

* * *

But even when the birth has been smooth and easy, and where the woman in child-bed seems completely healthy, the most active care must be taken to maintain her in the community. For although giving birth is something natural, and the state of a woman in childbed is not to be considered a real disease, Tissot is nonetheless right when he compares this state to the state of a gravely wounded person where a small mistake in conduct may easily have fatal consequences. Every day one can see country women in childbed, who, still feeling full of strength, get up in the first days after having given birth and return to their domestic duties. This proves that not all women suffer equally in childbirth. In addition, travel books reveal that in general among primitive people the women do not make so much ado with giving birth, and once it is over, they hurry without delay to the nearest river and into the water, whereupon they take up their occupation again like everybody else. A Kalmuck [Tatar] woman often mounts a horse on the second day after having given birth, and performs her household duties as before. This is where the exhaustion and deterioration of a good physical state among town-bred and pampered mothers makes itself felt most clearly. They are hardly able, without danger to their own lives, to bear the strain of the many muscles required during childbirth, without the consequence being a high fever or exhaustion: a cause which, as mentioned before, makes the mortality of town women in childbed much greater than in country women. On the other hand, however, the women giving birth in towns are safer than in the country because of skilled assistance by better midwives and accoucheurs. Yet despite of all this, the mortality of women during and after birth is far too high in most regions, and one cannot believe that the Creator stipulated this irrevocably. The experience of all physicians and accoucheurs confirms that at least two-thirds of women giving birth, who are in a bad way, could be saved through either a more appropriate way of life or more care. Thus the secular authorities should better heed the complaints of the physicians, and their inaction in this matter must certainly be considered one of the greatest sins of omission.

* * *

There follow expositions concerning the harmful consequences to women in childbed of christening feasts and other festivities.

§17

Further care of women in childbed

The police must provide that nobody causes a woman in childbed fright, fear, or annoyance. The sensitivity of women in this state is so great that if their lives are to be taken care of, not the slightest disturbance must be tolerated at such times.

* * *

There follow various recommendations to keep terrifying creatures (animals, human beings) and customs (tolling the death knell) from women in childbed.

In order to prevent all noise near and around women in childbed, a law was passed in Haarlem, Holland, according to which all commotion and turmoil in the neighborhood of women after birth is strictly forbidden. A sign is also affixed to the doors of women in childbed which, when seen by a city or town beadle, forbids him to enter such a house. "Such love," says Van Swieten, "is shown by the community to every woman who gave her country a citizen. The inhabitants, who are used to such a law and fulfill it faithfully, are thus taught already from the cradle to honor fruitful mothers and to keep all noise out of the neighborhood." How worthy of imitation is such a philanthropic law, and how important to everybody who knows from experience how often the life of the best women citizens on such occasion is sacrificed out of mere carelessness and unpardonable mischievousness! Even their rest must be respected, and for this reason, too, the nocturnal wanderings through the streets of drunken persons with noisy musical instruments should be stopped.

Since there is nothing, however, that so affects the minds of women in childbed as when impatient creditors insist on payment of their debts at such a time, it is only right that during six weeks neither demands for payment nor enforcement of payment be permitted, so that the fruitful woman citizen does not feel a detrimental effect on her health through lack of food, nor the newborn be in any way adversely affected.

* * *

Frank once more warns against using for statutory labor the husbands of women in childbed.

§20

But since some women in childbed are in great poverty, the most cruel abandonment and a lack of the most essential necessities is to be expected. It would certainly
be a grave mistake if the police did not provide the means to remedy such a great
and widespread shortcoming in the republic. Von Sonnenfels demands that if poor
women in childbed have no support, this should be reported by the midwife and the
priest, so that the police may receive the child gratuitously. The proposal is very
philanthropic, but I believe that it is better to leave the child with its mother until
such time when it needs her care less, and that the police pay her so much as is necessary to keep her and the child, at least during the first six weeks and until the mother
herself is able to earn money. The point is only to find how to do this in the most
useful manner.

* * *

*Frank describes, as examples, various institutions in France, England, and Germany;
then, he continues:*

Therefore how worthy of imitation must be the arrangement instituted by the
Grand Duke of Florence some years ago (1776)! This wise friend of the human race
and tender father of his people, touched by the misery of distressed women in childbed, had presented to every poor woman of his capital who gave birth some six pounds
out of his own income. Then provisions were made so that a salaried midwife was
appointed in each of the four quarters of the city. She was charged with the duty of
going as soon as she was called to a poor woman in labor in her quarter, without giving
preference to another woman in labor because of payment, and to assist with all
possible zeal in the birth. But for this, she was not permitted to accept the least in
return, neither as payment nor as gifts. In order that provisions were made for more
difficult cases also, special surgeons and accoucheurs were appointed for each
quarter of the city as well, and they also had to come free of charge to the assistance
of poor women in labor. On top of all these arrangements, the other accoucheurs and
midwives of the city are obliged, whenever it is demanded, to assist poor women
gratuitously. Moreover, in the Royal Hospital of St. Maria Nuova, all poor women
in childbed receive free of charge all the medicines which they might need in their
state.

It would be highly desirable, therefore, that every community take equally good
care of destitute women in childbed, and not remain indifferent to all the sad consequences of the hitherto obvious neglect of their needy female citizens.

* * *

A SYSTEM OF COMPLETE MEDICAL POLICE

Volume Two

Human Procreation and Marriage Institutions.
Preservation and Care of Pregnant Women, their
Fetuses, and of Lying-In Women in Each Community

PREFACE

The quiet, but public success which was accorded my first work on Medical Police (Medicinische Polizey) and, as I may say without the slightest suspicion of ridiculous complacency, the strictest observance of Horatius' Versate diu, versate nocturna! furthered the publication of this, the second volume. Considering that nobody before me had elaborated on Medical Police according to such a farreaching plan, I begged for indulgence if, as I myself easily foresaw, imperfections now and again crept in. Now I have even more reason to beg for indulgence without this request being held against me, since the importance and the variety of the material, the considerable difficulty of collecting at my own expense all the writings concerning this field in a place which is not very rich in books, and finally (almost inexplicable in our philanthropic times) the sparcity of outside contributions for beneficial sanitary regulations, all this must be a heavy, albeit not excessive burden on my shoulders. Not excessive in that my way of life is laborious anyway; so that I need not be compelled to blink anxiously toward the often indecisive word of command of some critics and humbly beg for indulgence. I do not seek more than to deserve well of mankind, so far as this can be expected of an individual citizen, without asking that all heads, including some strange ones, should nod and express their approbation and thanks.

Because this volume contains various subjects, there is little I want to say beforehand. Some subjects may seem not to belong to the realm of Medical Police in the strictest sense, but it might be useful to point out in passing to the prudent fathers of the Republic, who can easily influence others, some important causes of the great mortality among young people. When at certain times business is less pressing, a patriot may introduce by example and habit what does not seem to be so easily feasible by police statutes, even if it concerns only a minor matter. Thus, the things which some like (in a fit of weakness due to despair that any good will be done that requires some effort on the part of the humane representatives) to classify as pia desideria, will prove useful in a book which, at least by its title, will induce some persons in authority to leaf through a medical treatise which, without learned and tedious digressions, is devoted to the public health proper.

I began and ended the first volume of this work with considerations concerning the procreation of a new world citizen and his maintenance up to the time of his birth in connection with the police, except that, to avoid making the book too unwieldy, the consideration of extramarital procreation remained. This, however, cannot be easily separated from consideration of abortion and killing of the fetus; thus, this section of Medical Police includes all subjects concerning the human being from birth up to that age at which he himself enters the circle of procreating, or fertile, members of human society.

The third volume, the publication time of which depends on the approbation which experts will accord my past efforts, is intended to deal with preventive measures, of use to everyone, concerning useful, or healthy, and spoilt foodstuffs: the best beverages, their varied adulteration, general and special security, the special dangers apart from vessels in which foods are prepared and stored, the most desirable layout and mode of construction of human abodes, public cleanliness, etc. Here everybody will easily comprehend that these few headings may contain so much that it will be worth the effort to see these subjects treated in proper context by a patriotic physician with knowledge and constant consideration of the expediency of his proposals.

Since it behoves us at present to say various things concerning physical education and the best arrangement of the lower schools, with a view to the health of the children, and since it is difficult, at a time when so much is being written about such subjects, to utter something new, I want to point out that I intend to touch here only upon matters that have the greatest influence on the general health of young pupils, and where the police must contribute the most. Each father, of course, has much more good to follow that was expounded more suitably by others. A philanthropist will find here many things that either deserve to be repeated by me, or that are completely unknown or not so generally known that my considerations could not be useful.

In addition, I repeat my request most urgently, and direct it to all philanthropists, to the esteemed principals of the republics, and to public societies and colleges, whose task is the care of public health of the peoples, to generously support this undertaking of mine, which is so important to mankind, by contributions, by publicizing useful equipment, and by carrying out measures that have been found to be expedient—to contribute with compassion their stone to the great edifice for the public security of their brethren! I will not forget anything, nor deprive of the sure gratitude of future times, those who will enable me to make this work as perfect as possible.

Bruchsal, 20 March 1780.

PART ONE

On defense of public welfare for the sake of preserving unmarried mothers and their infants

§1

What should move us to compassion for unmarried mothers and their infants

Who is free of the prejudice which everywhere so embitters the fate of the people, who views nature as a whole, how from the monumental elephant to the tiniest Infusorian, and from the lofty cedar to the humble duckweed, all living beings in all corners of God's earth, each at its time, follows the fierce urge of procreation? Who considers how the passion of animals in rut sends them seeking each other despite all the elements, as assuredly as lightning and thunder, moved by a certain quality of the atmosphere, by the great stress of emotion which the Creator put into the common song of life when He had finished Creation?—Who finds from the history of mankind how much mischief has been caused by the diversity in reasoning on this matter among so many nations (with complete certainty that in this usually unplanned flare-up of recently matured beings, the procreation of each separate creature is intended as is also the continuation of species)? Here the legislator places the boundary stone of sensual urges far beyond that which nature demands and would now give the forces of both sexes unbridled licence, and soon subordinates the much lesser requirements of one to the debauchery of the other, and calmly interlaces into the political system freedom to arbitrarily plough under the field that which has already been sown and is in bloom; if the legislator wantonly sacrifices the certain harvest of a new seed, ... when elsewhere some would moralize that all mutual physical attraction of the sexes is an indecency offending human dignity, and degrades to the rank of imperfect beings the class which occupies itself with the procreation of God's creatures according to deeply ingrained natural laws.—Who sees the increase of expenditure everywhere, the general tendency to comforts, the proliferation of classes where a woman, if not always indispensable, sometimes becomes excessively lascivious, the natural equality of the sexes abolished, and the ratio of maidens awaiting to be provided for to the number of men who can or do consider marriage seriously dropped to at least a fifth?—Finally, who is convinced in his innermost self that no matter how often the storm of the most powerful of all passions has been weathered in a single unfortunate instant, the fall of the most innocent soul can be as terrifying in its consequences as the crime of the craftiest street-walker can hardly ever be?—Whoever considers all this with unprejudiced eyes, must be seized by a sad feeling when after so many opportunities given to the people to be wanton, and with a constitution in some regions which contradicts nature so greatly, yet a still curable member of society is branded with eternal infamy by an unfortunate remnant of barbaric laws, and a momentary transgression—errors of an often unavoidable rapture of the inner senses—is put in the same class as those vices which terrify nature when committed in cold blood.

§2

Intention of the following investigations

Far be it from me, in this work, to defend debauchery, and I shall describe here its consequences for the public well-being: it is certain that prostitution in each country should easily be considered the first plague, but I demand compassion and justice for the seduced sex and its unfortunate consequences for reasons which may make the source of child murder clearer and should show that the unnatural mortality of our sex and the complete derangement of numerous classes of people should be sought mostly in the contradiction between the laws and our nature and in the distorted assessment of the human heart. Great men, before me, have defended the rights of mankind against the frequently cruel treatment of the weak sex. I believe that medical science is able to supply additional reasons, and thereby I hope to make more comprehensible to every philanthropist the advantages of milder treatment of these wretched creatures. Perhaps in time these considerations will induce useful conclusions concerning the attenuation of a poison that for long has been devouring the entrails of mankind, the daily increasing spread of which has been so long an indomitable ill. Too long one waits for only individual acts of persons infected by it in the community, and neglects employing powerful means because, it seems to me, there is too much fear of the specter which is supposed to wander around where the real antidote should lie hidden, if one can hope for it.

PART ONE
Section One

On extramarital procreation in general

§1

On extramarital procreation

According to law the state of cohabitation is really wedlock: without it, it becomes concubinage or fornication. But since very few persons live without intimate intercourse with the opposite sex, fornication increases in proportion to the smaller ratio of marriages, and though such mistakes take place even among married people, when we speak of excessively free living the number of unmarried is the largest who so do.

§2

Disregarding the unlawful way in which a maiden becomes pregnant, and the advantages to the pregnant wife which the married state provides in various aspects, the state of pregnancy is just as estimable in the former as in the latter; both carry a citizen under the heart, and a divine creature which, independently of all human rules, grows up on every fertile soil where it is sown. Can the fetus be blamed that his father before his act of procreation did not publicly exchange rings with his too gullible mother, and did not have it publicly proclaimed that henceforth he would sleep with her? It is bad enough that love and marriage are not one and the same, and that first all one's property must be accurately added up and a perilous calculation has to be carried out before one can have both. . . The words "Go and multiply" apply to all maidens who feel that they are grown up. Those who, because of a special predisposition feel it most but at the same time are not able to make a man happy with their "yes," then commit certain exuberant acts the consequence of which, if everything takes its due course, consists after nine months of a child which, just as a newborn in wedlock, has all its straight limbs and the makings of a small or great man. It is unexpected when in our times the philanthropic endeavor to defend everywhere illegitimate children against the power of a prejudice, which produced so many child murderesses and choked many a talent, is called "a very unpolitic act of a newfangled philanthropy which rears its head at the expense of civic love," because through the proscription [legitimatio] of all extramarital children, and through lessening the disgrace of having produced an unfortunate child out of order, the strongest inducement for marriage is eliminated, that therefore the blemishes with which our ancestors designated the illegitimate births are reasonable and justified for the good of marriage. I ask now whether there is any basis in the law of nature that parents may bestow the natural gift of freedom on the child, or whether it is not an irresponsible action to punish an innocent creature because its parents were not innocent?—"But the question is not simply about the voice of nature and the rights of mankind when civil rights are in the balance". . . This may be so. But will a single man get married sooner only because the child which he might sire against his will may live as a bastard and be deprived of certain advantages in the community? Rather is not such a consideration the weakest protective wall against the torrent of incontinence of most people who, either because of lack of sufficient wealth or because they are too weak to struggle constantly against physical attractions and against the even more important consequences of debauchery, indulge in forbidden lusts? If even any effect has come from the contempt of a deflowered mother and its fetus in the community, it was solely the desperation of these two. For men have long since learned to take lightly the tender feelings in such events when things have come to such a pass that the first seduction of an honest maiden is deemed a mere gallantry. The language of experience and its most convincing proofs should be listened to: that exaggerated severity of the laws against an unfortunate mother and an abandoned child has probably induced many thousands of maidens to save their honor by murdering their child, who would have been unhappy anyway, or when this could not be done without incurring retribution, to look for an end to their despair in their own death against which the hangman's sword is deemed inconsiderable when a sensitive and agitated creature has such terrible prospects for the rest of her life.

But because of formerly divine and now human laws, extramarital cohabitation is a crime and the subsequent pregnancy has become a deleterious matter, it is natural that each community must take care that through this interdiction the number of legal marriages is increased and that the number of illegitimately procreated persons is reduced as much as possible.

§3

So much could have been learned everywhere in the world after several thousand years' experience, that a certain act cannot be so easily eradicated through which maidens become mothers without having to give express consent, and that all human restraint does not achieve any more than at best closing the shutters when the room seems to be too bright.

* * *

§6

And whether extramarital sexual congress is to be publicly tolerated

But the question is now whether it is right to inveigh against this debauchery with equal vehemence, or whether in view of the impossibility of eradicating prostitution completely, it is not better to keep it within certain bounds and let the police with all the powers at its disposal see to it that these bounds are exceeded as rarely as possible? Not that these debaucheries will forever be a great evil in every state, but they may probably decrease if at least there is order and some certainty in a matter which is not predisposed to be completely eliminated. If with all this, extramarital sexual congress remains a deleterious and vile act, it must be admitted that clandestine whoring is a much greater evil and the most certain ruin of the states.

§7

Disadvantage of clandestine whoring in the community

Clandestine prostitution is an insidious plague in every community, and one of the main causes of the degeneration and great mortality of mankind. Thus it was ever since man and woman were joined in matrimony by necessary laws and the work of procreation, which they jointly undertook, was sanctified. But another cause has made it much more terrifying in our days, namely venereal diseases. All the reasons that have been brought up in the defense of public houses of debauchery hitherto are weak if confronted with those that can be drawn from the source of the ruin of the population; assuming that by tolerating public opportunities for debauchery, infection could be prevented or weakened, which is difficult to determine.

Particularly because of venereal disease

Since its timorous inception, this pest has seized almost all the tarts who sell their bodies, and because of the enormous number of these wretches, public health in every state suffers more from it than from almost all the host of other diseases put together because it usually ruins the genitalia of both sexes and puts the nerves in complete disarray, the offspring is formed from poisoned matter, and the juices of several generations are prepared for the most terrible diseases. After what I have said elsewhere on this subject, I only want to mention the following: no remedy would be too expensive for the state to pay if it would be able to dry up the sources of this horrible pest, or if this cannot be done, at least draw it off.

From this point of view extramarital sexual congress is doubly a subject the cessation of which must be the joint wish of all patriots.—Let us take a certain number of men in one town or in a whole country, men who either cannot marry or, having a sufficient income, are deterred from such a bond by the difficulties of the married state, but who do not want to forgo intimate intercourse with the female sex. If we examine how many women are ready to lead such a life in this same republic and offer their love to the dissolute men, we shall always find:

Firstly, that the number of men as against the number of public women is always incomparably larger, and that in consequence, to one of these women there are always several men who in the same way at the same time seek their satisfaction; and that this represents complete polyandry which obviously is in conflict with the natural laws of procreation and with the true advantages of the population.

Secondly, that the public women always represent the most beautiful part of the sex, which of course must increase the loss to the procreation of a perfect human race.

Thirdly, that the young men enfeeble themselves infinitely more by extramarital procreation than would be the case if they were married. The libertine becomes prematurely weak and exhausted, whereas a married man, even by his indifference toward a certain act, finds a means for conserving his strength and consequently for making his procreative ability enduring. I know of no stronger proof against polygamy than the fact that through multiple enticement to marital acts the seed attains more rarely that ripeness which is required for producing a perfect being. A man who indulges in love with several persons finds in the variety of their charms precisely that which nature withheld from one woman alone, so that the procreative potency of the man is exhausted no sooner than the woman also ceases to be disposed to love and fertility. How is it that some men have to resort to the art of their physicians or to stimulants in order to be able to fulfill their marital duties? The reason is that in their unmarried days they indulged in the lures of variety and never gave nature a chance to rest, or else in the first years of their married life the fire of imagination dried up their nervous strength. How much must all this take place during extramarital procreation, where neither moderation nor order is to be expected, and where new forces daily offer themselves for repeated squandering?

Fourthly, that a given number of neglected women will endeavor by every means, even more than men, to prevent conception, partly because pregnancy reveals their faults even more, partly because through the discomfort and the nature of this state, as well as through giving birth, they lose a considerable part of their allurement, and finally, because the profit to be derived from their daily debauchery will be missed for some time and unaccustomed poverty must be feared. Therefore among 2,000 dissolute tarts there is hardly one who has two children.*

Fifthly, that an unfortunate tart, even when she begins to feel the first signs that conception has taken place, is far from ceasing to have intercourse with the debauching men. This not only prevents all hope of fruitful cohabitation on the part of the man; it also usually helps achieve the ungodly intention of deliberate abortion by the guilty mother, because as I have demonstrated, too zealous intercourse, also by a married woman, especially in the first and last month of pregnancy, leads not unfrequently to the destruction of the fetus.

Sixthly, that because of the large amount of abortifacients, even if they do not take

* Moheau, "Récherches sur la population de la France," T. II, p. 100.

effect, usually the health of the unfortunate women is greatly destroyed; many even pay with their lives, because of the severity of the medicines, the frequent evacuations, or through the external force applied parts of the body are deranged and through inflammation and the ensuing gangrene, destroyed.

Seventhly, that even lascivious men finally become disgusted with whoring. Experience has shown that after a long series of alternate changes, the attraction of the entire female sex is finally lost, and the taste for human congress is easily diverted to unnatural intercourse which must cause very severe injury to both the population and the public well-being.

Eighthly, that when all attempts to achieve their abortion have failed, the infants conceived outside marriage, nevertheless, seldom attain that maturity and strength which they would have achieved had they been born to a married couple because of the continuously untoward behavior of the mothers and the violent agitation felt throughout the pregnancy. It has been observed that love children are healthier and stronger than those born in wedlock. I believe this applies to those begot by a healthy and still unexhausted couple compared with the fruits of indifferent or otherwise enfeebled married couples, but it does not apply when the latter have an equally good predisposition or when the former commit the act of procreating casually and with the excesses that usually go with the whoring life.

Ninthly, that unmarried mothers usually have a miserable confinement where their ruin is advanced by the continuous feeling of their present and the future fate, as well as by the great lack of the necessary care, especially in the case of illness as well as lying-in.

Tenthly, that a person who, being single, has given birth to one or two children, is usually completely wiped away for the population because such a woman has neither so much allure, nor can she afford to be so bold as to adhere to her former way of life without exposing herself to the greatest severity of the law. This circumstance now forces her to seek her sustenance by becoming a shameless procuress seducing young beauties to a similar way of life. I cannot understand why Süsmilch commended the habit as a very laudable and Christian custom "that some artisans do not like a master to marry a deflowered person;"* as if this vice alone, or at least more than any other, deserved to be punished by the community with eternal penalties. As if in the married state, which in reality is a means of incontinence, an improvement were not possible and if, instead, it would not be commendable to win again a female citizen who had been lost, especially since not every maiden who becomes pregnant, because of exceeding fertility, out of love or weakness toward a seductive man, is necessarily a whore.

And finally, the fate of the innocents, born to unmarried mothers leading a whoring life, should be considered: the effect of infection by their debauching parents, or by

* "Divine Order," Part I, p. 240.

seed corrupted by either venereal disease or illness or enfeeblement, those who lack tender care by motherly hands in the first days of life, or the most essential support during their entire youngest and helpless childhood. The influence of a suitable education on the general morals needs thought also, as does the physical well-being of future citizens which depends to such an extent on a suitable education. It suffices to consider the great mortality in those houses in which the state receives the unfortunate fruits of debauchery and has them educated at great expenses, in order to prevent child murder. It is then not surprising that of all the illegitimate children begotten in one year, there is barely one third left after less than ten years, and less than one fifth after twenty years. This is an extremely high price for the state to pay in terms of the great loss of so many fertile mothers and the lower morals of a large number of persons.*

§8

It is not surprising, therefore, that all nations sought means against these disastrous consequences of debauchery, and it is worth the effort to name some of the foremost uses of the police against debauchery, and then to judge their influence on public health and well-being.

Even before venereal disease became widespread, most nations thought that inasmuch as there was no hope of rooting out the disease, it might be better to allot incontinence a certain place as on a ship in danger, part of the good wares are thrown into the sea. And taking knowledge of the human heart into account, disorder itself be brought into some kind of order. Therefore in each town, where there were extraordinarily large crowds, some houses were established, where the true means of stilling the delirium for some time and of bringing people back to reason was stored and made available at any hour, thus making married women with their daughters and sons secure from mad acts.

* * *

There follows a historical survey of the development of bordellos.

§9

Such a house, even if its necessity is admitted in very populous towns, large ports, and trading cities, must either raise the inducement to clandestine whoring and the occasions of infection with venereal disease, or else the police, by administering it, merely becomes a privileged negotiator.—Certainly, all the objections which could be rightly raised against debauchery with public women, apply doubly to the so-called whorehouse, if it would not be possible to use it for preventing a much greater vice in the state.

* * *

* See Part Two, Section Four, Of foundling hospitals and orphanages, §2.

§10

There is something to be said in favor of an institution which would serve the following purposes in large and sumptuous towns:

Firstly, that those who cannot support a wife yet, who despite their scruples, against all moral motivation, and despite impending civil punishment, are unwilling to restrain their passions, or who because of a special temperamental predisposition cannot easily do so without suffering consequences, could be induced by a certain, albeit enforced, admission of unapproved and possibly limited excesses at least to spare innocence, to respect the bond of marriage between others, and to look after their own health better. Not that the intention is thus to waive the punishment for vice which usually follows directly upon every offense including lechery, even if it is not venereal disease. The intention is to at least protect future generations from the unfortunate influence of a horrible heritage and to prevent even further innocent infections in the community.

Secondly, that the despicable public tarts, who now are scattered in large towns and who like rabid sheep among an uninfected flock in the company of innocent or still ignorant persons cause both moral and physical ruin, be isolated as much as possible and prevented from seducing inexperienced but righteous young men who can so easily be diverted from the path of virtue by so many snares, or even married men, in order to earn a miserable living and to indulge in their wantonness.

Thirdly, that just these public tarts, isolated from the society of citizens, be subjected to the strictest supervision and at the slightest sign of infection be more closely restrained, and up to the complete recovery of their health, be prevented from spreading further in the community the inherited poison.

Fourthly, that the fetuses of such incontinent mothers be protected by the vigilance of indefatigable superiors against all possible devices and attempts, in case of lack of supervision, and be maintained at the expense of the incontinent ones.

Fifthly, that thus the maintenance of mistresses, which costs so many citizens their fortune and their health, and is so vexatious to young people, be prevented in the community, since it is so deleterious to the health of many men and the population in general, in view of the great uncertainty in the behavior of a kept woman and the constant temptation to maintain herself barren.

Sixthly, that the errant husband, who indulges in an unfortunate passion, against all the duties of his married state, regardless of the dearest bonds that bind him to his family, at least be restrained from consorting with such persons who would communicate to him a poison with which he would plunge into extreme misery his innocent wife and a number of offspring.

Seventhly, that all men and women visibly infected by venereal disease be prevented from sexual intercourse with each other by strict supervision and examinations until completely recovered and able to give every possible security, because of the consequences threatening themselves and the fruits of such intercourse.

Eighthly, that venereal disease be recognized as early as possible in the public tarts, and immediately be suppressed in the initial stage by a suitable cure.

Ninthly, that the shameful way of life, once chosen by a heedless maiden, should not sever her forever from virtue. If her reputation were spared, there would remain to her, after having admitted her mistake, the possibility to revert to life and perhaps to a fruitful union without continuously adhering prejudice and without noise. However, this is usually impossible because of the spreading of the lapse, committed by a maiden, and this has forced many a tart to continue perniciously in her way of life.

I leave it to others to judge to what extent such an institution is feasible and can be justified against certain moral objections. It is only certain that every opportunity of debauchery is all the more deleterious to public health, the more it escapes the supervision of the police, and the more it is able to entice not quite mature young people; thereby, all the good predispositions for future procreation of a durable species are destroyed, and the best forces of the citizens are wasted to the greatest disadvantage of a state.

§11

The police must endeavor everywhere to reduce the number of loose women

The police must therefore endeavor very determinedly to pick up all public women as soon as possible and to keep them in penitentiaries and workhouses. But they should never let themselves be induced to leniency by the standing of their protectors if the tart omitted to take certain measures to protect the health of such persons, or because the way of life is less noxious to the community, for it seems at least to me that there is no way of preventing the evil consequences of extramarital procreation and fornication except by either destroying the vice of lechery at its root and thus at the same time to suppress venereal poison, or by allotting vice its own residence and watching it there as a spot which may develop into the most dangerous plague unless the most stringent measures are taken.

The regulations by the police against loose women and those who shelter them are ever stringent; but experience teaches that the implementation of these regulations is most difficult and never completely fulfills the intention of the law. Especially in recent times, the laws have harassed prostitution; according to them procuresses and pimps should be expelled from every republic and, together with their helpers, exposed to corporal punishment. Special supervisors of morals and commissions of chastity were even established; their intentions were always the best, but they never achieved everything that would have been desirable for the general well-being, and especially for the health of the citizens.

* * *

§15

But nothing so much deserves the attention of the police as that the fetuses produced in disorder in the community be protected at all times by a mighty arm against the daring attempt of their unmarried parents and the rights of the yet unborn citizens defended against the cruelty of raving wretches. The craze either to abort a fetus immediately after conception by all possible means or, if this does not succeed, to abandon, or even kill, the child immediately after it is born, is one of the most important concerns of Medical Police and therefore it deserves to be specially examined in the subsequent sections.

PART ONE
Section Two

Of deliberate abortions, exposure and killing of the fetus

§1

The effect of the passion upon the soul does not reveal itself in any other situation as powerfully as when an otherwise well-bred maiden feels for the first time that she carries in her entrails a living being which has been conceived improperly. This instant, so terrible for an unmarried pregnant woman, soon seizes her entire mind: shame, fear, terror, and desperation alternate, and even death becomes to this otherwise timid sex an object of the most passionate longing. I have mentioned earlier the cause of such violent storms: shame and imminent misery are the powerful mainsprings of such indescribable affects; both are the necessary consequences of our social system, which had to subject the right of procreation to certain rules and to punish their infringement.

§2

Under these circumstances, the greater the terror is, the greater is the instinct of self-defense against a threatening disaster and misfortune to the being which is still locked in and unknown to the world, whose presence often causes such an important, an unequal fight!.. Where is the maiden who has come to grief and, at least at the beginning of her dread, has remained idle, has not ravaged her own entrails, in order to get quietly rid of an enemy whose daily growth threatens her with ever more certain dangers?

> Quas non herbas, quas non medicamina—
> Attulit audaci supposuitque manu?

§3

The thought that abortions are widespread among all civilized nations, and what consequences abortion has for the reproduction and the general well-being and health in all states are self-evident. Nevertheless, one cannot help noticing in many nations a very depressing contradiction between the notions about the morality of abortions and the history of human thinking on such an exceedingly important subject; for who, without obtaining proof, should suppose that a deed such as this, even if carried out by married persons, would have ever had the protection of public law or would at least have enjoyed indifferent leniency?

* * *

There follows a historical survey of the forms and means of abortion.

§10

Of abandoning children and abortions

When all attempts at ridding herself prematurely of an embryo have failed, the unfortunate creature in her desperation is left with only one way out of her predicament: to slay her child by herself, or, if nature still has sufficient leeway to make a person hesitate before committing such a gruesome act, to abandon the child and thus leave it to an uncertain fate; for there are examples that such children, abandoned at deserted places, are not infrequently devoured alive by dogs and swine, but mostly perish miserably in some other way.

This entirely unnatural crime has the same origin as the deliberate abortion of an embryo, namely fear of disgrace and future misery; but it is useful to seek out other causes in the history of this murderous custom, in order to find an even better remedy upon perceiving how this mentality testifies to the baseness of human mentality, or at least in order to judge those remedies which occurred among the most notable nations.

It is very likely that the audacious undertaking of freeing oneself of a newborn child by killing it was based originally on hatred of the mother, on suspicion or the certainty of her infidelity, on the impossibility of bringing up several children in case of a migratory way of life or of feeding them because of lack of sufficient food. Martial nations, especially republican ones, had their special reasons for considering too great an increase in the number of their citizens as deleterious, and consequently for viewing child murder as less cruel.

* * *

Then follows a historic survey of the forms of abandonment of children and their killing and of the harsh punishments stipulated for abortion, abandoning and killing newborn children. On this we bring a passage from §14.

A merely arbitrary punishment was stipulated for abortion of a fetus during the first half of pregnancy. On the other hand, French law since Henri II has completely abolished all differences in punishment for abortion, and the finding that an unmarried pregnant woman had concealed her state, or had borne or aborted a dead child which could be neither baptized nor buried, was punishable by death.

* * *

There follows the original text of the edict which had been in force in France since Henri II up to Frank's time.

§15

Defense of the death penalty for abortions

Even in our days there are some scholars who endeavor to defend the death penalty for abortions against weighty objections. "According to the effect," says Sonnenfels, "it is irrelevant whether the child is killed by medicines or violence or aborted either when it really is born or still in the womb. If the laws distinguish between live and inanimate fetuses, and are more lenient in case of abortion of the latter, the legislation seems less than perfect."*

It is correct that the ancients' opinion of a child in the womb not being a human being was based either on prejudice or on mere dispute about words. There is no reason why I should deny a living creature, procreated by man and woman and endowed with human shape, the title of human being, merely because it is connected to the mother by the umbilical cord and requires her influence in order to mature completely, the lack of which influence, however, changes the nature of this creature as little as it can prevent a trunk branch that springs from an acorn belonging to the genus of the oaks. However, if one wants merely to say that in regard to civil actions, a fetus is not a human being,** nobody will assert the opposite.

Despite the generally held opinion, which is held even in most courts of law, a fact that does not need much proving in view of the now prevalent general conviction of all physicians is that a child is just as much a living creature before half the pregnancy is over, as it is after the first half.

* * *

Under such circumstances the abortion of the fetus is of course a greater crime, and in agreement with von Sonnenfels and others one may doubt: "whether the difference which the laws make in punishing abortion carried out during the first or the second half of pregnancy is justified or not." "The punishment" he says,† "may be viewed from any point of view, but it should mete out the same punishment for both kinds of child murder. If one bears in mind the damage which the state thereby suffers, the effect of this vice is in both cases that a human being who should have been born is not born, and thus mankind is robbed of a (still very doubtful) member. If the malice of the deed is judged, the mother savages her own entrails in both cases.

* L.c. ["Principles of the Police, Financial and Commercial Science."] §162, p. 210 ff.
**Paul. Zachias. "Qu. Med. leg.," Lib. I, T.I. qu. 3. n. 12.
 † L.c. §162.

The distinction between intention and result of vice (crimen affectus & effectus) has led to errors in legislation, and perhaps not only here. The intention alone, not the result, is here the subject of punitive justice: a raving madman who kills somebody is exempt from punishment; a man who is in full possession of his reason is a murderer, even if he missed while striking the fatal blow. This distinction can be of some use only in the case of a crime where restitution takes place."

§16

There are, however, many objections to this which seem to be justified

Even those cases are investigated by courts with the cooperation of physicians under oath where it is known that the perpetrator had animum occidendi. And if by the Visum & repertum of the physician it becomes clear that there is still a doubt whether the injury or a perilous disease, probably contracted at the same time, achieved the fatal effect, it seems to be a hard thing to treat the perpetrator in the same way as someone who cracked somebody's head. I have already said that there is no remedy of which it could be said with certainty that it aborts the fetus or that would as surely cause the miscarriage as would be required to base the sentence of death on it; on the contrary, it is certain that few of the remedies have much effect. On the other hand, most premature births are due to other causes, either inevitable or causes that do not seem so important and can never be counted as capital crimes. Since only extremely rarely can it be said that an injury inflicted by a mother on her child is absolutely lethal, it seems that, without distinguishing between the first and the second half of pregnancy, the sentence of death for abortions encounters great difficulties, and that there is always the danger that a girl, who is punishable by death because of her intentions, may in reality be punished for a mere natural defect, and thus the state suffers two deaths instead of one.

There were, therefore, jurists and other judicious men who held the opinion that a person who seems guilty of abortion and admits it, no matter whether the aborted fetus was alive or not, should not receive the death penalty, but on the contrary, banishment, or at the most, flogging. The depravity of abortion, says Balemann, should be punished not by the Pale but by the sword because we can never be certain that the abortion was caused by the remedies used, for there are hundreds of causes through which a fetus may die in the mother's body while the mother still feels life.

Does it not seem that punishment by the sword is too harsh in view of such uncertainty, and should one in our times have so little compassion with a maiden who acts in such a weak-minded manner out of sheer desperation?... I admit, it may happen now and again that a strumpet who really killed by aborting her fetus will thus be punished too mildly, but in view of the proven uncertainty and the always equivocal effect of abortifacients, there are always a hundred dangers that a gross injustice is being done. Here it seems that the accused must have the benefit of the doubt. I gladly leave it to philanthropic jurists to judge whether the position of an unhappy and desperate maiden is an additional reason for mitigating the punishment, if in the throes of the most violent passion she commits a deed against which her heart would surely rebel at a time of quiet,—whether such a person can be improved by some means, or whether there is no milder remedy available to make her weakness less dangerous to the state than execution, which people must never resort to if one of these conditions may yet be fulfilled?*

* * *

§18
On punishment for child murder and the exposure of children

The measures to be taken by the police against child murder and exposure of children merit the most painstaking consideration, for in all countries where the matter was handled by force, the results teach us that the gallows and the sword are unsatisfactory means of preventing such ills.** In recent times the strictest means have been too long applied to combat these vices. I say too long, not because child murder deserves the death penalty any less than other crimes, but that it would be better to think of means to make this vice as rare as adultery was at Sparta. For that, the law ordered that he who was caught at it should by way of punishment supply as large a golden ox as he was able, and by standing on a steep slope, give it to drink from a creek flowing in a deep valley. How is that possible? a foreigner asked . . . The reply of the Spartan was that it is as impossible as that adultery should be committed at Sparta.—Thus the skill of the legislator consists more in advantageous inventions how to prevent vices, than in exquisite ways of punishing them. Especially if he has all of nature against him and if the vice is such that greater strictness only induces the perpetrators to think of more refined devices. In this instance, they are easier to invent than the most elaborate laws for their suppression.

* * *

§21
Of a charitable endowment for unmarried pregnant women

It is thus absolutely necessary to think of gentler means, and here no better proposal can be put forward than that which was devised several years ago by the earlier and favorably mentioned Privy Councilor Reinhard at Baden, which was made public under the heading of "A Charitable Endowment of Special Kind for the Notable Advantage of a Mediocre Town."†

---

* "One is not entitled to kill a person, even as an example to others, unless he cannot be left to live without danger." J. J. Rousseau, "Contract Social," Ch. 5.

** For this reason, according to public news, child murderesses in Sweden are not punished by death any more, but only by the penitentiary and annual flogging, but the deflowered maidens are protected against all abuse by punishment. "Frankfurter Reichszeitung," No. 134. 1779.

† Mirabeau also put forward a similar proposal in "L'ami de l'homme," T. II.

The endowment actually consists of a gratuitous sojourn the enjoyment of which would be permitted for some time to various needy natives, but also to unfortunate foreigners, especially piteous women. Again I let this deserving writer speak his own words with which he indicated to the last-named their comforting place in the above-mentioned charitable endowment: "Part of my ultimate purpose is also the care of the innocent children, so that their murder is not added to the first transgression of the mother. This purpose would be largely achieved if such persons had a secure shelter and living some time before confinement so that the children could be born in security, and if, after the delivery, they could stay until they had the strength and found the opportunity of moving elsewhere and lodging their children. Thereby the lives of many children would be saved; especially, since it can be observed that when child murder is not committed in the first and most violent emotional shock, it certainly will not be committed later. A few hours suffice for nature to prevail. After that a reasonable state of mind follows. The misfortune is averted. For certainly every reproach which is especially desired or abhorred seems in the event always more pleasant or more terrible at first than it is in fact; little time suffices for the violent emotion of our mind, be it in pleasure or grief, to moderate and gradually to dampen.

"But in order to continue further in the footsteps of humaneness, all the foreign self-proclaimed loose women (against payment in advance) could also be admitted. On the other hand, they should not be required to state their place of residence, country of origin, or who the child's father is; after having spent six weeks there, they would be released."*

* * *

Frank then quotes various laws which stipulate that single women themselves have to report on their pregnancy.

* L.c. pp. 216–222.

PART TWO
Section One

Of protection during early childhood against special accidents and early significant failures of the common education methods which inhibit healthy growth

§ 1

Nature provided every newborn creature with such guardians, namely the procreating couple itself, as the greatest king on earth would attempt in vain to buy for himself. The tenderness of parents toward their children and young has something so appropriate that it is really the noblest of all the animal instincts and, after the procreative instinct, the most useful. Look at the weak and timid hen, with what penetrating cries she fills the air in order to apprise the terrible predator, still poised high above her, of her heroic vigilance, and her chicks of the magnitude of the impending danger!... She, the powerless, readies herself against the bloodthirsty, although certain of perishing, and who has not seen how she does carry out her intention and attempts to buy the lives of her young with her own life?—Thus all nature thinks of the maintenance of its newborns, and even man is not yet completely degenerated in this respect.

§ 2

Not yet completely!... I wish I need not have to reproach here the king of the animals by which I lower him so far beneath the class of lesser creatures! But experience teaches that with most parents neglect of the tenderest young under the greater dangers takes place, and the number of victims who succumb annually to this cruelty is just as great as or even greater than the number of children who die of really accidental diseases.

* * *

In the following paragraphs, Frank discusses measures to be taken in the case of newborns being apparently dead, as well as the dangers which threaten children when they are rocked, or sleep in the same beds with adults (smothering). Of fatal accidents in early childhood, we quote in § 15 those that happen to children without supervision in that they shed light on the social situation of peasants in the 18th century.

§15

It is similar in the country: when peasant women have to work in the fields, they nurse their children who are not yet a year old, and then leave them alone at home, without any supervision, either in the cradle or even crawling about on the floor, and they do not see them until they return home at midday or even in the evening. In the meantime, the unfortunate ones scream themselves half dead, and disregarding the effect of the fear and anguish caused by such a state, to which one- and two-year old children are also subjected, it is certain that this often gives rise to inguinal hernia or omphalocele in such children in the country. The disorder furthermore enhances the evil because the child is bound to suffer hunger and thirst, and must be half suffocated from filth before it receives nourishment and help, whereupon the food is devoured too quickly because of the previous excessively long lack of it, and this in turn is the cause of further consequences. To all these accidents, the children of townspeople who have been turned over to village wet nurses by their exuberant mothers, are also exposed.

All this is compounded by the fact that the mothers, before hurrying away, have to lock their rooms and houses well, and thereby prevent their neighbors from helping the endangered creature, or out of carelessness or forgetfulness they leave the door open and thus expose their helpless children to their fate. Repeated experience has taught that in the country small children who are too weak to run about, may be attacked and dismembered by pigs, dogs, and cats when the doors are open. As late as in 1777, on the 6th of January, a pig got into a peasant's room at Ottenau in the Eberstein region, and an 8-month old child had both its arms devoured after it had been thrown from the cradle; when the mother came home, she found the child dead in the corner. I remember at least five or six such mishaps which occurred within no more than twelve years in the Baden provinces alone and due to the same causes. This was published without any further comment in the Rastadt and Karlsruhe Weekly and Intelligence Journal. Children who walk about in the house but cannot yet look after themselves, often fall down the stairs which they were able to climb; they fall into open cellars, into the fire,* and into the liquid-manure pit or the well, both of which are fairly deep, in front of most farmsteads.

Measures must be taken against such disorder. It is true that there is so much work to do in certain summer months that sometimes there are fewer than ten farmsteads inhabited by adults, and all doors are locked. One can hear the cries of desperate children for hours from most such houses. It is neither expedient nor advisable to take very small children into the field. The parents, who are overloaded with work, cannot possibly watch their children to such an extent as would be necessary for their safety. If a child cannot walk yet, the coolness of the soil on which it lies is bad for it,

---

* For instance as late as 1773, a child who had been locked in while both parents were away burnt miserably to death on a very hot stove, without anybody being able to come to help.

or, if there is no shade far and wide, the sensitive creature can hardly be protected against sunstroke. If the child is old enough to run and play alone, then a nearby puddle, a creek, a ravine, or something similar are all causes due to which, as experience in the country shows, several children perish every year, without much attention being paid, as far as I know, to these frequent sources of the ruin of the hopeful children of the diligent peasant.

However, what can be done to facilitate the observation of two such great and often contradictory duties, that of maintaining life by unavoidable work, and that of protecting one's helpless young against mishaps?

I believe that the following measures should be taken, even if this entails difficulties.

1) No nursing mother should leave her child in the first year for longer than that she is able to suckle it in the first quarter [year] every two hours, in the second every three hours, and in the third and fourth quarters at least three times a day without the milk being heated, and to provide for all its other necessities.

2) No matter whether a child is still suckled or not, it should never be left alone at home without supervision by an adult person. Out of two or three households, depending on the number of dependent children, the mothers can take turns, or instead of them, a sensible adult person, to watch ceaselessly over the safety and feeding of the children. This woman could be obliged to do this work just as if the children were all her own. Otherwise the parents are responsible for the safety of their children, and mothers especially should not leave them alone without compelling reason, in order to attend to matters that should always rank far behind the mother's duties.

3) Dung pits and puddles of liquid manure should not be near dwellings and windows, even for reasons of public health; but in view of the children who drown every year in them in the country for lack of supervision, they appear even more deleterious. The police, therefore, must earnestly urge that these sources of accidents be removed. Equal care should be devoted to open wells, entrance doors to houses, and trap doors to cellars, neglected stairs, stoves, etc., which cost the lives of many children or at least turn them into miserable cripples. The laws concerning wells stipulate, therefore, almost generally that wells should be carefully covered and secured. German law says: "Whoever digs wells or pits (and also such [ditches] that serve for the draining of manure and, though often very deep, stand open in front of every farmhouse) is obliged to cast up earth so high that it reaches above the knees of an adult man. If he does not do so, he is to make good any damage that may be caused by it." Saxon law is even more explicit in this matter: "Wells are to be protected knee-high from the ground, otherwise the damage is to be made good by him who caused the consequences, whereby the word consequences is to mean whether somebody's cattle or even a person fell into the unprotected well and perished there." Friesen, therefore, maintained that every owner of a well into which a person fell and perished should be forced to make good the damage; but since

according to Roman law, the life of a free person cannot be valued or estimated, such an owner is to be charged with compensation for the damage according to another law.

* * *

PART TWO

Section Two

On the maternal duty to suckle and its influence on the welfare of the state

§1

The nutrition of newborn infants is not a matter of indifference to the state for it has the most obvious influence on the death and the life of the infants. If one sees that more than a third of people perish due to constant mistakes in this matter, it is obvious, I imagine, to pose the question: "whether the representatives of society will agree to deal with such matters as these?"

§2

The most natural food for the newborn is mother's milk. I do not think that our fathers could have foreseen this kind of depravity of their grandsons: that one day a mother would be permitted to dry up the full spring which flows from her bountiful breasts after delivery, the most dangerous time of her life; for her greater safety and as the most necessary nourishment for her child . . . that the terrible mishaps are caused thereby; that otherwise sensitive beings could not retreat in time from this dangerous path: "yet the grimmest animals bare their breasts and nurse their young."

As soon as the mother, who often became pregnant against her will, has given birth, neither her own danger nor nature's voice are able to assert its rights: she hurriedly withdraws from the weak being and turns it over to an animal or, at most, to a wet nurse who, as Rousseau says, is not a mother herself if she is base enough to prefer for the sake of a lump of money, a strange child to her own.

§3

The origin of this unpardonable practice is probably as old as it is innocent. If a child had lost its mother at birth or after birth, or if the mother could not nurse the child because of lack of milk, other nourishment had to be found. Sometimes a child could be seen thriving on the milk which a compassionate neighbor offered the thirsty and miserable child from her own breasts; perhaps these were for a long

112

time the only cases which could move the tenderness of our ancestors to take such a step.

Gradually some apparently lazy mothers lighted on to the idea to use this innocent invention for their own convenience. The rich, who had finally learned to have most of their duties performed by others in enforced labor, also gladly availed themselves of this opportunity to be rid of yet another burden.

* * *

Frank then briefly sketches the history of nursing by mothers, discussing in detail its advantages to mother and child. The entire Section 3 of Part Two deals with the institution of wet nurses.

PART TWO
Section Four

Of foundling hospitals and orphanages

§1

As long as extreme poverty is unbearable and such poverty cannot prevent a large number of children in very poor households, as long as debauchery among the people cannot be eliminated and an illegitimate child is an object of constant reproaches, it must be expected that redundant and disadvantaged children will continue to be exposed, especially in large cities where the number of unfortunates is always larger. See what has been said on this subject in Part One, Section Two, §§17, 18, 19, 20. Experience of many years has now taught most authorities that mere palliatives can achieve more than if the police with fire and sword seeks out and persecutes vice among the large masses, instead of endeavoring to save the lives of the exposed without endangering the lives of the mothers who expose. The police should even somewhat favor the inevitable exposure so as to prevent the worst choice of the unfortunate children even being secretly murdered.

"The judges have considered for a long time that exposure of children is a vice;* but the severity of the laws is always tempered by wisdom and reason, and the

---

* Meissner says: "This is very just, and it is desirable that things be left as they are." Two treatises on the question: Are foundling hospitals advantageous or harmful? Gött. 1779, p. 125. Strange enough, and as if the authorities therefore ceased for an instant to consider exposure a vice because according to a million experiences, they believe it to be inevitable, and therefore choose the lesser evil. Would it not be better if in a city such as Paris where every year more than 3000 illegitimate children are murdered and some of their unmarried mothers are therefore hanged, that the police not permit nor approve of the vice of fornication, but prevent its effect by measures that perchance are costly. Even if it were true that some maiden or other would therefore say yes to her seducer a few instants sooner, which she will not omit doing even if there were no foundling hospitals in the world, once the hour of seduction has come. In Stockholm, says von Hess, the clergy opposed the beneficial foundation of a foundling hospital for a long time: their principal reason was the pretence that the foundling hospital would make the city open and free for adultery and incest. As if these sins were not committed if there is no foundling hospital, and as if the authorities were not duty-bound to prevent murder when they cannot prevent adultery and incest. These gentlemen, instead of attacking these vices with their divine eloquence, demanded from the authorities that they prevent their expression and ignore it even if it costs many persons their lives. Commonsense and philanthropy eventually prevailed against prejudice and craziness. "Free thoughts on matters of state," p. 41.

persons in authority saw that exaggerated harshness entailed some very undesirable consequences. Among these unfortunate children some were sacrificed very cruelly as offerings to the false honor of their parents for a shame which, while deserved, is sinful in effect. Others, although born to a rightful marriage, were abandoned or even murdered by their desperate and wretched parents. Therefore, the authorities in Paris have shut their eyes to exposure. Now neither father nor mother has a pretext for getting rid of their children in such an inhuman way, and at present the life of their small children is safe.* Everybody was in agreement on the need to contribute to this aim. Nature always abhors its destruction, religion opposes it as an obvious abuse of divine laws, the state opposes it as an obvious loss of citizens, for the number of citizens makes for a state's strength and splendor."**

There were attempts, of course, because of the astounding increase in the abandoned children annually, in Paris, to extend to all foundling hospitals the reproach that they are not only increasing whoring, but that they are also inducing poorer parents to expose their own children. The number of foundlings in Paris increased between 1745 and 1766 from 3,233 to as much as 5,604 and it still increases every year. The total number of children born in Paris in 1772 was 18,713; of these, 7,676 were foundlings. But the Count of Buffon shows clearly that more than half of these were legitimate,† and this becomes even more obvious if one takes into account the number of years 1749 through 1755, 1764, and 1765. In all those years, the number of births in Paris was greater than in 1772, but the number of foundlings never exceeded 3,775; 3,785; 3,783; 4,127; 4,329; 4,231; 4,273; 5,560; 5,495, respectively.†† Also in Lyons in 1772, out of 5,320 children born, 977 were foundlings, thus one of five children was for the foundling hospital.‡

If, however, one keeps in mind that a girl who gives herself to a seducer (because of the thought that there is a foundling hospital in case she has a child) permits herself very little satisfaction from her passion, or who in case of extreme poverty, does not avoid the opportunity of fertile intercourse, one can easily see that the mass of unmarried people give little thought to considering "what will I do with my child?" and such plays very little part in the motives for a more religious way of life. This is proved most convincingly by the fact that loose women, who trade most with their bodies, are not the ones who most populate the foundling hospitals. On the contrary, with their inventiveness in preventing pregnancy, even if only to retain

* Since such a foundation has been established in Paris, practically nothing has been heard there of child murder. Dictionnaire Encycloped. Verb. Exposition d'Enfant. Etat de la Médecine, chirurgie & Pharmacie en Europe, pour l'année 1777, p. 216. The same was observed in Stockholm where child murder was nothing rare, before then. Von Hess, "Free thoughts on matters of state."

** "Tableau d'humanité & de la bienfaisance, ou précis historique des charités qui se font dans Paris," p. 64 ff.

† "Supplément à l'histoire naturelle," Tome 7, p. 517 ff.

†† "Recherches & considérations sur la population de la France," Tab. V. ch. 13, p. 280.

‡ "Meissner, l.c., p. 43.

their allure all the longer, they look down with a kind of contempt on their sisters who are less versed in vice and who are so awkward that they do not know how to avoid the consequences of forbidden intercourse. Like von Sonnenfels, I believe that one need not worry that the state will be burdened too much by the number of children exposed by married people. "Love will have a strong enough influence on parents who themselves can educate their children. And if they deny the rights of mankind to such an extent that they expose their child, then they are scoundrels, and by being with them the child's life and morals are in danger; it is, therefore, all the more worthy of general compassion."* Besides, if everywhere in the republic the signs of each pregnancy are observed, and of married women also, if the police will be more careful than hitherto in acquainting themselves with the number of children born in each family and to supervise their education from time to time, if the police will always require parents to account for their children as property only entrusted to them by the country, then there will be fewer errors of abandonment, even in large cities. This on the part of married persons, for in other matters, it will be possible to supervise details, regardless of the large number of persons, when head tax or other taxes are to be fixed by quartermasters and others in authority. But if this supervision is extended further, and if it helps the needy father over-burdened with many children, if the state supports him effectively and assists him in supporting his family, how could there be any possiblity that a mother not under duress would be willing to leave her child in strange hands, once she has embraced it lovingly for the first time?

§2

However, although I defend the leniency of the police toward the exposure of children, I have very little sympathy for the foundling hospitals in their usual state. They are reproached deservedly, as Schlözer often did, and which applies to all other hospitals, too, that in most places in the republic they poison the air and foment the spreading of infectious diseases. In addition to that, the mortality of the children in such houses is also very very great.

Calculations in various foundling hospitals showed that only very few children attain their fifteenth year there;** Baumann, with the aid of special lists demonstrated that in the House of Charité in Berlin, where unmarried pregnant women are admitted to prevent child murder, and are kept for six weeks free of charge, 10 out of 67 new-born babies had already died in the first month. The number of illegitimate children

---

* Principles of the Police, Financial and Commercial Science, §99. Such innocent and disinherited children only rarely have a father who recognizes them, and a mother who has the inclination and ability to educate them properly. If their lives do not end in early youth, they usually become idlers, beggers, or even thieves, especially if they are excluded from most crafts, as in the case in many places. Bergius, "Cameral and Police Magazine," Verb. Foundling Hospital.

** Meissner, l.c., p. 73.

who died there within one month is approximately twice or two and a half times greater than the number of legitimate children who died at the same age. Between 1771 and 1774, almost every fourth child died before the age of one month.* According to Moheau's tables, the mortality of foundlings in their first year is twice as great as that of children born in wedlock and brought up by their parents in France also. In the hospital in La Rochelle, 517 children were admitted in the course of five years; of them 286, i.e., 11/20, died within a year of their admission. In the course of the first ten years, the difference in the mortality of these two classes is not so great any more because the foundlings, after they have left the home and survived the first years of their lives, are now subject to general human fate. Even then, the mortality of foundlings is about one third greater than that of other children.** Although some such children in these houses make good, there are only a few among them which the country can count on, and it suffices to listen to those who are in charge of the education of these unfortunate children to realize how weak are most of these creatures who were begot by such seed and brought up in such homes.† According to ten years' experience in Rouen, the 27th part of the children at most who are brought up in the hospital attained manhood. Of these, however, at least 2/3 were in very bad health, so that out of 108 children, 104 died before their fifteenth year, and at the most, two of them could be counted among human society. According to Raulin, despite all the solicitude that is usual in such homes in France, in Grenoble, 25 children out of 100 died, in Lyons 36, and in Montpellier as many as 60.†† According to reports by von Justi, in the civic hospital in Vienna, despite its almost princely income, out of 19 children, hardly a single one survives.‡ Out of 13,229 foundlings who were admitted to the hospital in London between 1741 and 1774, only 2,353 reached the age of 5 or 6 years.‡‡

§3

There are various causes of this great mortality in such houses. The following deserve to be especially mentioned here:
1) Infection of children with venereal poison from their parents. Widespread venereal disease, especially among the illegitimate who make up the largest part of exposed children in most places, is one of the most important causes of their great mortality. This applies particularly to large and lascivious cities, and in Paris most foundlings are in such a bad shape that they die of venereal poison before they can be separated from the few healthy ones. But this is not yet the root of the evil. No matter whether

* Remarks and appendixes to the first two parts of Süsmilch's work, 11. I. §240.
** "Observations of a traveler through Germany, France, Holland and England," Part II, p. 108.
† Moheau, l.c., p. 222.
†† Meissner, l.c., pp. 78 ff.
‡ "Police Science," Volume I, §250, p. 213.
‡‡ "Jakobi, "Contemplation of God's wise intentions."

such children are kept in foundling hospitals or are sent to the country, they always infect their wet nurses, and through them sometimes entire families.*

* * *

2) Of the lack of mother's milk. Of this, I have mentioned much elsewhere. I want to add the following. It is difficult to choose a wet nurse, from among many, who will agree with the nature of children who miss their mother's breast. What is bound to happen if so many children are to be fed by so few nurses! In the large hall of the Paris foundling hospital six or eight wet nurses must manage to feed alternately a much larger number of infants. In other French foundling hospitals, too, the persons in authority are reproached for the situation in which one and the same nurse often has to take over two or even three children. It can be easily imagined how little is nature satisfied here, even if the nurses enjoy abundant food, and this is the real cause that such children, although not always venereally diseased, hardly look like human creatures. Finally, the attempt to bring up children on human milk in such homes has been abandoned, and other nutrition is being sought.

* * *

Frank then deals in great detail with the experience gained in Paris, Stockholm, and London with artificial feeding, and he reprints the expert opinion of the Paris Medical Faculty of 1775.

3) The uncleanliness of the air. Foundling hospitals have this shortcoming in common with all other hospitals. The former even surpass the latter with their unclean miasmas and frequent evacuations of very frail or even more grown-up dirty children. Immediately upon entry, one senses this difference most grievously, and despite all appearances of cleanliness, the repellent stench of urine penetrates everywhere. In a Paris foundling hospital it even causes inflammation of the eyes. I will deal especially with this important subject concerning the cleanliness of the air, the beds, and linen at another opportunity, and I confine myself here to point out that the consequences of the almost inevitable neglect in these matters must have a lethal effect on the very sensitive nature of the children.

4) The unhealthy location of such houses, their faulty construction and arrangement. These subjects, too, will be dealt with by me more in detail elsewhere. It is certain that when foundling hospitals are to be established, they are never suitable for large cities, where mortality is much greater anyway because of the more unclean air,

---

* See Part Two, Section Two, §20. For this reason no wet nurses at all are admitted in Aix-en-Provence to venereally affected children or children suspect of it.

and where it must increase excessively in foundling hospitals where the weakest and most susceptible creatures live together.* It is a matter of course that the location next to high walls and town moats, on swampy soil, and in streets where clean air cannot blow through, especially when the usual abode is allotted to the lower story of the hospital,** must be very detrimental not only to the lives of these miserable children, but also to that of the citizens who live in the vicinity.

Barely 30 years ago the foundling hospital in Paris was surrounded by old buildings, and was hemmed in on all sides by high walls. In 1739 a contagious disease attacked a large number of children there, and most of them lost their lives. The physicians proved that the disaster had been caused by lack of good air, and then, at last, several old buildings were torn down and the hospital was enlarged. This made the foundling hospital much healthier, but the rise in the value of the site in a large city always prevents even the best builder to build according to the project of those who want to see such houses built according to health principles; not to mention the fact that the higher price of all foodstuffs make the maintenance constantly much more expensive.

As regards the arrangement, nothing is as detrimental to the intention of bringing up the children in a healthy style as to lock them all together into one or two large rooms where the crying of one prevents them all from sleeping, and where the attendance that is necessary for everyone maintains a constant commotion. When there are often more than a hundred foundlings congregating in one room, how quickly must they transform the atmosphere into a steam bath, even if the room is large, especially at night when windows and doors are closed. Not even the strongest fiber can resist such an atmosphere, especially when care is not always taken to dry the diapers and blankets in a specially assigned place in winter. Since only very few foundling hospitals have their own infirmaries or sickrooms, every contagious disease is bound to spread quickly among all the children present. And no matter how simple the disease, it can easily turn into a malignant hospital or jail fever which must be all the deadlier here the less such small patients can be given the proper medicines, and the less their special needs can always be guessed!

5) Lack of supervision, greed, prejudices, indifference, and cruelty of the supervisors and lower servants. Important faults which greatly raise mortality in most hospitals! The first founders, full of zeal and philanthropy for the perfection of their foundation,

* Lüders believes that the repugnant skin diseases peculiar to the foundling hospitals would not originate there so often, or would be at least milder, if these establishments were removed to the country. "Diss. de educatione liberorum medica," Gött. 1763, p. 7 bottom.
** According to Goch's reports, in Norwich Hospital in London, more persons die in an upper room than in a lower one. Gött. gel. Anz. 1775. Appendix No. 63. The rooms there, however, are 15 feet high, airy, and very clean. This is rarely found in cities, where the lower stories of the houses are mostly closed to air.

of course provide everything that is needed for constant and good development: however, it is well known what most people are like! . . . Soon the selfishness and greed of hired leaseholders take a hand, and then the life of a hundred persons is as nothing against as many thalers, and soon the entire capital of the best founder is used only for paying privileged murderers in the community. What good is supervision by a sleepy steward at certain hours when confronted with the sly maliciousness of selfish servants to underage wretches whose drying out and exhaustion is the only excuse for approaching them!* In time I shall say more about this source of most unscrupulous administration of most hospitals.

But not even the misjudged worth of the unfortunate creatures, and an almost unavoidable indifference on the part of most attendants toward suffering mankind is all; sacred prejudices sometimes increase the mortality in foundling hospitals to incredible proportions. Ballexserd quotes a lady who expressed her astonishment at the miserable appearance of the children at a famous foundling hospital. A children's attendant, a devout nun, assured her most tenderly that these good children were all very happy to die in order to partake soon of eternal bliss, and that, anyway, it was desirable for the hospital that the children admitted did not live long; otherwise, its income would not suffice for maintaining so many persons.**

6) Lack of movement and excessively monotonous way of life. This cause has only a future effect; education in most houses, where so many children under a few supervisors have to grow up together, is mostly a monastic education where efforts are neither made nor can be made to let youth enjoy all the advantages of an active life. So, one expects some resistance against the influence of all the different objects encountered in human life, the various changes of air, etc. Pale faces and bloated, feeble bodies are here more often the result of too tender an education and the lack of wholesome movement than of the originally bad condition of these children. The excessive order and punctiliousness in all their rules of life, I mean in eating and drinking, in leisure and movement, in waking and sleeping, too much accustoms the body from earliest youth to machine-like punctuality, so that at the first entry into the [work] world the slightest deviation from the monastic regularity, which was absorbed in the first years, must astonish every child, especially a male one, when suddenly the hours are changed, work is transferred from the moderate room air to the field under the burning midday sun, nights are changed into days, and a good, warm bed into wet and cold soil. Most of them are unable, without loss of health, to withstand so many unaccustomed influences, and thus, for all its large

* Meissner says: according to the public newspapers of 1772, Luisa de Jesus, aged 22 years, was hanged in Lisbon for killing 33 children at Coimbra because for every child newly admitted she profited one bed, one cradle, and 600 reales or 1 Imperial thaler in money. L.c., p. 114.
** Ballexserd, "Dissertation sur l'éducation physique des enfants," p. 86.

expenditure, the republic has only brought up a band of useless weaklings half of whom are immediately felled by diseases upon their first appearance in the work world, while the other half helps in physically degrading mankind.

7) Guidance of children toward unhealthy handicrafts and factory work. That children who are to be dedicated to the learned class are made to learn the first principles of the sciences may be justified in time. But despite this, or precisely because of this, many of them learn the wrong occupation or become sickly creatures. But nothing can excuse the custom of teaching very frail children who are still growing, to learn arts and crafts which, as in most kinds of factory work, will entail the need to force them into unnatural positions. This causes very strange ailments even in adults, and necessarily prevents the good formation of the body, a healthy state of entrails variously compressed into too narrow a space, secretion of most necessary juices, and the regular deposition of new nutrients. I shall prove elsewhere that it is impossible to promote general health and a good physical state in citizens of a republic in any other way than by diminishing as much as possible the large number of very unhealthy craftsmen, or at least by stipulating more accurately the age at which young persons, who are still growing, may devote themselves seriously to such crafts. It is just this detrimental intention of turning foundlings into factory workers instead of bringing them up as useful farmhands or real peasants,* that the state could alter by alloting its waste land, with moderate assistance, as property or for use. Making factory workers of foundlings causes, in addition to the indigenous diseases of foundling hospitals, cachexia, scurvy, goiter, and also a number of such ills that are mostly at home in factories, as scabies and other skin diseases which usually originate from work with wool, hernias, narrow chests, consumption and others. These necessarily increase mortality in such [foundling] houses.

There are so many, and even more, circumstances which prevent the fulfillment of the noblest intentions concerning educating foundlings, and which at best, prolong the fate of these wretches, instead of improving it. Therefore, such foundations have always provoked the objection, which being based on arithmetical certainty is unassailable, that the state either loses its entire capital or can expect only such low interest that much more useful foundations which could be more profitable and would be a surer way for the state to invest its funds could be established in the community.**

* * *

* "Ephemerides of Mankind," 1776. Vol. IV, p. 197.

** Meissner, l.c. In a successful treatise on poorhouses which was defended in the ducal military academy at Stuttgart in 1779 by Equerry von Winkelmann, mention is made in defense of foundling hospitals that in examining the use or detriment of such foundations, one should take good care not to take accidental shortcomings for necessary and substantial ills. For foundling hospitals have always been judged onesidedly, always as they really were and not as they should and could be. p. 62.

PART THREE

Care of health of young scholars and the necessary police supervision in educational institutions

§1

Certainly the police has no subject that it must supervise more thoroughly than that part of public education through which we become useful citizens of the state, and get to know the relation of our duties toward God, the fatherland, all people, and ourselves. The number of teachers in our days is infinitely large, and everybody is now busy with the long neglected work of a better moral education of youth from all classes of mankind. But it seems that sooner or later much of what has been built too hastily will have to be razed again because in some places it was forgotten to take the measure of those for whom it was built.

§2

Whereas in former times too much or too little was done in this matter, for youth was seriously occupied with things that had little use for their future destination, now suddenly there is an endeavor to melt together all the four faculties in a small crucible—and from this mass, already in the first children's schools, to mold from weak beings theologists, judges, physicians and philosophers. I wager this comprehensive plan can be put into practice! But far be it from me to congratulate mankind on this. Such an intention can be put into effect only at the expense of public health and good bodily constitution, and just as it would not be advisable for me as a physician to invent a means of making beards grow on seven-year old boys, or to advance the power of procreation by ten years so as to increase the population, just so one cannot expect anything of the excessively early employment of the tools of our power of reasoning and of the unnatural strain on the weak brain fiber, necessary for various higher concepts.

§3

The police, therefore, has to see to it that no enervating system or a system that makes its fibers prematurely stiff interferes with the public education of youth.

The police must thoroughly examine the rules and regulations which guide youthful occupations, games and entertainments, their mental and physical exercises, and endeavor to prevent equally overexertion and neglect of the forces with which nature endowed the young body, and to ensure only uniform perfection of the whole. The police must indicate to each age its limits, and it must not anywhere promote the construction of vain hothouses of human reason, for it is impossible to make children into more than garrulous philosophers without damaging the perfection of their bodies, to the detriment of their general health and even of the sciences. The police must determine the duration of schools and their kind. It must even stipulate the number of those who may successfully choose a scientific career without being permitted to overexert their mental forces to the detriment of their health. It must indicate to the irate teacher or father reasonable bounds in their chastisement of unteachable or obstinate young people. It must endeavor to restore the lost spirit of joyful physical exercises and the skillful development of all the physical faculties, which is so necessary for youth, and it must deal altogether with the smallest details concerning the health and well-being of this important class of people.

§4

No matter how much has so far been written about education, I still believe that the commodity of health still receives least consideration in most public schools and educational institutions. Each of the subjects mentioned here deserves to be made up and to be reviewed from this point of view by a physician.

PART THREE

Section One

Of the disadvantage of too early and too serious an exertion of the youthful spiritual and physical strength

§1

We pay for the excellence of our reason compared with the so-called instinct of the animals by a very long-lasting childhood. Just as the growth of our body lasts for a third of the entire life span, our spirit, too, up to the completion of its development feels the influence of the imperfection of all bodily tools. There are few animals which are not all that they should be in a much earlier youth, whereas man approaches very slowly the time of his complete maturity.

During this time interval, there are very various mainsprings acting in our machinery in order to make it as perfect as possible. The most visible among them all is the irresistible desire for pleasure and variety, for hopping games and amiable fun.

An observation that deserves the attention of a philosopher is the fact that when one surveys all of nature and sees how all living creatures, from the enormous elephant to the tiniest mouse, the cruel panther and the terrible lion, as well as the earnest and long-suffering donkey, hop through an important part of their lives with equal abandon, and make fun throughout their youth without a care... Can one misinterpret the intention of the Creator of all and deny that the joy of youth and all blossoming nature's smiles are a condition on which the fate and flourishing of all individuals depend for the rest of their lives?

* * *

§3

Disadvantage of too serious a method of education

It can be seen from this that one works against the plan of nature if one tries to force the playing and laughing age to serious occupations and stiffening work, and by bold heating of the youthful juices, squanders the material for the future formation and perfection of the growing body. But there is no particular difference whether one overexerts the mind by too early brain work or the flesh fibers by bodily exertion before they have reached the required consistency. The damage always consists in that the nutritive juice needed for the advantageous growth of animal strength is squandered in an unnatural manner, and thereby the perfection of future citizens impaired.

* * *

§5

The age at which youth may start to study the sciences seriously must first be determined.

Together with language, children also acquire the ability to understand strange mental images and concepts, and it is natural to conclude from this that their receptiveness of different impressions also presupposes a certain physical disposition of the brain which makes it possible to accept and store in the memory without detriment a daily increasing number of words and images. It was found that the natural inquisitiveness of four- to five-year old children greatly increases the opportunity of creating in them such lasting impressions that these are in many cases decisive for their entire future lives, way of thinking, and inclinations, and can never be completely displaced from the initially allotted space in the mind.

It is understandable, therefore, why everybody endeavors to make every kind of use of this favorable time in the human age. And since there is nothing more important than the principles of religion and the sciences, everybody makes haste to stuff the brains of children with words, as if the entire art of education consisted only in training the tongue muscles to say and parrot every kind of expression, and as if the salvation of mankind were to be sought in reverberant sounding and learned words.

* * *

§13

Necessary selection of those who, because of better talent, may study

Just as I proved in §3 that a greater application of youthful mental powers usually greatly reduces the body's perfection, so must this occur even more to the heads of those who want to devote themselves to the sciences by all available means, without being provided by nature with an easy grasp and excellent talents. Either they never attain their aim, or they expend all their best forces early, and thus increase the number of persons, which is in our time quite considerable in any case, whose physical weakness is usually very conspicuous. These persons certainly are not an inducement to view science as a means of attaining bodily happiness.

The police, therefore, can render a real service to the population and to the perfection of the human race if it puts a stop to the parental craze of making scientists, or at least idlers, out of all their children. And if, to the advantage of the working class, they will reduce to two thirds the number of those who now want to escape from the peasant or burgher class by learned indolence, but having no particular predisposition, attain no more than increasing the number of the more than burdensome M . . . or useless schoolteachers and preceptors, or even half-starved rhymesters.

* * *

§14

Of heavy labor and crafts for which youth is usually encouraged

Finally, a law must see to it that rash or hard-hearted parents do not force their still tender or half-grown children into irksome and dangerous crafts which retard growth and undermine health in its first predisposition. Elsewhere I have already mentioned this subject, and the public well-being certainly requires that authorities everywhere see to it that the limits be stipulated at every age for the use of the youthful strength and that parents, attendants, and employers who put an inhuman strain on their children and servants prematurely and to the certain detriment of their physical state, be called to account. When I see that a half-grown boy in his twelfth year is apprenticed by his parents in all earnestness to blacksmiths, locksmiths, bricklayers, joiners, or conversely, like a galley slave to the rowing seat, is attached to the cutting table of the tailor to be kept there all day with bent head and in unchanging position, etc., it is easy to predict that both candidates will later be either crippled or sickly and feeble citizens in the republic. Not to speak of all those who died at their difficult handicraft of a constantly maintained excessive drive of the juices flowing in still weak vessels, of hemorrhages, of consumption, and of emaciation. While I am writing this, I have to treat a tailor boy who was of good health and sound body when he was made to take up the handicraft in his tenth year. Habit or short-sightedness caused the boy to tailor away all through his apprenticeship with his head hanging down, and the result was very bad; all his cervical vertebrae make a broad arch backward which presses the head so much forward that the chin cannot be raised without force more than one-and-a-half inches from the breast-bone. Ramazzini gave a detailed description of the cases which occur in almost every handicraft, caused either by a continuous unnatural position or by unhealthy material to be processed, or from the location where the work is sometimes carried out. But I do not know that he remarked how much more frequent and more certain are the illnesses of those craftsmen in every community where no law protects the still tender youth from premature coercion to this or that handicraft or trade that is detrimental to their health and proper growth.

When parents themselves teach their children and instruct them in their own handicraft, the danger that the weak creatures will be forced into detrimental activities is not so great, but even here greed and coarse minds often enough overstep the boundaries. If an affluent burgher likewise abuses his paternal power so badly that he sacrifices his sons' health and bodily perfection (in order to rid himself of his children early) to his wish to see them accepted in this or that guild—and thus helps increase youthful mortality so much—then, I think, a law would have the desired consequences if it stipulated the age, especially for crafts where the skill required does not necessarily depend on such early training. It should not easily permit weak children to be forced into heavy manual labor, and half-grown boys into work which must stunt their growth, and sometimes even cause incurable diseases.

It is even more irresponsible if the authorities allow vile parents to train their immature children as aerialists and tightrope dancers whereby the health and firm build of the entire body and its joints is endangered and at every instant their life is at stake, thus perpetrating cruel abuse on God's noble creature.

* * *

Similar supervision is deserved of street and church beggars who undertake to disfigure their children in all kinds of ways to produce conspicuous malformation that arouses general compassion, and thus increase their daily alms in this most abominable way. One should look in large cities, in front of the gates, on bridges, and in churches, to see whether the number of crippled children does not exceed all proportion, and then using experience as a guide one will be convinced that this class of parents often already in the cradle deliberately twist one child's limbs and bend them, there let another with a deliberately broken thigh or foot quietly heal in such a way that this limb must for ever remain useless, and there a third has his head or his lower extremities blown up to an unnatural size. Or these parents in some other secret way change and debase the human figure so that the natural perfection and formation of a large number of persons is thereby destroyed, and the class of useless cripples everywhere increased. Finally, there is also cause to add to those arts, the early learning of which is detrimental to the health and perfection of the youthful body, the art of playing wind instruments some of which are very bad for the weak chest of half-grown boys, and often cause spitting of blood, lung diseases, ruptures, and other illnesses. It is so that in a country where there is a general predilection for such art, a law precisely stipulating the number of candidates, their ages, and physical condition would be useful. It would be right to forbid all young men before their eighteenth or twentieth year the playing of the trumpet, the French horn, and the flute, which all require a considerable strain of the chest, and restraint and moderation of the air to be expired, which is detrimental to the bodily growth and the uniform distribution of the juices. And, since it can matter little to the state that some of the perfection might be lost when such art is learned somewhat later, it would be right not only to enforce this order but to see to it also that tender, full-juiced, weak-chested, young men prone to bleeding never be admitted to the learning of such art, and that all music teachers be forbidden to teach them without special permission by the authorities, so that the number would be reduced of those who, in order to provide a pastime for other persons, sacrifice their own belows and shorten their lives.

* * *

In the subsequent Section Two of Part Three, Frank describes the principles of good school hygiene. He deals most thoroughly, and in accordance with his liberal principles, with the subject of methods of punishment predominant in 18th-century schools.

PART THREE
Section Three

Of the reinstatement of gymnastics and its advantages in public education

§1

While excessive taxing of youthful forces through inappropriate work ruins the soul and the bodily health of infinitely many children, on the other hand, there is nothing so much opposed to the successful development of both sexes as when all free movement of young people is smothered by prejudice, comfort, and laziness. I have proved the incompatibility between constant restraint of children from all play and pastimes, and the intentions of nature, and I have freely revealed my thoughts concerning the monastic education of the female sex.* Further explanation of the damage caused by present-day, fashionable effeminate education has been postponed up to now, and it deserves the complete attention of persons in authority to whom the public education system is entrusted.

§2

Its disadvantages

I shall not waste time here by enumerating all the advantages of a coarser way of education accompanied by plentiful movement of the body: this has been done of late by several skilled physicians.** It suffices if one sees daily the difference between an effeminate and a freer way of education, and when a limb that has been used for various kinds of work ever since youth clearly excells by its perfection and strength. When city children with their pale faces, bloated skin, hardened glands, and weak limbs sink into a genteel state of anxiety upon the slightest movement, helplessly melt into sweat, and suffer from a thousand ills of which the peasant lad does not know at all; when all death lists show that the mortality of city children is so much greater than the mortality of the working masses; when finally, only the sons of those citizens can be usefully employed who had the good fortune to have received a less

---

 * "Medical Police," Vol. I, Part Two, Section Six; Vol. II, Part Three, Section One, §1, 2, 3.
** F. Hoffmann, "De motu, optima corporis Medicina." Hebenstreit, "Exercitationes adolescenti aetati salubres."—Krüger, "Children's Education."—Unzer, "The Physician."—Ballexserd, "De l'Education physique des Enfants·"—The Silesian Physician·—Tissot on the Health of Savants, etc· See also what I said on this subject in Part Three, Section One, §3.

128

tainted upbringing because of their lower rank, for all physical accomplishments requiring strength and persistence; then, I believe, it is quite superfluous to have recourse to reasons of medical science to prove the damage caused by modern, effeminate education. When the Royal Society of Sciences in Dijon, which in 1775 recommended investigation of the influence on the morals of physical exercises and public games current among the ancient nations now considers that subject as being among the most important questions ever posed by the Academy, then, a closer examination of the effects on the general health of the nations of such games must make every philanthropist wish what Tissot already wished so fervently: that these useful pastimes, the abolition of which was one of the main causes of the increase of lingering illnesses, be reintroduced, at least in places which nowadays are so often founded for the education and instruction of youth, that gymnastics and young people's pastime again become—as in former times—a subject for super-vision, and thus become a means of restoring the deteriorated elasticity in the sinews of all civilized nations.

* * *

In the following paragraphs, Frank provides a survey of the development of gymnastics since antiquity.

§6

Necessity of improvement

The great and beneficial revolution that has taken place in the educational system of many regions for several years now confirms my conviction that persons every-where are now beginning to recognize the advantage of busier and more natural instruction over the effeminate education under which youth must suffocate. If Locke, Rousseau, and the upright Montaigne who was an example to both, and some of the present directors of public educational institutions had no other merit, they would deserve infinite thanks if only for having endeavored to maintain their pupils in good bodily condition, and having searched for ways to unite health and sciences, sensi-tivity and nervous vigor.—It is high time that people have begun to counter the whining, sensitive voice of effeminate weaklings, and the yearning-for-pity choir of vaporous and convulsive virgins, and have rescued the honor of those nobler feelings which in almost all societies gradually were becoming such childish irritability that all objects that affect our senses seemed already to have lost the natural relationship appointed them by the Creator. Instead of calmly stimulating our powers of per-ception, they caused nothing but senseless distortions and madness, in short, exalted feeling.

§7

The laboring class of people has already been provided for by nature, and whoever of them has not suffered extreme misery and has retained sufficient natural reason as he had acquired by his way of life and his health will never want to exchange this treasure for the pernicious high living of the rich. But in order that those in the human race in this class and in many others, who either strictly pursue sciences or are otherwise obliged to devote themselves to sitting arts, do not sink even lower in its good quality, the police must take measures to make the mind of such persons take heed of the important part which freer movement and exercise plays in health care.

It does not suffice that young people who attend to their studies are granted certain days of rest and are given opportunity to enjoy fresh air. Efforts must be made in choosing games for each sex, for each age, and in determining what of each, and of all of them, is to be carried out. The damage which science and a sedentary way of life cause the general health thus can be prevented as much as possible at an age at which the body gains its bad or good disposition for the future span of life.

* * *

§10
Necessity of a public instructor for exercises

In all towns, which are the real seat of the idle way of life, the teachers of lower schools must either accompany their pupils without exception into free fields, arrange their games and supervise their exercises, or—and this I suggest most strongly— a special teacher for exercises is to be appointed who will supervise the whole system of exercises for youth. In accordance with all that I have so far pointed out, the post of such a teacher for the health of student youth certainly must be one of the most important posts which for the good of the state is required in places where the young of an indispensable class of citizens have been educated with great costs mostly to become sickly creatures who are of use only for a short time out of their whole lives. Besides, the establishment of such a teaching post would nowhere require any extraordinary expenditure: there is hardly any town so small that it does not keep its fencing or dancing master, and often a basically shallow and unknown foreigner derives greater advantages from such services that are so unimportant to the state, and often dangerous to it, than many another teacher. Thus, after a more prudent choice of instructor it depends only on the community to use such a person to better advantage and to entrust to him a more general instruction of the male youth in useful exercises, and to stipulate exactly what such a teacher would have to do with the young.

* * *

§13
Of public exercise places

First of all, a safe, spacious playground, commensurate with their number, must be allotted to youth at a certain distance from the city (so that a healthy change of air can be effected, and the boys, tired out from games, do not too quickly become quiet and cool down). If there is an opportunity to allocate a separate building where the young people can carry out their exercises in severe or stormy weather, this is certainly very desirable, and various agreeable activities can be devised for them here.

*   *   *

In the following §14, Frank deals with problems of safety posed by the games young people play. In this connection, he also touches upon the occupational disease of runners, and the damage to health which may be caused by dancing.

On the winning-post in foot races

Care must be taken that the winning-post in foot races is at the right distance in regard to age and sex, and that no one jostles someone else in order to overtake him. When the winning-post has been reached, all those taking part in the race must return [slowly] to the starting place in order that they do not cool down too rapidly. Lycurgus also let girls take part in this exercise which is so advantageous for the development of the body. Unfortunately, our beauties are not inclined to flee any more, and they received from their Creator only half enough muscles for this. At Bretten, a neighboring district town in the Rhenish Palatinate, there is a race of all the shepherdesses every year on St. Lawrence Day; it is arranged very ceremoniously and attended by large numbers of persons. The winning prize, for which all the shepherdesses race in light attire, is a ram and certain articles of clothing. The town clerk waits at the winning-post for the agile victor, and rewards her vigor.

Speaking for races here, I cannot refrain from saying a word about the runners whom noble persons everywhere keep for distinction, and to which task some parents encourage their well-built sons because this kind of servant receives a higher wage in general. The origin of runners or couriers goes back to the times when the postal service had not yet been as generally introduced as now. Then, special and confidential servants had to take letters and messages sometimes to very remote places, which nowadays the post-horse can and must do much better. The gentlemen took pride in the fact that their servants ran better than others; and thus the toilsome profession of runner demanded such exertion in order that the runner and his employer attain some fame, that many young men ran themselves lame before they could be considered skillful enough. A hundred bets were made between persons who themselves could not stand any longer on their own feet in the afternoon, wagers that one runner would excell over another, although it could be assumed that such experiments ran counter to human nature and that they had to have a fatal outcome for one person, if not for both. In large cities, where the number of houses with one or more runners is considerable, the number of runners is also considerable, and consequently this occupation is still enough in use to play an important role among the unhealthy arts and to be worthy of police supervision. How can the police calmly look on while so many well-built young men devote themselves to a profession that is so dangerous to life? How can the police be so patient as to permit that a human being can be driven by anybody who has a mind to do so, and can be made to jump slavishly in front of his carriage through mud and swamps, where there is no need for such harshness and mistreatment? There is a sensible reason for a reigning monarch to have his runners close by so that his orders may be sent out at any moment, when a rider is not always available, or it is undesirable to send him by horse. But that every country squire to whom fate has given several thousand thalers to spend annually, seeks such vain display through the fact that every year a person runs himself consumptive in his service or, in order to save the honor of the house, breaks his neck, obviously demeans too greatly man's character. The state, therefore, must determine who should be permitted to keep runners; wagers between employers, as well as between the runners themselves regarding their skill and agility in running should always be punished, because nature is always abused, and a citizen should not be easily permitted to put horses and persons in the same class, and to use the latter to announce unfeelingly to the world that one in full sweat is a weakling.

* * *

Rules of caution at public dances

As regards the exercise of dancing, I suggest various rules of caution. Because dancing causes violent movement of the body, it is least suitable in the hot summer when indolence firmly reigns, and moreover all animal juices indiscriminately incline to being so very stale. Liquifying perspiration and the desire to refresh oneself with a cool drink unite so that dancing persons are plunged into dangerous illnesses. It is advisable, therefore, never to permit a public dance at such a time.

A thousand experiences have proved that the female sex, when engaged in its monthly menses, ruins itself most by dancing. Of course, the police cannot enforce obedience to a law which would forbid women to dance under such circumstances. In addition to a general warning, however, the police can make the parents responsible for the consequences, for the state of their daughters cannot be unknown to them; and they should also make it evident that a bleeding maiden incurs a certain disdain.

Pregnant persons may take part to advantage in such amusements, but a mother who is past the first half of her pregnancy, and thus certain of it, should never, under pain of strict punishment, be permitted to expose herself and her embryo to the danger of falling or of a strong concussion due to violent dancing. In this connection, see what I have said on this subject in the first volume of Medical Police.

In that the rapid transition from rest to violent movement and from the latter to the former can always have the most critical consequences for people's health, Unzer's suggestion that all balls and dances should begin and end with minuets, is certainly worthy of every consideration.* No dancer, male or female, should be permitted to leave the dance floor before a quarter of an hour has passed after the

* "The Physician," Chapter 100.

last dance, in order that often lethal colds may be prevented as much as possible by such caution. Of course, such a careless sweat-drenched dancer will catch cold just as easily when he must wait longer in his undervest, but the large mass of people will benefit from this rule. Nocturnal balls which last until daybreak, when the winter cold is harshest, cause colds to occur much more often, and it is most important that the police does not give its consent easily to such affairs.

Among all dances, the healthiest must be those danced by country people in open fields, under shady linden trees, where neither great heat, nor much dust, nor the exhalations of so many persons spoil the air as it does in narrow rooms. However, dancing under the open sky is forbidden in Saxony. Other reasons must be found there that dancing in houses is commended. In consequence of that policy, a respected citizen could help remedy all hardships if he would attend such amusements as a witness on behalf of the police.

Permission should not be given for every kind of dance to be introduced everywhere at will. Physicians note daily that the so-called shuffles and waltzes are detrimental to health, especially to health of women. Certain English dances also drive body movement to excess, and a number of minuets must follow before a ball ends, if bad consequences are to be avoided. In the bishopric of Würzburg, shuffles and waltzes have been prohibited forever by a general law of 18 June 1765, and a princely rescript of 1767 in regions of the Principality of Fulda repeats this law.

* * *

After discussing fencing, riding, and swimming, Frank touches on the healthful effect of walking, and he condemns acidly the bad habit of that time of using a carriage for going even the shortest distance, and he regards the carriage as a status symbol.

§15

Necessary promotion of walking

Walking is a very good means of luring idle city dwellers from their caves, and a shrewd police will promote it, even if some persons should be tempted thereby to abuse this good action. In moderately warm countries, walking is a very beneficial movement for all classes of people, be they weak or healthy. Of course, the Persian laughs when he sees the European wander about the streets without having any business, and he laughs even more when in answer to his question as to why this is done, he is told: I walk to have some movement, for the inhabitants of hot countries are usually lazy and sluggish, and they spend most of their lives sitting, because the intense heat causes to be secreted spontaneously through the skin that which we must work to expel.

* * *

In towns the maintenance of so many horses and carriages has long been considered an important cause of exaggerated expenditure and a source of exhaustion for many families. Attempts were made to remedy the malady from the merely political view by certain taxes which in some places, such as London, now yield immense sums, but they did not pare down the luxury. As for the effect of this taste on the health of the nobility and the upper middle class, much more effective laws should be devised. What differences (I cannot say this too often) can be seen in the same nation barely three and a half centuries apart!... Once, kings, princes, and women were still on horseback: the foremost duties of armored nobility and of its courageous and manly cavalry, the most lowly, and of all classes, incurred movement on foot and a strong and manly body, the honor and ornament of the young German man, and gardening, kitchen, and domestic work gave the blue-eyed maiden of cedar-like straight build, sinewy arms and nimble feet!... Today, everybody who wants to be distinguished from the rabble, is drawn in cradles by horses... Fifteen thousand carriages in Paris, and relatively as many in all large cities; where barely 200 years ago the monarch of this kingdom himself informed his confidant by a letter written in his own hand that today he could not drive to him because his spouse intended to use the carriage for herself,... today Germany's hero sons with effeminate features, their feet in glittering white silk, their bodies swathed in the finest embroidery, with knitted brows, a hat instead of the paternal helmet, now worn under the arm, roll gently back and forth, to the musical comedy and to the card-table where they get only acquainted with the names of Alexander, Hercules, Charlemagne, and Lancelot upon loss of their fortune and their health. They are barely strong enough to hold the silk parasol toward the sun which dares shine into the face of the dainty male doll, if he ever leaves the shiny carriage and hops across the street like an articulated toy!... The future mother of the defender of German honor and name, with pale cheeks and withered white breast, and thickly painted over in red, wearing fishbone armor, all day among insipid little men she lies immovably fettered to the seductive sofa ... a declared enemy of all domestic occupation and a future, ruthless, half-mother of sickly sons,—all this only because of the murderous prejudice that it seems less gentle to do what keeps the common people in good health, and that he cannot be counted among nice people who has not forgotten everything including walking, and yet can make large steps in the world!...

Certainly, these considerations deserve the serious attention of the police to heal this dangerous illness of the state, much more so than considerations of a general excess in expenditure. The number of carriages that were made only in order that reciprocal boastful visits can be made almost without shaking the body, testifies more to our weakness than to lavishness, depending whether one considers it a sign or a cause. The following is the means of teaching a noble people to walk again: to make it difficult to be driven comfortably; on all occasions where it is possible to do so without great fatigue, to use the tools allotted by the Creator for improving one's health, and by prohibiting all games which do not employ the body predominantly; at least to young people, that weaklings and idlers in the republic meet with deserved disdain; and that young men who excel particularly in public and healthy exercises meet with honorable distinction; that the erection of public buildings for various health-promoting games and exercises be favored. Order and the police should be supported in this, and even to eradicate in the education of the female sex the childish, the enervating dallying, and the eternal sitting, in short, the monastic education. This was depicted already in the first volume of the Medical Police, since it maintains in such an unforgivable way the more beautiful half of the human race in a state of paralysis. This must gradually degrade the manly character of most nations, fill all the provinces with invalids, and extend the rule of the physicians over the entire globe.

* * *

A SYSTEM OF COMPLETE MEDICAL POLICE

Volume Three

Food, Drink and Vessels. Laws of Moderation,
Unhealthy Clothing, Popular Amusements. Better
Layout, Construction, and Necessary Cleanliness of
Human Dwellings

PREFACE

I deliver the third volume of Medical Police (Medicinische Polizey) in the confident hope that if the content of the previous two parts attracted the attention of the learned public, this will apply in even greater degree to the subjects dealt herein. I only wish to have in every district, no matter how small, at least one philanthropist in authority to be an interested reader of the considerations submitted, for the truths that are being expounded here are mostly so striking, and the gain from and necessity of obeying them so convincing, that it would be difficult even for the envious to doubt the possibility of putting them into practice. It will, at the least, seem disgraceful for the indifferent observer of human needs to disobey generally beneficial rules and to publicly reveal what little respect he has for the physical well-being of society.

However, I would like to draw the attention of the people in authority to one circumstance. I mean the effect of excessive oppression on the state of nutrition of the ordinary people. Here I do not want to overstep the boundaries of my profession and moralize, putting forward the often repeated complaints of mankind. I only wish to make it generally understood that just as the health of individual parts of the state determines the general usefulness of that great body, so does it enhance the ease in acquiring the necessary sustenance, and altogether the good physical state, of the working class and the longevity of individual citizens, and consequently the worth of the population of a country. The paucity and extreme shortage of digestible foodstuffs under which the lower classes now groan have the effect that this important part of mankind really suffers from a kind of emaciation which cannot be cured by physicians if the compassion of the great does not cause either the sources of foodstuffs to be increased or the value of things to be again brought to such a level that the relative wealth will be such that the lower class is protected from lack of the most essential foods. If only several great men, inspired by the spirit of the unforgettable Henri IV of France, would make a noble plan and help the food situation of their people in such a way that the diligent peasant would again have hope that he with his children, as the great man wishes for his subjects, could consume a chicken in rice! This would certainly be a greater achievement than no matter how many large towns are decorated with no matter how beautiful hospitals. It is always more deserving to procure food for the masses of the poor than to let the consequences of extreme want be cured for a short time by physicians in a very expensive manner, in a hospital filled with thousands.

I see with pleasure that lately several skillful men enriched Medical Police (Medicinische Polizey) by their public contributions, and thus assign to this important part of our science the place it deserves. Mr. Uden of Berlin, the deserving author of a work that greatly enriched forensic medicine, will be of even greater service to mankind if, according to the plan, he will found a magazine for Medical Police from which future times will be able to supplement what may be lacking in the present work.*

Those who believe they are in a position to determine in practice the value of my opinions, may judge whether I overstep the bounds of the legitimate police if I view each subject of it not only as a mere physician but also as a regular member of human society (who, regardless of that character, also has to make his voice heard when advice is to be given concerning public matters). The way I went to work is this: I myself remarked that in some imperial city and in small districts some proposal or other may seem impossible or really may be inapplicable, but the important point is always whether this impossibility is caused by mere prejudices the duration of which, fortunately, is not forever when enlightened men are willing to fight them resolutely, or whether the cause of their inapplicability really lies in their very nature. At least I already have the pleasure of really seeing a not inconsiderable part of my thoughts, hitherto expressed, to have been realized in various states, and more than I dared hope, but I do not want to be so immodest as to ascribe the desert to myself. Sometimes a regulation is obeyed better in a foreign country than where it first appeared, and this should be an encouragement to make proposals even at places where there may be doubt as to their usefulness.

The assumption that the state must take up any matter to which society is not indifferent, and that the ignorant must be under the tutelage of the more reasonable, is not a bad principle, no matter what objections are raised**: and considering that no proof is needed of the need for a good policy in general (for this cannot be conceived to be in pieces) in every well-ordered community, I do not understand how a health ordinance, the most important part of a health policy, can be thought to be superfluous or even be felt as unbearable tutelage or odious coercion. Who would be tempted to choose Constantinople rather than Vienna for his permanent abode because there anybody, according to his own discretion, may leave feces lying in front of his house as long as he wishes. Or because it is not forbidden there, in case

---

* I just received the first number of this useful magazine for forensic medicine and Medical Police, and the public will certainly eagerly await the continuation.

** Examination of the presumed necessity of an authoritative Collegium medicum and of a medical coercive order. Hamburg 1781,8.

of any pestilent disease, to be infected and in turn to infect other unsuspecting honest people!

The amicable foreigner, not excepting the sensitive Yorick, will less resent the police in Paris, whose eye watches the citizen's every step, once he is acquainted with the country's system, than the boisterousness of the London mob where anybody, only somewhat differing by his foreign mien or clothing, is called a French dog and is exposed to all sorts of mischievous maltreatment. This mob, when in the throes of mad religious fervor, violates international law and storms the church of a respectable ambassador, while the police is unable to stop the disturbance; this mob is even permitted to treat its own regent and ministers, if it feels like it, in the most unrestrained manner.

That in Paris, in spite of all the supervision, there is still such disorder as cannot be found in London or Amsterdam, is probably not due to the police (although about the latter two as stinging a parody could be written as about Paris), for each country has its customs that cannot be completely eradicated, and everywhere much happens even if the police does its utmost. My abode is open to everybody who is invested with authority and seeks the perpetrator of a heinous act. My conscience tells me that I am not able to commit such an act; this is my justification and the justification of every honest man. Is it pressure if one lives under fair laws that are derived from nature and from social life, the advantage of which must be obvious to every unprejudiced person? Is it freedom if one is permitted to undermine lawlessly one's own well-being as well as that of other citizens? In such case I do not have the right notion of pressure and freedom, or I admit that I was born to be a slave.

But if to a single one of my readers it should seem that I could ever abuse the admittance of the necessity of a medical ordinance so far as to state that in future no man be allowed to marry off his daughter without examination by the honorable faculty, or perhaps even no man be permitted to sleep with his wife, the "mistake" (although I was well understood by almost everyone) on my part lies more in the lack of a clear definition of my real concepts, not that the true substance of the matter was sacrificed to the pleasure of a comical representation of a proposal that had never been uttered. The prudent police will never meddle in a household as long as it does not disturb good order, and one can sleep placidly, alone or in twos, where there is equal submission by all citizens and consequently public and personal security.

It can be easily proved that I am not asking too much when I demand that on public occasions pregnant women are to be restrained from excesses. Only a few months ago, at O, a place 4 hours from here, a young peasant woman in the eighth month of pregnancy appeared at a public dance. The midwife, who saw her hurry to the dance, warned her not to have too much movement: but the rash woman waltzed for over an hour with all her strength, as far as her large body and the crowd permitted. The consequence was that she soon suffered very fierce abdominal pain and labor pains; she immediately ceased feeling her child which up to then had been very lively. Then there was bleeding, and finally on the third day she bore a dead boy, whom she presumably would have carried the full time and born alive. This and other examples of pregnant women, who in their venerable state indulge in everything that they indulged in when single, are not rare. In the rarest of cases is the police able to defend the unborn child: but where it can easily do so on public occasions, it should not do it? . . . . Why? . . . . .

Whoever is deterred by the multitude of my proposals concerning public health should consider this: a prudent lawgiver must have a large number of rules in his head which he, without edict and public printed regulations, is able to bring into use, either by giving a good example, or by some other means that are imperceptible to the public. And then most has been achieved when the old abuses stop and a new order has been introduced.* Nowadays we do a thousand things the introduction of which once required special laws, of our free will and without orders by the authorities. It will be the same with a health regime that is founded on natural principles.

After all, I speak with a public of whom only a few are physicians. I therefore must endeavor to make myself understood by nonphysicians, risking that my colleagues will be bored when truths known to them are mentioned. The work therefore is somewhat extended thereby, but so far the physicians have not been able to eliminate the evil. They will therefore permit me, since I have the good fortune to be read by many forthright persons of authority who otherwise are not used to reading medical treatises, to carry out my plan which has found general approval.

I have often considered the thoroughness of the Mosaic police laws which certainly far surpass any public health measures taken in any state, and I compared with admiration our times with those olden times, when the great lawgiver dealt with the lowliest detail to such an extent that he even ordered that every Israelite in camp should have his little shovel with him, with which to cover carefully his excrement with soil.** Nowadays much more important proposals on medical matters immediately evince sayings such as: "Well, yes, how can this be done?" "This is too petty for the police to bother about it! . . . ." "That way everybody would have his hands bound, etc." However, basically, we are simply too lazy to do good, and we value too highly every step that is required of us for the sake of the public weal.

The present part [of the book] contains everything that I considered worth saying about human nutrition. No matter how much there seems to be, I hope that no page will be found that I could well have crossed out. In some sections I found various

---

* "Toute idée patriotique, je me plais à le croire, a un germe invisible, qu'on peut comparer au germe physique des plantes, qui longtemps foulées aux pieds, croissent avec le temps, se développent et s'élèvent." "Tableau de Paris," Préface. The reader is requested to peruse what I said about this in the preface to Volume II of "Medical Police," pp. 89 and 90.

** Deuteronomy 23:12, 13.

points that previously had been elaborated by other physicians, but from a modern point of view there was little. I endeavored to put everything in order, always indicated the sources from which I drew, and I always endeavored to contribute so much that it was always easier for me to add my own thoughts than to insert extraneous matter, since I do not want to seem unjust either toward others or toward myself.

In the present volume I could not deal with public security, one of the most important parts of Medical Police, because the book would have become too large, and I save this for the subsequent volume; on the other hand, I believe that the treatise on public cleanliness institutions can be rightly incorporated into the section on human abodes in general.

Moreover, I believe I owe the coming century, which is so highly praised by this one, the following explanation: publicly and repeatedly I asked for foreign contributions of useful medical ordinances, but in this undertaking, which was approved by Germany, I found support in only very few places. In spite of that, I intend to continue my effort to elaborate this vast subject on my own: and this, I hope, should ensure for me future indulgence of the thinking public of this and of future times.

Bruchsal, St. John's Day, 1782.

PART ONE

Of healthy nutrition

After all terrestrial creatures came into existence, the kindness of their great Creator was mindful of their maintenance. The interaction of so many bodies made it reasonable to expect that the parts would soon become mutually disarranged and that certain sizes and shapes would soon be eliminated, and this would in every respect disrupt the intention of Creation. But the Almighty gave decay a purpose; He devoted even decay to the maintenance of His creatures, and made the dust of one into the mother of the other. He allotted to the mineral kingdom a place for their growth where suitable moisture flowed through. To the plants, to most of which He had given life without power of locomotion, He gave the milk of the earth as food, and like infants, they could nourish themselves from this general mother's breast. To the animal kingdom, whose destination was more extensive, He gave prudently as companions two feelings: hunger and thirst; then He bade them look for their livelihood and stipulated the firm rule: the more numerous He let them be on earth, the more would they compete for each place and thereby be forced to seek some other place; that not only the largest animals should live on prey, otherwise they would soon remove all the smaller creatures from the surface of the earth, but that certain species should seek only certain nutrition, and that each species was to find its own, without eternal strife with other animal species.

And thus we see how in the great household of God, the food dispenser Nature allots a table to each creature and cuts the requisite morsel.

Among the hungry whom nature has to feed daily, man should be most easily satisfied for almost everything is a means of quietening his stomach. That is why our table is the best stocked of all, and the entire plant and animal kingdom delivers its tithe and tribute to us, the handful of dust the form to which we eventually revert as we return to Mother Earth and decay in order to fertilize the roots and plants which in our lifetime we nibbled on. Not even the mineral kingdom resists our teeth completely; it is known that certain nations in Africa choose certain soils for their food and that they fall ill if they have to do without it for a long time. Adanson saw in

Portugal and further afield that the Negroes ate some kind of soil to which they were so used that when they are taken from their country to America, they are greatly affected by its loss. It is a kind of reddish yellow *Topfstein* (Fr. pierre ollaire) which in Martinique is sold in public markets as a foodstuff under the name Coanac. Other nations mix a fine soil with flour and this serves them as food.

§3

Our forefathers were not ungrateful for this generosity of nature. Their palate required even less stimulation and the stomach was not, as in our days, the tyrant which now quickly succumbs under the eternal business of digesting, turning into a wholesome nutritive juice the foods brought here from all parts of the world.

Once luxury had won the upper hand, the rich left the vegetables, and especially garlic and onions, to the poor, while apples, almonds, and similar fruits are now served only as dessert, until things went as far as they are now.

* * *

§9

Therefore the police must endeavor more than in any other matter to see that nothing gets lost of what mankind has to learn necessarily at such a high price. It must search the history of all times and nations in order to have that assurance which usually suffers greatly because of the attractive and deceptive appearance of some foodstuffs which through the avarice of the vendors and the greed and ignorance of the citizens cause so much damage to society. The police must concentrate all its attention to see that the people's choice of various foodstuffs suitable for their nutrition is not made more difficult and that the various foodstuffs are of unobjectionable quality. It must take accurate stock of widespread diseases and investigate what are the main kinds of food that each class consumes, whether on one side or the other too much of some food or other does not yield the material which to one province, more than to the others, imparts a certain property to the blood and a preponderant inclination to serious endemic ills and to a greater mortality. The police must not be content to think of a better arrangement of the nation's diet only when a dangerous epidemic threatens; long before then they must determine by fatherly examination the quality of each ordinary foodstuff, and also mutual relationships and influence on the present and future inclination of the public health, restrain Jewish grain dealers who could harm health, endeavor to detect and punish poisoning of the most widely used foodstuffs, enforce cleanliness everywhere, and keep a watchful eye for all the consequences of infringement and against unforeseen accidents.

* * *

PART ONE

Section One

Of the procurement of meat

§1

Taste, fancy and origin determine in all regions those animals which have to yield their flesh for our preservation.

* * *

§2

It is most remarkable with what care the Jewish legislator went to work here when he stipulated which kinds of animal could be eaten in its entirety and which partly by the Israelites. It is only to be regretted that the reasons for so many stipulations concerning clean and unclean animals, permitted and forbidden parts of them, which often seem quite unimportant and contrived, are now almost entirely unknown; yet, it seems certain that the Egyptian and the Jewish dietary laws, which in many respects seem to have been similar, must have been based on experience with the certain advantage of such detailed restrictions on the appetite of a people exposed to certain epidemics.

* * *

The Jewish nation had 28 regulations touching on foods forbidden to it. Among them were four special [positive] orders; the remaining 24 were actual prohibitions. Among these, were nine which concerned meat. Michaelis developed beautifully some of the reasons for the dietary laws of the Jewish nation*: but it seems to me that the main rules are based on experience which is lost to us. The most important prohibitive laws were:
1) Neither a piece of cattle nor a wild animal,
2) No unclean bird,
3) No carrion,

---

* Mosaic Laws. §203.

146

4) No meat from a stoned ox,
5) None from a mangled ox,
6) None that had been detached from a living ox,
7) No blood,
8) No fat from an unclean animal, and no sprained tendon, and
9) No meat boiled in milk is to be eaten.*

The remaining prohibitions concerned fish, reptiles, worms [creeping things] and the plant kingdom.

The Jews were permitted to eat ten species altogether of all the created animals: ox, sheep, goat, hart, roebuck, fallow deer, wild goat, pygarg, wild ox, chamois, and all the subspecies belonging to them which have cloven hooves and chew the cud were permitted to be eaten.

Of birds 24 species were forbidden to be eaten;** these were the eagle, condor, sea eagle, ossifrage, ospray, vulture, kite, and all kinds of raven, owl, night hawk, cuckow, hawk, little owl, cormorant, great owl, swan, pelican, gier eagle, stork, heron, lapwing, bat.†

* * *

§3

But since in our days and in the temperate regions of Europe many animals may be eaten without harm, whereas in a hotter climate certain diseases would not permit this, not all of the rules which these old nations evolved in regard to this is still applicable. Yet, everywhere we find traces of such care of the healthy nutrition of the citizens that puts us to shame, and we find also many other things which have either been introduced in well-policed towns or which, in view of the circumstances, should be introduced. Just because cattle-breeding today is only the business of the lower class, and slaughtering is no more the act of an individual family head, who in the auspicious glut of better times chose the healthiest of his lambs and threw away with distaste as unclean everything unnatural that he found in the entrails of his cattle, who consumed the blessings of his herds with his children, just for this reason I say a reasonable police must now take his place, and with watchful eye put an end to the base avarice of unscrupulous butchers.

* * *

*   Rabbi Mos. Maimonidae, "Tractatus de cibis vetitis."
** "Which birds were forbidden by Moses is sometimes impossible to determine because of lack of knowledge of the ancient language, and the Jews who still believe themselves obliged to observe the Mosaic law, are in the unpleasant position of having to observe that which they do not understand themselves and have to interpret at random." Michaelis l.c. §204.—But is not this the fate of all nations which derive their laws from times long past?
† Deuteronomy 14.

PART ONE
Section Four

Of the procurement of vegetarian sustenance

§1

Vegetarian sustenance, as the first and most natural nutrition of all, deserves a special article because it is so widespread and because it really constitutes the people's greatest sustenance. I pass over the largest part of the history of the bits of nutrition that were gradually accepted from the plant kingdom, partly because it is known only in fragments, and every part of the globe has its own history, partly because it is not so closely connected with Medical Police.

§2

If it is necessary that the police see to it that there is never a shortage of meat in towns, this applies even more to foodstuffs which the bulk of the population requires almost exclusively for its maintenance. The public, if necessary, bears with lack of meat long enough, but if there is only a suspicion of imminent lack of bread in large cities, the people permit themselves every unruliness toward the police. On the whole, meat may be viewed as a mere supplement; when starvation is mentioned, everybody understands by it the lack of grain and the ensuing lack of bread to be made from it. Starvation and epidemics are inseparable ills, and history is everywhere full of devastations brought by lack of grain. Then, one can see entire hordes of miserable people driven by voracious hunger, hurling themselves on raw food, roots, herbs, and green tree fruits, and filling their stomachs with indigestible things.

* * *

§27

After everything has been said as to what the police has to take care of in regard to grain, milling, and baking of bread, there is still something to be said concerning other things connected with the plant kingdom. The main thing is: in large towns a supply of sufficient vegetables must be ensured; among them, everything poisonous and suspicious must be destroyed; and in cooking, all that could have an adverse effect on the health of those who partake of it should be avoided if possible.

§28

Ordinary people in towns, like the peasants, live mostly on vegetables or plants and fruit which they grow themselves, in addition to some milk. To prevent future shortages, everybody has learned to see to it in time that he has stocks for the winter, when plants do not grow. No fashionable household can exist without vegetables, roots, and fruit. The police, therefore, must take care that there are always sufficient plants and vegetables for sale at low prices especially in towns: people cannot be assured of good health without adverse effects if they live exclusively on meat.

§29

The selection of different plants and fruits, which are on sale for general nourishment, is no less important. Here it was often proved by the saddest occurrences how dangerous it is when ignorant or greedy people are free to bring to market whatever they want. Most animals know, due to some wondrous instinct, how to distinguish very accurately on the pasture the poisonous plants from their healthy fodder, and having complete freedom amidst a mass of plants threatening instantaneous death, they pass them by without having a teacher to warn them. They carefully pick out every herb that they like and leave the poison untouched; it is rare that an animal is poisoned, except sometimes when some animal driven by hunger devours something deleterious together with dry fodder. Only man either never had the natural gift or lost it gradually because of his social life which completely changed his taste and the other senses, so that every year there occur cases of poisoning by plants that were mistakenly eaten, and their number is considerable in every community. Here I want to mention the most prominent items which caused special accidents, either because they were eaten out of folly or because they were thought to be harmless foodstuffs, or they were eaten knowingly in the rash hope that they will not cause any harm. Here I cannot list all the poisonous plants which cause harm but rarely, and because of some unlikely confusion. Haller, Guérin, Gmelin, and Paulet gained special merit in this matter because they described plant poisons of their countries accurately and lucidly, and thus warned the public of various dangers.* The police everywhere should have such useful works translated into the mother tongue, have them provided with good clear illustrations, and have them communicated free of charge to every public country school, so that the citizens are acquainted in time with the causes of terrible accidents, and will learn to counter them as quickly as possible.

* * *

* Halleri, "Historia stirpium indigenarum Helvetiae." Guérin, "Dissertatio de venenis vegetabilibus Alsatiae," Argentorat. 1766. Joh. Friedr. Gmelin's "Abhandlung von den giftigen Gewächsen, welche in Deutschland und vornehmlich in Schwaben wild wachsen," Ulm. 1775. Paulet, in den Mémoires de la Société Royale de Médecine, année 1776," p. 431–460.

PART TWO
Section One

On the care of the drinking water and the wells

§1

As people do with all other things when they deem themselves in full possession of them, they do not appreciate the value of good water. Yet all human societies, before they settled anywhere, always made the first condition a constant supply of potable water, and unless forced to do so, they did not dwell in places where nature denied them an abundant source. Most people therefore chose the banks of large rivers, and stretches of fifty or more miles of country remained as uninhabitable deserts, given over to animals, because people cannot, like animals, wander about for days, and when a source dries up, hunt about for uncertain puddles. Domestic cattle, without which a society cannot exist for long, also had to be considered every time. The Scriptures relate in several places the history of famous springs for the possession of which bloody battles were often fought in regions poor in water. Knowing the place in the desert where a cool spring bubbles is by far the most important part of geography for the Arab who wanders about the hot sand; and the horde which manages to maintain possession of such a spring is the one which, in hot years, lays down the law over long distances.

* * *

§2

Most springs, wells, and rivers owe their water to dew, snow, and rain which penetrate through the surface of the earth, and again well up from the depth after shorter or longer sojourn. But the earth is not uniform everywhere; it contains the most varied components not all of which are able to resist the dissolving power of water; therefore, it is understandable that the waters often have medicinal or poisonous qualities, depending on the regions through which they passed.

* * *

150

§3
Necessity of having a good police for wells

Therefore the police entrusted the physicians with, at least in our times, the duty of examining the wells and springs that are to serve for public use. In view of the fact that we are not short of means of determining its main effects in advance, either by chemical examination, or from accidental occurrences, or from the region and the known constitution of the given soil, or finally from analogy, it would be absurd to learn only from uncertain experience what can be accumulated only over many years. Already the ancients, therefore, dealt with this subject, and among the publicly employed physicians there is not one who did not, or according to the precepts of his art should not, in the first years of his medical practice diligently study this part of natural history of the district assigned to him.

* * *

After Frank has expressed his opinion on the various characteristics of potable water, and dealt with spring-, rain-, and snowmelt water, he sums up the utility of these considerations and then discusses in the following paragraphs how to keep wells, cisterns, and rivers clean.

§13
These observations may suffice to enable everybody who has to look after the well-being of a human society to judge society's requirements concerning potable water, and in case there is a choice, always to make the best choice. One will be able, without the assistance of physicians, to determine in advance and fairly accurately, and from the difference in the available waters, their future influence on public health, and learn to explain naturally the usually very general causes of endemic cases in certain regions, such as the soil and the position of a village, its air, its foodstuffs and drinks, etc. By now it happens that experienced physicians and chemists are charged with thoroughly examining the different available springs, wells, and other potable waters, and thus determine the natural contents and advantages of each. The purpose is that the same water does not have the same beneficial effect on everybody, and therefore, that the inhabitants be enabled to make the best choice. Nor should the police be satisfied to have in stock only as much water as seems required to satisfy the most pressing needs where it is feasible. The police must provide abundance and freedom of choice of this natural product which is so decisive for health.

* * *

§18

Keeping rivers clean

As regards keeping clean rivers and ponds from which people and cattle obtain their drinking water, the police justly sees to it that near human habitations and in places where water is drawn for internal consumption, there are no discharges of latrines, cesspools, tanneries, dyeing shops, soap factories, slaughterhouses, etc., and that no dead animals or other foul objects are thrown in. This care is extremely important only in the case of small creeks and slowly flowing waters and rivers; in the case of large and rapidly flowing streams, this matter is not so important. For either the foul bodies that are thrown in remain on the bottom, or they are carried away by the flow. In the former case, the depth of the water, the rapidly receding waves that are immediately replaced by fresh ones reduce the ratio of the rotting parts to the fresh ones to a degree that is not dangerous to health. In the latter case, the disadvantage is in any case reduced in a short time.

* * *

In Section 2 of this volume, Frank deals very thoroughly with the production and treatment of beer, wine, and brandy, as well as with the quality of drinking vessels and eating utensils.

PART THREE

On moderation in general

> "Je vous laisse en mourant deux grands Médecins: la diète et l'eau!"
>
> Du Moulin.

§1

Human beings have cause to envy the luck of all other animals in regard to the constancy of their well-being and unlimited readiness for every vital function. But we are very unjust if we blame Mother Nature for this important difference between us and other live creatures and do not look for the cause to which we have to ascribe this fateful disinheritance of such important gifts of nature. Up to this hour all animals, except man, still walk quietly along the path assigned to them at the time of Creation, without any claim to a better fate, and they reach the end of their lives with an assurance only rarely disturbed by external accidents, compared with which the ordinary mortality of human beings, living together in large societies, could be called a persistent pest. Our intemperance and the power of our passions have cruelly robbed us, probably forever, of the noblest gem which the Creator gave to each creature immediately upon its origin, and it is our fate to suffer pain and illness from the earliest years of our childhood, which we pass with groaning under the hands of ignorant or too clever educators, up to our premature old age. The most reasonable physicians admit that nature has the smallest share in all the accidents which beset us now, and that most diseases are nothing but the result of nature defending itself against our continuously exaggerated passions and their attacks. Let us deduct impartially from the sum of all human failings all the accidents originating from intemperance; the number of the remaining illnesses will amount to a few physical ills which are made necessary by our transitory body and its different destination in nature.

§2

This occurrence of nature has taught us to think of remedies the invention of which may on the whole cost humanity dearer than the ill itself. How many victims did humanity suffer before the art of healing self-inflicted diseases achieved that medioc-

153

rity which entitled it to be called a science! Thus humanity now had two ills instead of one: diseases and physicians; both are children of intemperance and increased luxury. However, it is incorrect to curse this art of healing as well, since it has already been produced with so much pain, and it is wrong to reproach with Rousseau the Faculty, if such bad material is supplied for its handiwork, and if it is supposed to build a strong edifice of health on its wantonly ruined viscera. It is a fact that we hold unlimited sway over a race which prefers to be humiliated by this rule rather than forswear its lust: what can be said against us? Perhaps that we should attend more diligently to our science, that we should abandon hypotheses and study nature more thoroughly! Well! Perhaps people want to say that they wish to have medicine without physicians? And thus, jurisprudence and theology, welcome, no matter how many times both of them have been at loggerheads with mankind!

§3

For a long time physicians were forced to defend themselves publicly against charges of selfishness by loudly teaching the foundations of their science, to their own disadvantage, and by unanimously warning the public about the daily causes of the most important diseases. If people do not want to hear this, why do they continue to blame the physicians and to call to them with Pliny: "Well, now! They live on our downfall! . . ."?

§4

But if the public is unable to recognize where its advantage lies, there are authorities to whom the physicians may turn. And with this intention I submit the following paragraphs for their consideration, with a feeling of calmness which should also serve as justification for all my brethren in office. The public intemperance, the excesses of an entire nation, and the shortcomings of unhealthy clothes that cripple the bodies, all these are not anymore the mistakes of an individual citizen; their consequences, therefore, cannot be damped with weak measures. They require the stronger hand of the official physician who, though he may permit a member of society to drown himself in wine in the dark, nevertheless cannot suffer a whole people to lose all its natural good qualities by debauchery. I therefore consider the following points as important enough to recommend them to the attention of the police authorities, and I believe that if there is no intention to dry up as much as possible this source of misfortune in a republic, all other activities of the police in regard to public health would be of little consequence.

PART THREE
Section One

On intemperance in eating and drinking

§1

After dealing with what the police has to put in order in regard to various foodstuffs, the consideration of measures aimed against gluttony in eating and drinking follows automatically. I certainly cannot presume to present my readers with a treatise on what and what not to eat. It is only my intention to explain to the state that though it may be less damaging for a single citizen to overeat, if this thoughtlessness becomes a fault of the entire nation the entire society cannot remain indifferent, that temperance laws on a large scale are something entirely different from the dietetic prescriptions of the physician, the violation of which prescriptions sometimes goes unpunished. The physician, who preaches temperance to this fellow citizens, is in the same position as he who preaches wisdom but himself is not wise. Although one being of youthful physique and in a moody fit may deride both, yet often after a few years some people have the unexpected occasion to feel what they did not want to believe: that the mistakes of the teacher do not make his teachings mistaken or untrue.

§2

Let me have the most valiant nation, its health like that of the first human beings who, like animals, ate plain food and suffered few moral and physical ills; before the end of my natural life, I am sure that the sinews of this nation will be slack and its best predisposition will be turned into the worst if an enemy of this race has found an opportunity of suppressing the natural plain nutrition and has replaced it by general and constant gluttony. It must be confessed that the largest empires always came closest to their end when luxury, and especially wastefulness in food, reached their peak. Not that the greater expenditure alone accelerated the fall, for though a glutton consumes more than a decent person, and an intemperate nation consumes its annual provisions twice as fast as a sober nation, it is the poorer class that suffers more misery and deprivation to the extent that the glutton wastes, and by their hunger they make up for part of what he has devoured. But it is the enervation of those who with their courage defend the fatherland, or at least have to lead its defense, the degeneration of those who need a healthy body in order to use their mental powers to the benefit of the state, and finally the pampering of all those whose existence is closely related to the well-being of the community, these plunge entire empires back into their former nothingness and turn the sons of conquerers of entire countries into the most miserable slaves of the physicians.

* * *

Diseases are inevitable wherever debauchery holds sway, and although our forebears, despite their bent toward drunkenness, enjoyed good health and were able to put a stop to the Romans' victories, this should not be used as an excuse for immoderateness. Our way of life has changed in every respect, and this has also changed the influence of such errors on the health. Ancestral intoxication from an innocent kind of beer, such as the one the ancient Germans drank, cannot be compared with the effect of the liquid fire which we now gulp down like water, all the less so since we also infinitely exceed in solid foodstuffs what our forebears consumed, both in quantity and quality.

* * *

Surfeit smothers and overwhelms the forces of the stomach and the intestines. The juices that have been only half digested go over into the blood in the raw state, accumulate in the fine vessels and glands because of their viscosity, curdle in them, and become the basis of tenacious constipation, swellings, hardenings, and dropsies of which innumerable persons must die in their best years. Daily and appropriate movement of the body could prevent some of these consequences; however, debauchery makes people lazy because all the vessels almost burst with thick juices, and the brain (until finally these people have the apoplectic fit that is so characteristic of them) is under pressure from the blood that is obstructed in the lower body and thus flows into the head. Who does not know that gout is a disease of good living, and in recent times it has become as general a household implement of noble persons as the spider in the hut, as expressed poetically but very truly. Nervous diseases, do they not hold sway over everybody from the great lady to the lowliest chambermaid, and from the canon with five sinecures to the lowliest schoolmaster? How does it happen that hemorrhoids are as common among city beauties as they ever were among men, and among men more common than ever before? I have already mentioned in the introduction to this work, that all this is due to our completely changed way of life, but especially to increased luxury in food and drink. Of course we do not think that this is to be feared, but our palates under the eternal stimulus of highly spiced foods eventually assume a cartilaginous hardness and insensitivity, and a subtle sharpness destroys at the first least opportunity, without being noticed, the entire mass of our juices and brings to a halt the whole machine, and unfortunately this, moreover, is transmitted as a sorry legacy from parents to children.

* * *

§6

The progress intemperance has made in Germany up to the middle of the present century is still too fresh in memory for me to have to tell its story here, to the shame of my country, although now the civilized people at least generally abstain from this vice. Suffice it to say that at courts, in monasteries, and in all public societies in the past, few persons even in the afternoon knew to which genus they belonged, and that a drunken hero everywhere was thought to be the man who belonged in first place. Thus, it is easy to imagine the general state of the nation and the influence of this vice on morals, state administration and health.

* * *

But the imperial laws that had been passed against drunkenness were obeyed so little and were treated so contemptuously that even persons of nobility publicly toasted each other: "To you and the Government's dismissal!" It is not difficult to guess the cause of this, for even the German Diets were tainted by this vice. The German laws, therefore, were called the morning language, because what was undertaken in the afternoon was so influenced by the cherished wine and beer that it was considered incorrect. At that time it was said mockingly: Comitia Germanorum sunt lenta & vinolenta. And the ambassadors were not only full in the afternoon, but in the Mainz Office they also used to put the wine bottles on the neighboring table, so that the clerks did not suffer thirst when penning what had been given ad dictaturam.* Ferdinand I, therefore, admonished the ambassadors of princes and imperial cities: "Remember that you did not congregate because of food and drink, but because of public affairs of the Empire. Therefore, flee with all your might from the loathsome intemperance from which soul and body perish, and follow your profession!"**

* * *

§7

Effect of intemperance

On the other hand, among the common people and among unrestrained youth left to themselves at universities, intemperance is still a widespread vice which robs the state of many useful citizens and destroys the ablest young men in the bloom of their age.

The number of those in every somewhat larger state who die annually of this cause is certainly considerable. According to the lists of London, the following numbers of drunkards died on the spot while engaged in drinking: 11 from 1686

* Von Ludewig, "Learned Announcements," p. 238.—Casp. Klock, "De aerar." Lib. II Cap. X. N. 25 ff.—Stryk, in V.M. ad ff. Tit. de extraord. crim. §17.
** Carpzov, "In Prax. crim.," P. 3. p. 146. N. 19.

to 1690; 5 from then on until 1695; 6 until 1700; 3 until 1705; 2 until 1710; 12 until 1715; 53 until 1720; 76 until 1725; 110 until 1730; 248 until 1735; 223 until 1740; 201 until 1745; 130 until 1750; 57 until 1755; 20 until 1758. Within a span of 73 years this amounts to a sum of 1,157, to which must be added 2,233 who were found dead in the streets in the above 73 years. Süsmilch says that they were not murdered; if one assumes that a few died of stroke, what else but drinking could have killed the rest? And this does not include the number of those who died gradually of drinking. If it were possible to record all the young men either at universities, on journeys, or finally on their travels where in the wine countries there is no end to drinking, who contracted the disposition to incurable consumption or other fatal illnesses through misuse of strong drinks, of brandy, of so-called liqueur, punch, bishop, wine, spiced beers, etc., if one were able to determine accurately all the moral and physical consequences of drunkenness in the country and in towns, and its inevitable influence on the community, if one added the cases of poisoning by adulterated wine, brandy, beer and similar such synthetic beverages, the state would indeed recoil because of the terrible number of persons killed by the misuse of a mere beverage alone, mostly because of the authorities who show so little earnestness in devoting all their attention to a vice which, albeit not eradicable, could yet easily be reduced.

* * *

§9
Measures by the police against squandering foodstuffs

Altogether it is more difficult to put a stop to squandering foodstuffs than to drinking: the police cannot count the dishes in households, and not everybody is willing to obey a law without supervision or coercion, no matter how just this law is. But in public and in ceremonial banquets, a prudent authority can and must stipulate certain rules against waste, and must punish their infringement, without being reproached for harshness.

The so-called baptism treats must be greatly restricted if not altogether abolished; I have already mentioned several times their unfortunate effect on the health of women who recently gave birth. In my opinion, a common or middle-class family should not be permitted such expression of joy about the birth of the child until the six weeks which are a critical period for every mother in various respects are over. What good is it all, but especially what good are expense and the noise for such a newborn child who will perhaps already be buried within the coming eight days, for most of the children who die in their first year perish either at birth or soon after, and give up their ghost while the guests drink to their health? . . . What good are the foolish expressions of joy in a house and at a time when the woman, exhausted after difficult labor and childbirth, so fervently wishes for quiet, and is so easily and dangerously affected by any noise, or by any vexing news (of which there is always some at such congregations), by every premature exertion connected with the preparation and arrangement of things which a peasant woman or a woman citizen without servants must make herself, and which endanger her life? Once the sixth week is over, such activity is less critical, and the waste occurring thereby is merely a simple object of the moderation laws that are required in every state.

According to such laws, a certain order could be stipulated for them and for wedding meals and funeral repasts, which nowadays have been abolished in many countries anyway. According to these it would be forbidden to serve more than a stipulated number of dishes or to raise the price of the entire feast above a certain limit.

* * *

A large number of male cooks in a state always indicates immoderateness and luxury among the inhabitants. The female sex is really born for the kitchen stove and a female cook always has in her favor the fact that she supplies cheaper and, at the same time, healthier foods. The male sex is in the kitchen, as everywhere else, more enterprising; and the health of the guests is the last thing which these persons consider when engaged in their cooking. In my opinion, a cook is a privileged poisoner, and I believe that it is real carelessness if these persons in the community are not subject to certain rules just as other guilds, rules the infringement of which should be brought to the attention of the police. A physician or apothecary must give an account if his prescriptions have an extraordinarily violent effect and that is just. By what right, then, has my friend's cook to dispatch me to eternity with his kitchen arcanum, or even by mistake, without being taken to account? Were any part of the system of sustenance to be taxed, I would place a substantial levy on the maintenance of a cook. Whoever among private persons, for this discourse is not about courts, is so highly learned in food matters that an ordinary female cook cannot cater sufficiently for his table? He has, to be sure, so much regard for humanity that he gladly takes upon himself a larger part of the public burden and proclaims he will gladly bear the cost for those who cannot possibly afford so much for eating.

§10

It would be ridiculous to take to account everyone in a community who once enjoyed wine in merry company until he was slightly tipsy, and who prefers to be cheered by this effective means rather than by the bitter poppy juice with which the Turk dispels his gloom. But it is no small matter that in our country every village, no matter how small, has at least six or eight taverns, and often more, which only wait for every penny of the ever thirsty peasants; that fifteen-year old boys vie with men in tippling and ruin health and morals with wine and brandy; that the little money the country folk have, instead of being used for the maintenance and education of the women, and children who starve at home, is thus chanelled into the pockets of an often fraudulent wine merchant. Too, entire communities can indulge in ugly intemperance to the advantage of a small class of people, without any other punishment than the reproach of their preacher; that most taverns in the towns, even in the morning, are full of people who do not leave until they have lost all control over themselves, and, to the general annoyance, find the broad streets too narrow; that through these and similar excesses, the state annually loses as many persons as it would in the worst plague epidemic that might strike every twenty-five years. For many unfortunate ones, after having committed their error, are immediately attacked by fatal illnesses, and moreover, most of them, suffering from chronic diseases, are a burden to the state for many years to come. Whoever would venture to deny the necessity of better supervision and stricter laws of moderation, would, I am afraid, already have drunk so much that he has lost part of his reasoning power.

* * *

PART THREE
Section Two

Of healthy clothing

§1

When I consider the history of the human race and I see on God's earth innumerable nations, one of them up to the nose swathed in furs and animal skins, the other as it was born by its mother, naked and bare; one protected against sun, cold, rain, or wind solely by simple blankets hung on them, the other decorated with colored feathers, shimmering silk, shining gold, with stones, pearls, shells and bangles; one with its color corresponding to the climate, the other painted, the whole body soaked in oil, with ineradicable, mysterious, or else insignificant lines drawn on the face, or the face even cut up and made to look like an embroidered wallpaper; finally, when I see among so many nations, that one is comfortably and at the same time daintily dressed, whereas the other is swathed like an Egyptian mummy or, like the Mordovian women, half suffocated under clothing that is as heavy as a horse's harness,* to the detriment of its good physical build, and who often merely because of the difference in color or fashion of the clothes hate each other in earnest and would even kill each other, I am always tempted to think that the royal animal is far below its fellow creatures in its ridiculous pride and not exalted over them.

Nature compassionately assisted the other animals, provided them with a hairy and less sensitive skin, and endowed them in winter with a specially grown fur which enables them to withstand the cold. Man appears naked and bare in the world, and even in his wild state is protected from the cold and wetness by only a little hair. Fortunately, the Creator provided him with the ability to become a permanent inhabitant of both the cold north and the hot belts of the earth, and with proper education, being able to adjust himself to his climate without depending completely on his invention of clothes.

§2

Nowhere does man need so much covering

Whether modesty or other feelings first made people cover their nakedness and

* Pallas, "Travels," Voi. I, p. 36.

thus lay the foundation for all future clothing, is irrelevant here. In our day, there are still innumerable nations whose inhabitants go about naked without any feeling of shame. And even the difference in temperature in the regions inhabited by such nations teaches us that cold and heat alone never determined the kind of clothes worn. If one goes back as far as possible into the history of all known nations, one piece of clothing after the other will drop off their inhabitants, even off those of colder regions, until we see man covered at best with an animal skin, even on snow and ice, thus justifying the goodness of Creation which apparently only at birth deprives us, but lets us gain abundantly by habit and custom what the other animals are born with to survive in the harsh climate.

* * *

§3

Effect of clothes on our moral and physical character

The physical and moral effect of gradually increased articles of clothing on those who have replaced nature's clothing by artificially covering almost their entire body would be a beautiful field of philosophical contemplations; but I choose only those garments which have a direct and important bearing on the people's health and on the state of our posterity.

The attraction which the nudity of one sex induces in the other sex is incontrovertibly greatest when certain parts are covered so as not to be seen by the interested party. This sentence is so true that the prospect of hiding natural attractions from the searching eye of the young man and letting him guess at something that one does not want to consider lost, has become an art of the fair sex, and a net in which we sooner or later are caught.

* * *

I have elsewhere described the invention of a great African woman regent who saw that her young men became cold toward the female sex and sank into abominable passions; she successfully stopped the almost incurable ill by instructing her sex to wear short skirts which covered certain parts that had previously been bare to the eye, and these were now furtively visible only upon greater movement.

Therefore thanks be to the honest veil which, instead of throttling the urges which the Creator intended to incorporate in our makeup, was able to engage our senses in a manner which (with regard to the effect of beauty on our heart) put the expectation above the enjoyment itself, and thus ensured the mutual affection aroused by each new kind of clothing and the new guise in which that which is hidden is presented. For cogent reasons I value this advantage of clothing very highly. I also view with a glad heart when the unfeeling and wanton old bachelor, who thought to leave nature and found loathing in its venal enticement, is suddenly drawn back to a healthier feeling and a happier relationship by a treacherously half-hidden virginal bosom.

It is desirable that these effects of clothing should not be accompanied by others whose consequences destroy our healthy build, the beauty of our figures, and our ability to carry out continuous and often unavoidable motions. But, unfortunately, . . . the tyrannical guild of French ladies' outfitters and tailors has decided that we Germans have to lose our health and all the advantages of our manly limbs in their tight fetters! Just view with me for a moment the constraint of today's clothing; observe how all parts of our body are confined and deprived of the ability of any free movement from our head to our toes.

Either we bind our hair tightly together on the head or we strap all the veins in our heads tightly under a coif. Our neck is encircled by a miserable string which can have been invented only by a surgeon who wanted to tie the jugular veins awkwardly and then open them. Our shirts confine our necks and forearms, a tight doublet armours our trunk, a pair of trousers encompasses our groins, straps encircle our knees, and we force our feet into shoes which, in addition to any feeling, choke off almost all movements!

* * *

From all this, the physical influence of every type of clothing on our health can be easily explained. As soon as man made clothing more than a mere means against bareness and inclement weather, dressing became a business which mostly hindered frequent cleansing of the skin. In the past, every country kept for long periods its clothing which was suited to the climate there. But since the French have become unrestricted rulers over the clothing of all European nations, at least of all educated persons, we see the cold north in silken robes almost approaching their original nakedness; and as ever since our young days we have protected ourselves, as if we were foreigners, against our country's air, and have assumed in the center of Germany the daintiness of an African skin, when we suddenly expose our bodies, when the calendar so orders, to the influence of all the changes of the fairly harsh weather inherent in our climate, we contract a thousand illnesses by our ridiculous caprice of trying to enforce summer by wearing light clothing.

Such effects of clothing certainly deserve the consideration of the police, who so far always dealt only with the mere moderation of pernicious expenditure in clothing, without considering the most important aspect of the entire matter, namely the influence of different kinds of clothing on the health of the citizens worthy of their attention. The ancient Romans allotted their special clothing not only to each sex, but also to each class and each age, and the censors carefully supervised the preservation of this custom. In our country, everybody wears whatever he pleases, and when a senseless fashion shapes our youth to cripples, makes our pregnant women miscarry in droves, and makes consumptive creatures of our daughters, the laws observe deep silence. It is not superfluous, therefore, in a work dealing with Medical Police, to show how wrong such quiescence is.

* * *

§5

Of the detriment of too many hairdressers

It may be all the same to the state whether we wear our hair straight or curled, and as long as inventions of the hairdressers do not cause any worse misfortune than the destruction of the natural proportion between head and trunk, our beauties may look out if they think we have a taste for the unnatural. But it seems to me that it is an entirely different question whether the police may remain indifferent when the number of wigmakers increases so rapidly and, therefore, a large number of well-built and healthy young men are dusted into consumptives within a short time and under the worst morals. I am of the opinion that this unimportant handicraft which rarely leaves its man healthy for long, should be entrusted only to such young persons whose faulty body does not admit of any nobler destination in the community. Twenty thousand wigmakers in a large state of whom two thirds of our healthy young men are transformed in less than twelve years into emaciated, panting creatures who barely live to their thirtieth year, either through the large amount of flour dust they inhale, or through the irregular way of life intrinsic to this company. This deserves the supervision by a philanthropic regent who knows how better to employ so many well-built young men for the sake of their health and who should not let the most beautiful youth devote themselves to this unhealthy craft, only because of its unrestrained way of life. This remark does not relate directly to clothing, but it was impossible to miss this opportunity to touch upon a matter that, in my opinion, is not unimportant when head adornment is being discussed.

I do not say that the police should prescribe laws because of the curling of hair; and although Schmucker remarked that since the ladies have been using so many hairpins for their head adornment, and the hair has been molested with so much pomade and powder, sebaceous cysts and lipomas are much more widespread than in the past; . . . and although, finally, our women must be more prone to head trouble since the habit has grown of carrying a thick forest of strange hair, or even a cushion, on the head, whereby the head is kept too warm because the juices are conducted to it more, and at night, when the burden is taken off, catching cold is almost unavoidable. Nevertheless, I believe that one cannot deprive the becurled public of the joy of being tortured by wigmakers, because of a seemingly petty cause without much fuss about the infringement of public freedom; although in our days a wise king forbade his subjects on pain of one hundred thalers' fine to let themselves be used by anybody for the curling of hair or dressing of wigs.*

* * *

§6

Of make-up

A much more dubious soiling of the skin is the make-up of the face and of other

* Adolph Friedrich, King of Sweden, in the cited decree of 26 June 1766, art. XII.

parts exposed to view, which is so beloved by our beauties. The wish to please is so natural to this sex that there is no wild nation whose women in particular do not paint their faces with special paints, and the whole difference consists only in different notions of beauty.

* * *

If making up among us would have remained the business of the women whose facial features were such that they were entitled to complain about nature, this endeavor to replace by art what nature withheld would be excusable. But that a beautiful face is deliberately painted over and thus, ungrateful to the Creator, denies all taste of nature and true beauty, that is really punishable and indicates either little reason or slavery to fashion.

Experience has long justified the voice of physicians who described the painting of the face, the chest, and also of the forearm, i.e., a considerable part of the female body, as very unhealthy. For the exhalatory vessels are clogged by such a covering, and as the paints usually consist of vermilion and various white leads, it is only natural that the unnaturally shrunk skin begins to wrinkle, the retained exhalations assume sharpness, and various stimuli act on the nerves of the head and especially of the eyes; and mercury, which is hidden in the vermilion, causes glands in the skin, and especially in the eyelashes, an unnatural influx and distention of the excretory canals, their inflammation, and subsequently, dripping eyes.

The police not only have to supervise public health but also have to stop all senseless customs and excesses of good taste, especially when such customs mutilate nature and destroy prematurely that adornment of creation, the agreeable facial features of useful women citizens. This is so, because, in the long run, the unhealthy customs only suppress the affection of the two sexes for each other which nature, by the excellence of female beauty, wanted to ensure; women thirty years old go about looking like grandmothers and are soon loathsome to their husbands. The police, I say, must put a stop to the excessively increased use of make-up for these important reasons, the use having penetrated even to the middle class. A pale face may by a slight tinge with harmless paint sometimes help nature, when a husband approves of this endeavor by his wife to please him, but that our maidens are covered with lacquer like carriages, and out of sheer caprice, brush away their health and natural good looks every day, against this a prohibition would be to the honor of the authorities' just mentality.

* * *

§9

Of corsets

In regard to corsets I have elsewhere remarked much concerning the female sex, and therefore I have little to add. The thoracic cavity was not created by the Creator to the taste of us Europeans: as is known, it is similar to a truncated cone the base of which is formed by the diaphragm, the sides and front by the false ribs and the tip of the breastbone. Its obtuse end impinges on the neck, but close to its adjacent parts, such as the shoulder bones, and the arm and chest muscles. Especially in females it obtains a seemingly larger volume by the two breasts. A skeleton, freed of all these parts, proves clearly that the thoracic cavity is wider on the bottom than on the top, and as is known, in living persons, breathing in is effected also by moving the lower, more mobile ribs upward and outward, and by the descent of the diaphragm, whereby the thoracic cavity provides a larger space for the distended lungs inhaling air. There the Creator should have . . . I stop in order not to blaspheme, but such is the language of those who defend corsets or extend their utility to the beautification of our waists. Approximately and equally clever, is the reasoning of the coal black Byaos on the Island of Borneo: they have almost all their front teeth pulled out and gold teeth put in their place. The first corset was certainly a surgical invention and only intended to make a hunchbacked creature straight again. Because of its success, it was eventually believed that no child could grow straight any more without a corset, although there was the example of a thousand nations in the whole of Asia, in Africa and America, who are not so silly to let themselves be confined so tightly, and yet excel by their beautiful bodies. The pressure of a stiff corset is strongest at the lower part of the thoracic cavity and around the stomach region; thus, it acts exactly against nature's intentions which wants them to be able to carry out alternating free movement. But since the upper part of the chest is also firmly incarcerated, one sees children confined in corsets, who keep one shoulder always higher than the other in order to provide some relief for themselves, and this unnatural formation often is then assumed by nature. The lungs, prevented from completely distending, resist for long the blood that is sent to them by the heart; eventually, upon but slight heating of the juices, they lose their equilibrium, and the consequence is spitting of blood and a consumptive state which usually costs the most beautiful maidens their lives. The ribs themselves, and the spine, which in no human being is in a completely straight vertical line, as a corset always attempts to keep them, often assume an unnatural sinuosity, and this cripples people instead of protecting them from such a state. The entrails of the lower body, under constant pressure from the ribs, also assume an unnatural shape, and this in turn, has a powerful influence on the other parts of the body.

* * *

There is no doubt that absurd corsets are to blame for the fact that among affluent women there are few who have full breasts. In some regions, the degeneration seems to become so general that the upper body of most beauties cannot serve any more for distinguishing the sexes. I, for one, consider this shortcoming more important than it would at first appear. The greatest damage consists, of course, in the fact that because of this many young mothers cannot nurse their children. For although a fat breast need not necessarily be the richest in milk, it is obvious that no great abundance can be expected from too meager a source. This important part of the female charm, with the kind permission of the moralists, has been formed on purpose so beautifully by nature and deliberately placed where it cannot escape the male eye and cannot easily fail in its effect on him. But I wish it would not be so neglected in the physical education of girls, and thus gradually deprive the fair sex of an important part of their natural claim to our external senses, for they always have a say in the mutual relation of the sexes and in the consequences of the mutual attraction. But nothing is as decisive for the female appearance as the shape of this spongy body.

* * *

In the subsequent paragraphs, Frank deals with other excesses of female fashion, with military uniforms, and with an instruction for merchants dealing in second-hand clothes.

PART THREE
Section Three

Of popular amusements

§1

An entire nation, like an individual person, can be viewed from the point of view of its actions; and just as the physicians in the past said, according to their hypothesis, that man was governed by one of the four temperaments, we see this in nations even more pronounced and on a large scale, regardless of all the previous mixing of the most varied races: in the Spaniard, earnestness and cruelty, and love of bloody animal fights;—the Englishman, self-sufficiency and disdain for other nations, and philosophical pensiveness;—the Frenchman, hopping about and engaged in witty pleasures;—the Italian, vindictiveness, distrust and slyness, using other people's weakness and assurance;—the Dutch, cold-blooded, calm, calculating of future profits;—and the German, now more than ever without his own definite character, imitating all other nations in his way of life and enjoyments. For all wishes and acts of such varied nations are determined by their original predisposition to climate, laws, and education in such a way that any deviation of individual natures cannot disturb the national temperament or obliterate its inclinations and characteristic features.

§2

Accurate knowledge of a nation's natural bent prepares the way for a philosophical regent to direct the large body, and the history of the human heart helps him draw up the important plan by which the nation's passions must serve as the primary mainspring of its most decisive moves. No nation is so faulty in quality that, given the right direction, it cannot achieve great things. There is no passion, in either individual person or the large mass of people, which cannot be subdued by another passion that is still sleeping but can easily be awakened, and the same nation which jokes light-heartedly with a serious face, lets itself be made to think, and even to cry, and be given direction, from the stage, and often through the mouth of an actress. Certain events, special occurrences, improved instruction can change a nation beyond recognition even within one life-span (of course, always maintaining their original predisposition), which is not really surprising, for of all persons living simultaneously in every state, about one half are female and unsteady, two thirds of all persons are children and easily won, and only one third of all have taken by habit the direction toward good or bad which is difficult to change.

§3

The persons in authority in the state therefore must treat the nation according to its natural tendency: counter passions with passion, and like the pedagogue, playfully set right the large crowd of children. A melancholy and sullen nation, like the individual melancholic, borders on desperation or insurrection without special cause; and the national spleen has the same sad consequences at certain times and on a large scale as the determined suicide's weariness of life. At certain times idleness, monotony of life, domestic troubles, weather, a thousand causes weigh as insufferably on mortals on a large scale as they do on mortals individually so that a regent who does not devise a means against that most natural and general illness of every nation, namely boredom, and in an idle hour does not make the nation forget itself and its really bad or imagined fate (for on the whole this amounts to the same) by beautiful games, and beautiful shadow games on the wall, shows a serious lack of care for the public health. At first, the Roman emperors knew this art perfectly, and they must be commended, with a view to the character of their nation, for the choice of the games they gave their people. If someone makes me forget my adverse fate for half my days, I am only half as unhappy as I would be without that. My health suffers much less under the burden of the hardship, and I am once again much more able to attend to various activities when I have found something that absorbs my pain. Without poppy-juice I would not want to be a physician, even though this palliative does not often remedy the cause but only the effect, and although, when applied at the wrong time, it sometimes even makes the illness worse!... In the hands of the experienced man who weighs every fact, it will be the greatest remedy that nature provided for mortals in their distress. Joy and pleasure, as well as sleep, flee from the unfortunate, but a deceptive slumber lasting only a few hours pours balm on his wounds; at last, he forgets his state and gradually gets well.

§4

It is said that distraction makes people thoughtless, opportunity intemperate, intemperance sick.—Thus a father who is worried about his only son may speak out, but the regent who has to make an innumerable family happy, does not make his entire nation sleep in the open because only one careless boy fell from the third floor of a house and broke his neck. He knows that even the most diligent of his subjects must sometimes relax, that constant tension of the bow causes the string to break, and that premature exhaustion is the lot of overzealous workers. Therefore, he orders popular amusements to be held, and allots each of them its limits and purpose; he lets every class partake in them, and watches over their security and well-being. And he fears the vices committed in the dark more than the weaknesses which originate only indirectly from public amusements and which, because the occasional cause is known, are more amenable to quick help. In France all garrison officers are obliged to subscribe to the theater stage, and Caesar and Brutus are performed for the common man. The cause can be easily guessed; with a cheerful and wide-awake nation, and with a class that cannot be subjected to any monastic order, the object is not that no mischief at all occurs, but that abominations and unnatural crimes be prevented through less questionable pastimes.

§5

Arrangement of popular amusements must take morality and health into account. An entire nation always moves like an uncontrolled flood, and if a dangerous overflow is to be prevented, every movement must be studied; all causes increasing the danger must be foreseen and checked by a strong dam. Enjoyed without moderation, all great pleasures are poison for the health, and the highest bliss cannot be increased another degree without being called pain.

In my opinion, it is best if the state itself looks after the citizens' amusement, and caters at common expense for larger, popular amusements and pastimes. If this cannot be done everywhere, the police is at least the natural authority and Maître des Plaisirs of the large crowd. In several states the police, against certain payment, makes the funeral arrangements for every dead citizen, thereby stopping all squandering on these occasions. A whole company of soldiers eats together and thus eats incomparably better than the low pay of each would permit separately. Equally, public amusements could be enjoyed with considerable savings if care were taken that not every citizen in towns has to devise a plan of his pastimes himself and pay for it all by himself. I would be straying here if I were not certain that such arrangements are the surest means of preventing wild instincts from causing people to attain their own pleasure at the great expense of society and of health, and that the police alone could thus take a stand appropriate to the importance of the matter and diminish suitably the excesses occurring during public amusements.

§6

The amusements to which people are still receptive for their recreation after tiring work delight either the mind only, or also put the body into moderate motion. In the former, the police must endeavor by every available means to prevent excessive pampering; let us thank science that has mellowed the coarseness and wildness of our behavior, and enabled our soul to seek truth with fine feeling, and to be touched by the beautiful in nature! But when visionary heads abuse them, and lead our esthetes to a langorous "Wertherish" tone which has the tendency to stretch even more the highly strung fibers of our female listeners, of both generations, then I lament from the bottom of my heart the fate of our posterity which, born of such weepy parents, must be composed entirely of woes, alas.

* * *

§7

Necessity of theater plays in large cities

Among the most agreeable pastimes for the mind in a large city are theater plays and music. In order that the people may be kept occupied during the long winter evenings, there is no better pastime than theater plays, if only the police observes that which has to be observed with a view to the moral effect of the plays. I do not want to argue at length whether or not morals are compatible with the stage. The matter has been decided in favor of the stage, once the police knows the power of such plays over the human heart and has banned all impertinence from the theater. But little has been done as yet for the public health in the theaters.

* * *

§11

Influence of [stage] performances on our body

As regards the themes which are dealt with on the stage, I want to draw attention to something. On the one hand, it is natural that predominance is given to the performance of such plays as are written according to the public's taste and may expect greater applause than any others. The formation of the taste which a nation gradually gets for some kind of theater play or other, however, depends to a great extent on that which is performed without the nation's being prompted by the actors' company. He who knows the powerful influence of the stage on the human heart must admit that an important part of city education depends on the frequent performance of certain actions under this or that color, i.e., on the taste of some play or other. This is all the more so because youth, which is still amenable to modification, constitutes the largest part of the audience. Thus a good actors' troupe makes a city laugh or cry at will, and the point is, which of the two now happens more frequently, so that the public assumes the mood which was given it on such an occasion.

I do not know what has been gained by too refined a taste having gradually dislodged from the stage almost everything that is lively, and by entertaining the public with so many tragedies, so much murder and death. In the past, in the times of a Molière, the stage endeavored to convulse the diaphragm of the spectator (who in the world at large, and even at home was sufficiently provided with sad performances) as often as possible and to feed the spirit of pleasure which is so necessary a feature of the people! I do not fail to appreciate what is noble and majestic in a tragedy, but the feelings which it arouses in the spectator's mind should not become commonplace feelings, and their repetition should not influence our minds so that they produce a particular predisposition to sadness and dark feelings. It is very flattering for the author of a tragedy when a tear rolls down from the eye of a sensitive beauty, or even down the earnest cheek of an amazed man, but what a difference is the effect on our entire state of mind afterwards depending on whether the tear had been due to crying or to hearty laughter! ... When three times a week I hear in all corners of the auditorium nothing but general sobbing, and the spectators walk home, quiet and dazed, with red eyes as if sand had been thrown into them, as a friend of poetry, I commend the skill of the author and the ability of the actor to affect the heart of their listeners; but, as physician, I curse the effect of their excessively active art. Like thunder-clouds which only rarely cover the entire sky and bring into healthy motion the air that had been robbed of its elasticity by too long a rest and the sun's constant smiling, this art should stir the human heart only at certain times. Instead it does not cease assaulting it, and soon it has conquered all power of imagination in order to soften the heart of the audience and set all nerves into poetic motion. In England it has long been the fashion that the author had at the end of every tragedy at least five or six persons murdered on the stage. That reflective nation liked these sadly cruel performances, and without noticing it, its predisposition to melancholy and dark grave-yard thoughts increased. In France, suicide has never been so much in evidence as now that every week on a public stage either a tenderly loving deserted beauty thrusts a dagger into her own breast or an unhappy hero ends his life in order not to suffer any longer. Sadness gradually settles on this land since there is no end to the whimpering on all stages, and thus that constantly singing, vivacious nation has its jewel and most beautiful property, namely joy, squeezed out of its heart by its actors. Although we Germans have a lesser propensity for laughing, we still laugh at our clown whom our neighbors chased from their stages many years ago. We were certainly wrong to tolerate the ill-mannered buffoon for so long against all the rules of good taste; nevertheless, laughter should not have been banished from the stage with it! In a large theater among a thousand persons seeking distraction, there are barely fifty who do not need very badly this life-giving balm, this cheering up, and borrowed joyfulness.

* * *

§12

The police, therefore, should give as much attention as possible to the taste of the pieces to be performed and to the contents of each new play, also as regards the physical aspect of so many spectators being present. The moral feeling of a nation has a great influence on the public health, and every great deterioration in it cannot but cause the machine to run too slowly or too fast. The theologians quarreled among themselves about the admissibility of the theater stage; a physician could remark much on that subject, no matter which decision was taken. I, at least, believe as follows: if the theater does not give us what we seek after tiring work and what we need most, namely a healthy diversion and invigorating strengthening of mind and body, then nothing can compensate us for the loss of time with such dallying, and for its influence on patriotic customs and mentality which cannot always be prevented, even with the strictest supervision. After sad plays, the actors always give the public a sop that is intended to make them immediately forget the violent emotion, for immediately after them, they serve something that makes them laugh. This procedure proves that the art of acting has not gone so far as to represent a final purpose, and the thoughtlessness of the respectable public cannot be mocked more than by promising publicly, as is done on the placards, that the whole crowd will be made to laugh and cry in one breath. If the moral that must be contained in every play is to make an impression on our minds, the minds should not be leveled immediately afterward, and if the good that could be done by so many tearful plays is not appreciated by the people returning home, endeavors should be made to put the fault right.

§13

I do not want to indulge here in a eulogy of the power of music over our hearts, but it certainly constitutes a substantial part of the balm which has been provided by Providence to the human race against illnesses of the soul. Physicians have recorded in their diaries several cases of illnesses which were healed by the magic of music, and its effect on sensitive nerves is so obvious that the circulation and exhalation, which had been put into disorder and been impeded by the convulsive state of the solid parts, were put in order by it within a short time, much to the body's relief. But the power of awakening passions, with which the remotest age has credited music, must make us use this divine means with discernment. Orpheus of the ancients, who was far from being a "Lolli" or a "Raf," is supposed to have defeated the underworld by euphonious singing, and David conquered his king's fury with his lyre. All nations mix singing into their divine services; the Catholic church raises the devotion of its believers by solemn music; and as a residue of this sacred habit, a touching morning song, accompanied by sacred trumpets, penetrates the hearts of the inhabitants of Protestant towns in Swabia and various other countries. Our forebears handed down to posterity the story of the heroic deeds of the German nation in songs, and in songs they were also able to lampoon effectively the faults of the great.*

The police, therefore, must see to it that this great means of encouragement and popular amusement is not lacking in large cities. It must provide in large cities good musicians who satisfy the ear of the listeners, and who drive out the devil of sadness in a sad hour, and, moreover, who are able to provide sound instruction in this

* Schmidt, "History of the Germans," Volume II.

art for the lovers of music, thus filling in many a gap of human life to the advantage of public health. But just as excessive effeminateness in composition and sensuality in songs must be avoided in order that no untimely and detrimental passions are aroused in the community, it cannot be permitted with equanimity that weak-chested young men learn to play difficult wind instruments to their detriment.*

* * *

* "Medical Police," Volume II.

PART FOUR

Of human dwellings in general, and of their management

§1

If the healthy situation of a place were the only criterion decisive for the settlement of a human society in some region or other, the physician—who would use all his experience of climate and the confluence of unfavorable physical causes of exhausted nations, as well as the principles of a rational knowledge of air, water, and soul— could stipulate many beneficial rules according to which people should act in founding new towns and establishing new colonies. However, it is known that things are not like that, and that necessity or lack of a better choice, provision of food, commerce, and many other causes have contributed to the laying of the first stone in the oldest towns, and presumably will always do so, no matter what objections a physician may raise. Moreover, in Europe most places that are in the least usable are occupied, and human abodes have already been given such a layout that a great, or at least complete change or improvement is out of the question.

* * *

§2

Even though the position of a place cannot be easily improved, however, much good may be expected within a relatively short time regarding the construction of human abodes. Towns which even 25 years ago showed the most outdated taste, are now beginning to become lighter, and good progress in all sciences extends its influence into every corner of the private house, unless old rights and prejudices larger than the buildings to be erected stand in the way.

* * *

§4

It follows as a matter of course that in this case it is not irrelevant how people live in different regions. I shall have opportunities of showing more in the following sections, but many predispositions can be greatly improved by human intervention, and just as the physician at the sickbed struggles against individual diseases, the political physician must seek out endemic ills at their source and dry them up. Many regions, previously almost uninhabitable because of innumerable ills, now compete with the healthiest regions, and Germany itself was once in its entirety a puddle if compared with the cultivated and healthy country it is today.

* * *

PART FOUR
Section One

On the best layout of human habitations

§1

The nature of the soil on which people come to live is determined by the nature of the water, and mostly by that of the air. These two are the great solvents of almost all natural bodies, and what they accept from them and retain changes their character so much that it often seems that we have to deal with a completely different thing, without any change being apparent in the exterior aspect. Adolphi, therefore, says that the healthiness of air is a very dark matter, and that it must be tested not by theories but with the aid of experiences, such that a region which because of its position seems to be the healthiest, is often unhealthy, and conversely, a seemingly badly situated place is the healthiest.* Therefore the judgment of physicians concerning the position of a town and its physical influence on the public health often completely contradicts the observations obtained from the lists of births and deaths in regard to this place, no matter how much arguing there is about each little village and even about the position of individual houses.

* * *

Frank then deals thoroughly with the advantages and disadvantages of dwellings on mountains and in valleys, and when discussing dwellings situated in swampy regions, he deals in §10 with the corruption of the air, and in §12 with the danger emanating from stagnant waters.

Pollution of the air is due mainly to the combustible substances which flow out of spoilt waters; moreover, the rotten volatile character of exhaling bodies endows it with an irritating and caustic property detrimental to our lungs. It is known that swampy soils are a mixture of constantly rotting plants, insects, etc., producing both the combustible and this volatile alkaline substance in abundance and mixing it with the atmospheric air.

---

* "De Aere, aquis & locis, *Lipsiensibus*," para. 2., pp. 5, 6, 7.

These exhalations of swampy regions, therefore, are rightly given a special name; they are called bog air.

* * *

Therefore, it is not surprising that on hot, calm days, with increasing rotting of the bog, its increased exhalations fill the atmosphere over a large distance with combustible and rotting effluents, so much so that the air thereby is made less suitable for breathing, or for many persons becomes quite unusable (not to mention what damage must be caused to our bodies by the inhalation of such deleterious vapors).

* * *

§12

Disadvantages of slow or still waters

The disadvantage of slow rivers, creeks, stagnant lakes, ponds, etc., is now easily explainable, nor was it a secret to the ancients, either. Seneca says of the Maeander:

> —Super aequales
> Labitur agros piger & steriles
> Amne maligno radit arenas.*

And this may be said of most waters which flow almost imperceptibly, never properly flush out their bed, and are overgrown by many reeds the roots of which, like a screen, retain all impurities, serve millions of insects for an abode, and rot with them while emitting an unbearable stench. How much do fortified towns suffer with their stagnant, mostly still waters, half filling their many moats in hot seasons, and how unhealthy are the houses adjacent to them! In the canals which dissect Amsterdam in many places, the water is mostly stagnant, and since the wastes of the entire city collect in them, the water rots, is covered with a green film, and emits such a horrible and unbearable stench as soon as the days become warm, that a foreigner cannot walk in the street for more than a quarter of an hour without having an unbearable headache and pains in the eyes. It stinks as much as in our country in the fall in places where rotted flax has been taken out of the water and put up to dry.—On the other hand, Amsterdam, too, is a very unhealthy place, and the air in all seasons is filled with watery and pungent vapors to such an extent that metals are rapidly corroded by rust; silver, no matter how well hidden, immediately becomes black; and the clothes in cupboards and closets mold and rot. Dropsy, cold fever, and greensickness are at home there.** Thus such creeks and moats can always be considered liquid bogs, and their effect also differs little from the effects of swampy soil.†

* * *

---

 * L. Annaei Senec. "Phaedra."
** "Observations by a Traveler through Germany, France, England and Holland," Part III, p. 365.
 † Adolphi, "De salubritate Silesiae," §XII.

§15

The necessity of drying out swamps

Drying out excessively moist and swampy soils, therefore, is always a very important matter for the police, and in various countries, land prizes have been given for each drained stretch. On 14 June 1764, the King of France decreed that all really swampy regions that were drained by their owner would be freed of all tax duties, even the tithe, for twenty years. Moreover, the authorities were empowered by the king to give special rewards for the reclamation of swampy regions. As late as 1776, the Senate of Venice granted an honorable patent of nobility to the head of the military academy at Verona, Colonel Lorgne, who had most successfully been in charge of the great task of draining the old town of Adria and its surroundings. It is known what sums the present Pope, Pius VI, expended on the draining of the Pontine Marshes. And everywhere, by draining barren swamps, the emerging spirit of better agriculture has begun improving the healthiness of human abodes.

Increase in the number of fortified towns has always been detrimental to public health in some respects. Therefore, let us express our thanks to Joseph II, the German Emperor who, to the real benefit of his happy people, had all expendable fortifications of his great states converted into peaceable dwellings, the swampy and rotting moats filled in by razing the walls and ramparts that hindered the influx of healthy air, and thus provided freedom for the incarcerated citizens, and, so to speak, let beneficial grain grow from the graves!

* * *

§17

Application of the previous considerations

Among all the regions which people may choose, or have already chosen, for their future dwelling, the swampy places of the earth that are always loaded with humid air are the most dangerous. Many other dwelling places are also detrimental to the health or security of the citizens, however, §§4, 5, 6, and it is the duty of the state police to give their main attention to them when new towns or human dwellings are founded, and as far as circumstances permit, always use the best situation for them. From what has been said so far, it is clear that a prudent choice is necessary, and that some regions are preferable to others, and it will also become apparent that the art of economy, which directs us to cultivate diligently even the smallest still unused area, also promotes public health, for cultivation always makes a region healthier. America now is no longer an unhealthy country since the diligence of its inhabitants caused the moist earth to be dug up, the extensive swamps to be dissected by drainage channels, the flowing of the rivers to be expedited, the thick forests, which always maintained dank air and resisted the passage of healthy winds, to be thinned out.*

* "Recherches philosoph. sur les Améric." T. I, p. 52.

It depends on us that, according to sensible principles, our new dwellings are laid out or, in the case of those already built, such measures are taken that the well-being of the citizens will be better served. Of course, even with all the detrimental properties of the air, people in all parts of the world are healthier than might be supposed. This is so because we gradually get used to any weather and any climate, especially when we were born to it. Yet, says Zimmermann, it has been often found that there are certain well observed causes why there are places in which an illness is more frequent than another one, why there are seasons of the year in which otherwise dangerous illnesses are mild, or otherwise mild illnesses are highly dangerous.* These causes must be reported to the state police by all their subordinate districts, from which it becomes clear why correct topographies, supplied by art experts, and those collected by Hautesterk and the Royal Society of Physicians in Paris, are such an extremely important contribution for those who have to look after the health and well-being of a country. Every publicly employed physician or district physician should supply the medical description of his region as accurately as possible, and compare every change in weather, every phenomenon concerning the healthiness of a place, with his site so that the science of the influence of human dwellings and the climate of each country becomes better known. By inducing the physicians in all places in Baden and the Palatinate to carry out accurate observations of all natural phenomena in their respective districts, the promotion of weather science in the County of Baden and in the countries of the Palatinate must have an excellent influence on the healthiest arrangement and layout of human abodes in time, and by such philanthropic endeavors, one will gain eternal merit among our posterity.

However, it does not suffice that the foundation of a town is suitable for receiving a human society. It may be converted into a very unhealthy place by wrong construction of the dwellings themselves and by some carelessness of individual citizens. In the following section, therefore, I have to give some rules which are worthy of the attention of persons in authority.

* Zimmermann, "On the Experience," Vol. II.

PART FOUR
Section Two

Of healthy construction of human dwellings

§1

Every animal in its early youth chooses its cave in which it seeks quiet and security from stormy weather and foreign attacks. Nature gave each of them its own niche, following which its future dwelling will be built, and the simple building always corresponds perfectly to the intention of its builder. Comfort for itself and its small family, security and cleanliness are the main features of all animal dwellings because no passions become mixed with the mortar there. It was left only to the inventive human being to improve the natural construction of his dwelling, to make a palace out of a hut, and to make a small world, i.e., towns of several hundred thousand inhabitants out of a small number of congregating family members. Now, protected by thick walls and sitting behind the stove, we defy the stormy north winds, but we stiffen and feel the consequences in all parts of our bodies when we are forced to leave the warm place for an instant. We are now certain that the flimsy hut will not collapse at the slightest opportunity and bruise us until we are black and blue, but a blunder in an ell, a slight earth tremor, brings the proud edifice down upon our numerous family and turns it into our grave. Now we have a place of refuge from the deadly spear and the murderous club of our hostile neighbor, but his thunder turns our dwellings into a heap of rubble, blows up the remainder, and finally gives up only when in possession of the churchyard;—thus we could rattle on of the consequences of luxury in dwellings which increasingly gives proof amounting to the greatest certainty that increased mortality in towns is found everywhere, and the greater the ratio of its towns to the country, the higher the expenditure on building construction rises, where every inhabitant is so much concerned that his neighbor does not cut off by building or poison the little air that he needs for breathing, so is that country all the more unhealthy.

People, therefore, will be all the more amenable to listening to the thoughts of a physician concerning a healthier way of building, since we have now advanced too far to return to the forests again, and since we really can no longer do without the many comforts which our larger dwellings afford us. Only a prudent way of building can protect us against the worst consequences of living together in large numbers.

* * *

§12

The large number of persons who have been moving from the country to towns since increased luxury, arts and sciences, comforts, etc., have made towns their seat, causes a shortage of space there which people believe must be relieved by making the houses higher, five or six stories high, and thereby building in effect several towns above each other. This general mania to make half a town dwell under one roof found the approval of the more affluent class all the more quickly because this class thereby attained what it had long wished for, namely, that they become masters of that part of the atmosphere, its share which nature gave every creature. Then, this class was able to force destitute citizens either to rot away in the depths or, while still alive, to pay a certain rent. One can usually recognize from the laws by whom they were made, and particularly so in regard to high buildings of which a Saxon legislator said: Everybody may build on his ground as high as he wishes and does, even if it is to the detriment of others.* Thus every street is turned into a vault in whose depths one almost needs a light at noon;** the exhalations collect and create a stinking aerial bath which cannot be put in motion by any wind, and like the uncleanest pond deposits its sludge in the lowest basin. If our fate were as hard as that of the fishes, and if like them we had to serve as food for an even more cruel species of animals than we are, the inhabitants of such bog air, because of their muddy taste, would be valued as lowly as we value fish which are brought to our table from oozy ponds. Since the streets are in no relation whatsoever to the height of such piled up buildings, no beneficial rays of the cleansing sun ever penetrate through the unhealthy fog, and thus the lungs inhale the constant loathsome atmosphere of the horrible reservoir. If one considers the effect of so many excretions of thousands of people and animals, the loathsome exhalations of various remains of used or spoilt foodstuffs, the smell of death from full churchyards, the offensive vapor which rises into the atmosphere every hour from the workshops of so many tanners, factories, soap boilers, dyers, chemists, and from various infirmaries and hospitals, etc., one can easily see the disadvantage of building construction in such a manner which, by cutting off access to all favorable winds, demeans a large city to a level below the unhealthiest bog, and in case of an epidemic, at least promotes contagion in the most incredible way.

* * *

* Sachsenspiegel, Volume II, Art. XLIX, p. CCLXX.
** Les maisons d'une hauteur démesurée sont cause, que les habitants (de Paris) du rez-de-chaussée & du premier étage sont encore dans une espèce d'obscurité, lorsque le Soleil est au plus haut point de son élévation. "Tableau de Paris," Tome I, p. 38.

PART FOUR
Section Three

Of public cleansing institutions and other habitations in towns

§1

Of the influence of cleanliness on the well-being of the state

In dealing with this important subject of Medical Police, I must refer to all that I have said elsewhere about necessary cleanliness of the air, of the various degrees of its spoilage, of the malignant exhalations of bogs, of stagnant waters, of large towns, etc., so that now I can lecture on pertinent matters, without digressions and without having to convince the public that strict supervision in this part of public health care is necessary.

What but an unclean person is in the eyes of well educated persons, the same, and even more so, is an unclean nation when judged by a civilized nation. Although now and again a prejudice penetrates into the ideas which we have of the cleanliness or uncleanliness of a thing, and although the history of so many incredibly dirty yet healthy nations, the Hottentots, the Greenlanders and others somewhat softens the judgement of a nation's uncleanliness, nevertheless, it is certain that even though an individual person may wallow in mud and slime without detriment because he has been hardened by habit and a completely animal-like way of life, a sociable nation cannot continue with such individuals without the well-being and health of the whole having to suffer enormously, especially in times of epidemics.

It suffices to see how the terrible plague originates mostly in eastern countries, and how terribly quickly it spreads among the unclean Turkish and Greek nations! How on large ships, which after all change their atmosphere every instant, uncleanliness promotes scurvy and malignant putrid fever, how in hospitals and camps the slightest illnesses often deteriorate into the gravest diseases and end in death! . . . On the other hand, look at the Dutch nation, living in the midst of a formerly inaccessible swamp; yet, it is tolerably healthy in the eternal fog only because their cleanliness (of course, pushed to the extreme but appropriate to the unfortunate situation of their low dwelling place) exceeds that of all known nations so much that, as Lord Chesterfield said, the streets in Holland are cleaner than the houses in London.* And because this commercial nation clearly knows the power of human diligence against the influence of an unhealthy region! Just look how the solid Cook sailed around the earth several times with so small a loss in human lives only because he enforced punctiliously the strict cleanliness of his ships and his people!

I may assume here that no more detailed proof will be required of me to substantiate the sentence: that uncleanliness is one of the foremost causes of most diseases of people; and that these largely could be healed better by police measures than by physicians, or at least prevented. Thus, I shall not even ask my philanthropic readers for their attention in regard to the following remarks.

§2

But there is such a number of public cleansing institutions that their investigation may easily lead to confusion. Now if I consider the pertinent subjects in the order in which the lectures on institutions of public cleanliness are arranged, with a view to the requirements of the country, the human dwelling, and finally, the citizens themselves and their handicrafts, nothing of importance should be excluded from such a classification. As regards institutions for the country's cleanliness, they comprehend the unhealthy treatment of the soil, the concern for cleansing the atmosphere by utilizing healthy winds, draining swamps and ponds, preventing frequent floods, and consequently also conducting water in secure beds and promoting its flow. However, as far as could be expected of me, I dealt with most of these points in the previous parts. Therefore, I have to report here predominantly on cleanliness in towns and other human societies. For the towns contain in concentration on a moderately large area all the causes of uncleanliness which are only very dispersed in the country. These causes, therefore, deserve the preferential attention of the police authorities. Here we have to consider the essential cleanliness of the town's exterior, of its streets, of its public and private buildings, etc. Among these, the influence of unclean crafts on the health of the inhabitants, and their own cleanliness, naturally offer themselves for consideration, but even these subjects must be treated partly in other articles because of the context and the order of arrangement chosen.

§3

Cleanliness of rivers

The oldest nations recognized the necessity and the great benefit of large rivers or other rapidly flowing waters next to human dwellings, and Oribasius said, rightly, that on the whole, all towns lying near streams had moderate air.** It is known that the air near any rapidly flowing water is constantly more in motion, and consequently less stagnant than elsewhere. The exhalation of clean water improves the foul and

---

* Letters to his son, Vol. I, p. 12.
** "Collectan.," 5. Chap. 3.—Hebenstreit, "Anthropologia forens." sec. I. Cap. II, p. 54.

dirty warm air, and foaming, rolling water exhales incomparably more and cleaner particles than any other. A river flowing past human dwellings flushes the collected impurities away every day, and even nearby swamps become less harmful through the drift which their waters obtain from the more rapid river.

* * *

Thus one can realize how necessary it is to use all flowing waters for cleansing human dwellings, and how contrary it would be to common sense if it were permitted to throw all kinds of impurities into the rivers, whereby their flow would be impeded and the waters polluted.

§4

I have spoken elsewhere of the maceration of hemp and flax, and its unhealthy effect on drinking water, and it deserves double punishment because it pollutes the less rapid and quieter creeks, and especially stagnant waters, as well as polluting the entire region with abominable exhalations. Ramazzini ascribed important diseases among the country population to this cause;* and the Royal Society of Physicians in Paris considered them sufficiently generally harmful to recommend its correspondents to pay special attention to it.** The foul vapors of the soaked hemp, which are deleterious to the nerves anyway, and the corruption which contaminates the water also spoil the air and are the reason that numerous ills may be expected even from the air. This, therefore, merits the full force of the decrees issued against it and quoted elsewhere.

§5

In many towns it was thought that the so-called town moats, which in the past had often been laid out for the protection of the place, should serve in the stead of rivers, and even now they are maintained next to fortresses. These moats are usually filled by a river, specially conducted there for the purpose, but in the case of small towns, where no river flows past, they are fed by inconsiderable and slow waters. Such moats are usually overgrown with reeds and rush and serve as abodes for a mass of insects and water plants. In the hot season they dry out by half or more, and then have all the effects of unhealthy swamps. Thus, several Egyptian towns have plague-like cases in summer due to the exhalations of the nearby lakes which are filled with reeds and mud and are dried up, but in Alexandria itself, the river Nile rises at the beginning of summer, flows into the lake, flushes the rotting mud away, and beneficially counteracts its exhalations which are poisonous elsewhere.†　However, in this country, the town moats are mostly the repositories of all a town's

* "De morbis Artificum," p. 627.
** "Pièces concernant l'établissement fait par le Roi d'une Commission ou Société Correspondence de Médecine," p. 17.
† Strabo, "Geograph.," Lib. V. XVI.

rubbish; the latrines drain into them; rubbish, dead cats and dogs are thrown into them; and the drainage ditches of the town, and many filthy puddles, etc., all flow into them. Yet it is rarely that someone thinks of cleaning these moats, and such cleaning sometimes is even dangerous to the inhabitants, especially when carried out in the warm season, for it has the same effect as slow flowing waters.*

Now that the danger of attacks by marauding irregular troops is much less, the police must have the numerous useless moats around every inconsiderable little town dried out and planted with healthy plants if there is not a nearby stream with which the moat can be cleaned. Or, if this is not feasible, the police can insist that the inhabitants at least keep the moat strictly clean, and speed up the passage of water through it by the construction of ditches and locks. If this is not done, a town surrounded by a moat is, as it were, buried in a swamp, and in the hot season is exposed to the most terrible epidemics. Petrus Salius Diversus says of Leiden that the stinking exhalations of the moats there caused the most dangerous plague-like fevers every year, but they usually disappeared once these mud holes dried up.

* * *

§8

On paving the streets

I come to consider now the cleanliness institutions required in towns and other places inhabited by people. The first thing that attracts attention is the necessity of paving the streets without which the constant driving and the dirt from the draft animals, the water stagnating in the ruts and tracks, etc., turn the soil of a town into an unhealthy and impassable bog. Paris, which presumably received its former Latin name (Lutetiae) from the large amount of muck on which one had to step, must have been the unhealthiest place in Europe in the past, until Louis XIV restored the cleanliness of the streets with strong paving, as far as the nature of the soil and the large number of persons permitted, and better assured the health of the inhabitants.** Lund ascribes part of the malignant diseases and putrid fever among the country people in Sweden to the unhealthy vapors which rise into the air in many Swedish villages the streets of which are still unpaved despite all the available stones.† Therefore, it can be easily concluded what influence the dirty streets of London, which are such an annoyance to foreigners, must have on the health of so many people.†† The Romans built their highways, as well as the streets of towns, with baked stone, thus preventing excessive accumulation of street mud in winter, and large amounts of dust in summer.‡

---

* "Histoire de la Société Royale de Médecine," A. 1776, p. 222, 223.
** Lancisius, "De noxiis paludum effluviis," P. I. c. IV.
† Murray, "Medical Practical Library," Vol. 1, p. 628.
†† "Remarks of a Traveler," l.c. p. 367.
‡ Guid. Pancirolli, "Rerum memorabilium sive deperditarum pars prior, commentariis illustrata ab Henrico Salmuth," Tit. XXI. p. 61.

The dust of our streets is an important cause of eye and chest diseases of travelers and townspeople. The inhabitants of Malabar easily become blind from the strong sunlight and the fine dust in their region.* Habermann says that in Vienna many cases of consumption are due to the dust in the always sandy streets.** In Malta, as well as in Egypt,† and also in New Spain, and especially in Mexico blindness caused by the flying sand that is constantly suspended in the air is something very common.†† The town of Valetta on the island of Malta has all streets paved with white squared stones; they cause much dust, and they are so harmful to the eyes that most people there have very bad eyesight.‡

The police, therefore, has to supervise both subjects very thoroughly. Wherever circumstances permit, the streets should be provided with proper paving in even the lowest village.

* * *

§9

Cleaning the streets

Cleaning the streets requires special care. The uncleanliness of towns is largely due to the fact that wastes from all sides are often brought and thrown into their streets. I do not want to speak of the disadvantages of such foul accumulations now; I shall only refer elsewhere to what I have said concerning this subject, and consider now the various kinds of defilement of the streets and the means of preventing or remedying this.

Everywhere there is very little order except for having house owners sweep together on certain days and at certain hours the rubbish which has accumulated in the streets. This is then removed from the streets to a special place, either at the public's expense by special carters, or by the owners themselves. No matter which way is the best to achieve this, the rubbish swept together must not remain longer than a few hours because the heat and fermentation causes an exhalation, the stench and danger of which increases greatly; negligent carters must be strictly held to perform their service. According to the street regulations in Hamburg, enacted in 1710, the carters who have been ordered for loading the street rubbish, must drive slowly through the town with covered carts, in the months of May, June, July, and August at 5 o'clock in the morning; in the subsequent months at 6, and in the months of the shortest days at 7 o'clock, and thus keep the town clean daily.

* * *

* "Eastern Travels," p. 815.
** "Treatise on Harmless Funerals," 16, p. 23. The same is confirmed by von Wasserberg, "De Haen praelect. pathol," T. II. p. 203.
† Thevenot, "It. orient," I.C. 5. it. P. II. C. 80.
†† Gottfried, "Hist. antiq." P. III. p. 608.
‡ Brydon's "Travels through Sicily and Malta," Part I, p. 272.

Of dung heaps and liquid manure pits

The dung heaps in front of houses and the liquid manure pits from which a stinking rotten lye constantly flows are too important a cause of atmospheric pollution to be tolerated any longer, no matter how small the towns. The police are so dishonored by the mere sight of such sources of putrid fevers, that I need not give many reasons for removing these dung heaps, beyond what mere good manners demand and what one owes the foreigner's eyes. It is only elementary justice that if someone wants to keep a dung heap, be it even in his own house, and its exhalations and foulness are obnoxious to the neighbors, he is made to remove the dung heap. Digging a liquid-manure pit next to a common wall so that the neighborhood suffers from the stench is not to be permitted.* It is even less permissible that someone leave his rubbish on a public street, or next to a city wall next to other persons' buildings.**

But it is better if endeavors are made to keep the streets clean by instilling in the citizens from their youth not to act contrary to this, and if every contravention is strictly punished. One easily gets used to throwing out of the window into the street everything that one wants to remove, and there are still towns in Germany where one cannot walk at a certain hour through the streets without the danger of being befouled with the contents of a chamber pot. Not to mention the detriment to the clothes of passers-by and various injuries stemming from this and similar nuisances, through such freedom which lets streets become common sewers, and no amount of cleaning suffices to keep the air of the town clean. "In Paris and London the streets are turned into public latrines, and the house owners must invent special devices and place iron obstacles in front of their houses, so that the Doctores of Scriptures, as I saw with my own eyes in Oxford, and as happens in London every now and again, do not p--s on their windows. Filthiness in the London streets is a real nuisance."† In several French towns in narrow streets I saw ten to twelve soldiers and other men engaged in such soiling of the streets without shyness and with uncovered faces, without having noticed that such shamelessness is viewed as something out of the ordinary. The stench in such regions is insufferable in summer, and the side streets are cleaned more rarely because the vehicles cannot always get through them.

Such filthiness must be prevented by all means by the subordinates of the police, and since it is not always possible to arrange one's natural functions in such a way that one is at a certain hour at the right place in a large city, care must be taken that there not be a lack of public latrines in such towns.

Throwing out dirty and harmful objects

Unfailing punishment must be specified for persons depositing dead animals,

* L.I. §1 and 2 ff. de Cloac. Speckhan, Cent. I. qu 10.
** Georg. Engelbrecht, "Discursus juridicus de peste & juribus circa tempus pestis," Of what is right in times of plague. Helmstad. 1693. §XVIII.
† "Observations of a Traveler," Part III, p. 367.

cats and dogs, in streets and next to public paths, even throwing broken pots and glass out merits punishment, for in addition to polluting the streets, injury may be done to pedestrians by such objects. The authorities can forbid persons to flush out barrels or other vessels in which badly smelling substances were kept and pour out such water into the street from their own homes.* Even someone who has a privilege [Servitut**] and may throw something out of his house therefore is not entitled to throw out urine, human feces, and similar ill-smelling things.†

* * *

Cleaning of market places

In public market places, the gardeners, herb merchants, etc., must be urged to keep the waste from their vegetables and foodstuffs in special baskets, and every time the market is over, that space, that has to be used by so many persons, must be cleaned.

* * *

§10

Of street sluices

Street sluices and their maintenance, therefore, are one of the most important aspects of public cleanliness. Herein, Tarquinius Superbus gained everlasting merit in Rome; for the benefit of the public and the health of the citizens, he had underground sluices and secret passages made which removed all the garbage from the streets and conducted it by seven converging creeks of water running down a steep gradient into the River Tiber. This extraordinary work was done so perfectly that a man on horseback could go through the brick canals and could always easily clean them.†† This is also the reason why the position of a town on a somewhat elevated spot and near a river is so excellent, and can be compensated only with much effort and cost, whereby the varied effluents of a town are afforded the necessary gradient.

But such street sluices must be cleaned often by specially appointed persons so that the stagnant, foul matter's abhorrent exhalations are not permitted to rise to the detriment of the entire town. On the other hand, care must be taken that the cleaning of such canals is not undertaken in summer, in hot weather, and even more so in daytime.‡ This important article had already been provided for by the Romans,‡‡ and we find several examples of such enactments in juridical writings.°

---

* Caepolla, "de servit. urb. praed. sub rubr. de Cloac." qu. 5.

** [Servitut—legal term, meaning the privilege to use another person's property for certain purposes.]

† Idem dict. tr. rubr. de servitut. projiciendi, qu. 4. 1. un. ult. ff. de via publ.

†† Tit. Livius, Lib. I. 56. Lancisius, "De adventitiis romani Coeli qualitatibus," P. II. C. 2. p. 67.—Zach Platners, "Treatise on Cleanliness"; pp. 12, 13.

‡ Plaz, "De sanitatis publicae obstaculis."

‡‡ Plutarchus, "Quaest. Rom. in Oper." T. II. p. 285.—Dionis Cassii, "Hist. rom." Lib. III. p. 750.

° Glos. in C. XXI. I. ff. quod vi aut clam. Caepoll. de servit. rust. praed. Cap. XLIII. Ripa de peste; C. 4. de remed. praeservandi contra pestem.—Adolphi, "De aere a. & l.," Lips. VII.

Good care must also be taken in the maintenance of the various openings of the street sluices necessary for receiving the inflowing water, both for public safety and to prevent the penetration of various coarse bodies, which might clog the canals. They and the drainage channels which lead from the houses into the streets must be well provided with iron gratings.*

§11
Collection place of town rubbish

At a certain distance from all human dwellings and public roads, and if possible at a place from which the wind may not so easily blow into town, every town must maintain several reservoirs for the rubbish brought there from the town. In Paris, two kinds of receptacles are filled, one with real excrement, the other with other objects easily subject to rotting, dead animals, entrails, blood, rotten plants, etc. The drivers conveying such materials must be strictly instructed not to empty any of these on the way into rivers, depressions, or onto fields; that they load the rubbish without delay at night into well closed barrels, and drive off before daybreak, after having previously swept clean the place where the loading took place; that under no pretext do they stop on the way and dirty the streets, etc.**

Such reservoirs are best planted with poplars or small forests on the side leading to town, for the trees not only keep the infected air away from town, but also greatly improve the air by their exhalations. After a number of years, when all the rubbish has been well rotted, the material in the reservoir is released to the country people for fertilizing.

* * *

§15
Uncleanliness of private apartments themselves

At this point, I advise on what is to be ordered for the sake of cleanliness in the apartments of the citizens themselves. I have already said that a prudent police does not meddle in matters of the interior of households, and if this regent of the nations eventually is misused as a spy, she degenerates into a tyrant of human societies and a disturber of the public peace which she should protect. However, in things on which the happiness of the entire society depends, every reasonable citizen submits to the law of public security without excepting any area, no matter how privileged. And who would state that he could reasonably intend to pollute only his share of the town atmosphere, without his neighbor having the right to object to such an attempt?

* * *

* In Brunswick open gutters and drainage channels without grids have been generally forbidden. Bergius, "Cameral and Police Magazine," Vol. III. "Of Street Cleaning," §11.
** Ordonnance de la Police de Paris, du 31. Mai. 1726.

§18

Latrines

In a great many houses there are no latrines at all, and entire families use certain receptacles for as long as possible in order to avoid the discomfort of frequent cleaning. The place where all the evacuations are collected is either a dung heap enclosed in a narrow courtyard, perhaps even the public street, or finally a nearby town moat. In the first case the air of an entire house, especially in wet and warm weather, is filled with abhorrent exhalations from which the entire neighborhood must suffer; and in the rooms in which the soiled receptacles have stood for a long time, such foul air is inhaled that its detrimental effects may be compared with the deleterious air of graves. In the second case, the streets themselves become a loathsome cesspool.

Many households in towns are provided with latrines, but these are sometimes not lined with stones, and all waste is conducted in wooden canals or canals consisting of boards nailed together, often even along the exterior wall of the house, into an adjacent dung heap below. Thus a whole side of a building is soiled, and the wooden hutch exhales a stench that is unendurable, even far-off. Other houses have proper latrines, provided with the required caldrons, but they are situated either in the center of the building or near the living rooms and bedrooms, so that the inhabitants are forced to breathe mephitic air day and night. Even when the latrines are well arranged, their necessary emptying is so long delayed after several years, or the owners are so unclean in their natural evacuations, that it is almost the same as if these facilities were not in the house at all. Even in the most respected households, I have often been startled by this matter; whereas, in the living rooms everything was sparkling and clean, and perfect order in every last corner, on the other hand, I found incomprehensible uncleanliness in the latrines. The open urine pools make the exhalations so pungent and biting that one nearby is in danger of suffocating, and in whole corridors the air is saturated with such volatile foul vapors to such an extent that even silver and copper become tarnished and turn black when exposed to them.

And thus, in a large city, there are few private apartments in which, in one way or another, the bad arrangement or care of latrines is not the foundation of the pollution of the common atmosphere. This subject, although loathsome, certainly deserves everywhere the best care by the police, both in order that no building be constructed without sufficient latrines, and that these be situated in reasonable places, built according to sensible rules, and maintained in a clean state.

* * *

No matter how much effort and care the private person expends on the good arrangement of latrines, the individual citizen's power in a town is rarely sufficient to maintain the necessary cleanliness regarding them. For not in every part of a large town is there flowing water which could help prevent the rapid filling up of the cesspools. This, then, is the place where the authorities, according to the example given by the Romans, can use the income of a large city to the greatest advantage. Strabo says that the Greeks were particularly skilled in rapidly putting up beautiful buildings. The Romans, on the other hand, concentrated all their attention on things that the Greeks considered too petty: the building of roads, water conduits, and street sluices in which all refuse of the town was conducted into the Tiber. These sluices were lined with hard stones to such a height that a cart had room to pass through, and the entire town, as it were, stood above the water which flowed through many subterranean canals so that its sludge might be removed. Dionysius says that three things in which he admired the greatness of the Roman people struck him mainly: the aqueducts, the public roads, and the latrines. One can conclude what expense must have been incurred in building the latrines, when, according to C. Aquilius' report, a thousand talents were expended on the mere construction, or their repair when once the waters could not flow freely any more. In our times, we endow an infinite number of useless and sometimes luxurious foundations, while neglecting irresponsibly the greatest requirement of a populous city!

* * *

§19

Of unhealthy trades and crafts

No matter how much a good police insists on the cleanliness of towns, it will not be able to completely attain its aim, as long as all the trades of the inhabitants are permitted to be carried on at undetermined places. Then it is always impossible to supervise accurately the occupation of individual citizens dispersed throughout the town and without such supervision, there are many trades and activities which particularly pollute the town air and thus injure the public health of the inhabitants. The craftsmen who cause loud noise and work with fire have been rightly directed to places in town where they do not trouble the citizens who require certain quiet, and where the danger of fire to the town is not so great. With a view to the well-being of such a town, however, there are still several trades and craftsmen who should be directed for certain of their activities, even if not altogether, to such places where they will pollute the air less and it will be likely that the air will be made less unsuitable for breathing.

First of all, slaughterhouses should not be tolerated in the center of the town or in places where the exhalations of so much blood, wastes from so many animals, even animal vapor rising from the meat, pollute the atmosphere so easily and so much.* Zimmermann says: "The town of Cork in Ireland is the place where from

* The noxiousness of even freshly slaughtered animals upon their opening and hanging up, the rising odor of the animal which quickly begins rotting, was publicly recognized in the past by the medical faculty in Leipzig. B. Ammani Med. Crit. Cas. 82.

August to January more than a hundred thousand head of cattle are slaughtered for the English fleet. In the northern and southern suburbs of Cork, there is a large number of slaughterhouses with deep pits next to them into which the blood and the useless parts of the animals are thrown. When the incessantly rainy weather appears, this quickly decomposed blood emerges from its morass and flows from the hills down into the stream. This foul matter not only poisons the air in general, it even poisons the otherwise beneficial north winds which blow from that side over the town. Thereof Rogers, an excellent physician of that city, remarked of the smallpox in the years 1718, 1719, 1720, and 1721, that many more persons who lived close to the slaughterhouses died. The fury of the diseases prevalent there, and being mostly of the foul kind, lasts as long as the slaughtering of the cattle, and usually ceases in January.* According to Rogers, the alkaline and stinking smell of the shambles made the air in the entire neighborhood so unhealthy that the smallpox rampant in the town became more plague-like there.**

From this it can be easily concluded that slaughterhouses in a large city may become the source of great evil, especially if proper cleanliness is lacking, of which I have already spoken elsewhere. Flowing water is almost indispensable for them, in addition to a somewhat remote position and free access of wind, if possible on all sides. Also, the slaughterers should never throw the animal wastes into shallow water because the water only partly flushes them out, and the rest is pulled out by dogs and pigs. They should be thrown into deep pits and well covered with earth. The many skins of slaughtered animals, especially those obtained through the knacker from cattle that died, must first be well dried at a raised place far from the center of the town before the slaughterer may be permitted to hang them up in his loft where, without this precaution, they spread the most abhorrent and noxious stench.† The same applies to the preparation of violin strings from the intestines of the animals; while they dry, they emit unhealthy vapors.†† Altogether I repeat that the slaughterers should be enjoined not to slaughter in their own dwellings, but in places where the police can watch, through appointed persons, over both the required cleanliness and the quality and correct distribution of the meat.

What has been said about the disadvantage of drying animal skins even more applies to varied treatment they receive at the hands of the tanner. It is known what an unspeakable stench a tannery causes in the neighborhood, how many foul volatile exhalations fill the air, what stinking sludge fills the nearby water from the soaking of the skins and the discharge of the rotting lyes, and finally, how impossible it is to make tanneries observe the cleanliness required in a populous city!

At Frankfurt-on-Main, as in other health-conscious towns, the slaughterers and

* "Of Experience," Part II, Book 4, chapter 5, p. 201. 2.
** P. 47. Haller l.c. T. VI. p. 211.
† Screta, "Tract. de Febre castrens," sect. 2. C. 3. p. 189.
†† Bern. Rammazini, "De morbis artificum"; op. omn. p. 532.

tanners are directed to remote places to carry on their crafts.* Such an arrangement is even more necessary since it is a temptation to bring cattle to drink in low places where the tanneries do not take up entirely the lowest part of the river, and where the water may be infected by certain epidemics from the effluents of the skins which often come from animals that died; even people may come to harm by using water from the creek that is saturated with rotten parts. There was an epidemic at Beauvais in 1750 of which the public notices said: "Because of the last epidemic at Beauvais, the King had the real cause investigated, and His Majesty was told that the tanners and cordwainers of this city, when processing skins, they soak them in fat among other things, and afterward they press out the fat and again boil it, which causes an insufferable stench and infects the air. Therefore a decree was given: the first time such boiling was carried out at less than the stipulated distance from the city, they were to be fined five hundred livres, and even more upon repetition."** The Romans in their time had already removed the workshops of the tanners and fullers from the city and beyond the river Tiber, for the fullers clean the woolen cloth with a vapor of sulfur and corrupt urine.† When the town air in Jena at one time was filled with many stinking vapors because of much slaughtering, in both the streets and the houses of the butchers, so that the streets were always covered with blood and dirty water, Duke Friedrich II of Saxony in 1551 ordered the slaughterhouses to be removed to beyond this city and to the bank of the Saale River.††

By the same token the blacksmiths, barber-surgeons, and surgeons must be forbidden to pour into the streets in daytime the blood often let from people and horses, as the warm water that is colored by much blood from bleeding immediately begins to rot. In bloodletting, the blood from several persons should be collected, and it should be removed in covered vessels at night.

Even more deleterious in a town are the candle factories, the glue and soap shops, and the dye-works because of their frequent loathsome, foul or acrid exhalations. When he investigated the unhealthiness of some parts of Warsaw, Tralles rightly put the blame on the insufferable stench of boiling tallow used in soap-making,‡ and van Swieten considered this trade one of the most detrimental to populous cities.‡‡ Therefore, in Paris an order was made that stated: animal fat in large quantities was to be boiled exclusively outside the city and at a remote place where the consequent stench would not annoy anybody.° Paul Zacchias insists especially on the

---

* J. Ad. Behrens, "The Inhabitant of Frankfurt-on-Main, Regarding his Fertility, Mortality and Health."

** Ant. Platz, "Treatise of Some Obstacles to Public Health," p. 16.

† Artemidorus, "De somp. interpret," Lib. I. C. LIII. Martialis L. VI. Plinius Lib. XXVIII. C. VIII. Lib XXXV. C. XV.

†† Adolphi, "De aëre a. & l," Lipsiens, §9. XII.

‡ Vera patrem patriae sanum & longaevum praestandi methodus.

‡‡ Commentar. T.V. p. 174.5.

° Ordonnance de Police du Châtelet de Paris du 10. Juin 1701.

removal of the caldrons needed in the manufacture of tallow for candles because of the deleterious consequences of their abhorrent stench.* At this opportunity I must recall to the reader that verdigris, which in many regions is mixed with the tallow to make the candles burn as if they were made from wax, may have most deleterious consequences on long winter evenings and, therefore, its use should be forbidden. Even the washhouses, in which soap is constantly dissolved in large quantities, combined with the dirt of the black laundry, and is driven upward by the warm water vapor, are a not inconsiderable cause of the pollution of a region, especially if the rotten soap-lye is afterwards poured into the streets on a hot day and slowly flows through the streets. "For it often happens," it is written, "that when laundry is washed, the soap or rinsing water is stopped and used for cleaning other things. It would be better if washing were done in courtyards and open squares, and the unclean waters poured out in good time."** The dyers and others use many dyes, some of them suspicious colors, the volatile ingredients of which are often deleterious not only to the craftsmen themselves but also to the neighborhood.† This is especially so as the cloth coming from the vats is hung on long rods which reach into half the street or even across the whole street, and dried there. In France, the dyers are permitted to hang up such cloth only under the condition that the rods do not reach halfway across the street, and that the lower edge of their cloth is not less than three spans above the ground.†† Through the black effluents of their dye, the milliners spread an unbearable stench in their whole neighborhood in summer, and I do not know what good the dye of the hats can do to those who have to wear them.

The production and exhibition of foul-smelling cheeses, the exhalations of herring barrels, of waters from fish and various other smelling wares, often spoil the air of an entire street, and they should move the police to at least admonish the grocers and merchants of these foodstuffs not to exhibit such wares in front of their houses at least and thereby perfume the whole street. A written, or if required, a painted board can explain to every passerby what is on sale in the house, without making half the town vomit because of the loathsome stench of piled-up cheeses, etc., and without poisoning the atmosphere.

The various factories, manufacturers, workhouses, penitentiaries, and orphanages, because of the many persons who all sit together in a small space all day and pollute

---

* Quaest. Med. Leg. I. 5. Tit. qu. 7.
** Prophylaxis of the City of Frankfurt-on-Main or Prevention of Epidemics, p. 7.
† Pigmentarii, dum variis coloribus coquendis, miscendis, indeque diversis, supellectilibus parandis operam dant, praetereuntibus haud levem, vicinis vero quotidianam maximamque pariunt molestiam. Nunc enim sulphure arsenicali praeprimis, impraegnatae terrae, cujusmodi est auripigmentum & cobaltum, ignis vi sunt subigendae, nunc bovino sanguine quaedam miscendae, nunc calcinandae, igne aperto comburendae, oleo aut vernice coquendae, nunc acidis spiritibus jungendae. Ant. Plaz, "De sanitatis publicae obstaculis," §IV.
†† Code de Police; l.c. Tit. VI. §III.

the air with their increased exhalations, deserve to be removed from large cities, even if economic reasons do not speak in favor of such a separation.* But, in addition, since such houses are occupied with work the influence of which is obviously unhealthy to the town air, as demonstrated by the smell which one meets upon entering, there are certainly the weightiest reasons to transfer such buildings and occupations to the country, where the workers are much healthier and will carry out their tasks with greater zeal.**

Silk production is now carried on to advantage in many regions, but in some Italian towns this spoils the climate. The scalded cocoons and the pupae rotting in them emit an unbearable stench, and weak persons living in the areas of manufacture are often bedridden for some time toward the end of spinning.† An occasional cause of a dangerous epidemic at Villeneuve-lès-Avignon was also held to be the well known abhorrent stench of large numbers of silk cocoons which the inhabitants let remain in the street or rot in a nearby swamp.†† All this confirms the necessity of greater cleanliness in such occupations in all private dwellings, but especially in public workhouses. The burning of pit coal causes a thick, suffocating smoke which, like a thundercloud, remains well in the atmosphere above a large city. In London it blackens all houses and implements, and it can be very deleterious to sensitive lungs. It was found that the damage done by this smoke is not so great in the open air as in closed rooms, where it often causes suffocation. This is an inducement that pit coal be well desulfurized before its use as is usually done in England, and thus relieve it as much as possible of its noxious basic substance.‡ As it is, countries that have no wood have no other recourse but to burn peat and pit coal, even if it is often detrimental to health. Custom, however, often checks inconveniences that are unavoidable to the unaccustomed.

Such craftsmen as coppersmiths, tinsmiths, blacksmiths, coopers, wheelwrights, etc., who fill the streets with pungent, and suspect smoke should be removed equally from the center of a large city and transferred to places which are more exposed to air and are not filled by such a large number of sensitive persons. Thus, the goldsmiths, brass-workers, armorers, etc., in Vienna are no longer permitted to work with noxious mercury or lead vapor in front of their houses; they must carry out such work in regions where the air is less enclosed. Only blacksmiths are tolerated in the city because they cannot be easily dispensed with there.

* * *

* Von Sonnenfels, "Political Treatises."
** "Of Ways of Making Such Houses Healthier." See article Medical System.
† "Additions to the Latest Travel Descriptions of Italy," by Joh. Bernoulli; Vol. I, p. 68.
†† "Histoire de la Société Royale de Médecine," a. 1776, p. 218, 224.
‡ Priestley proved that the pit coal vapor does not really kill by suffocation, but by its effect on the nerves, and I shall have more to say on this subject in the article on public security.

A SYSTEM OF COMPLETE MEDICAL POLICE

Volume Four

Public Safety Measures as Far as they Concern
Public Health

PREFACE

I published the first three volumes of Medical Police (Medicinische Polizey) under circumstances which would have deterred many from writing as freely as I did, even at the danger of becoming a martyr of medical truth. In view of my lack of talent for such holy vocation, I did not succeed in this. Nevertheless, my undertaking did have an effect which ended in propelling me as far as Italy, where, because of the numerous new occupations involved I had to forgo the continuation of this work for some time. But I never abandoned it completely, as was thought now and again. I believe that there is no better way for me to convince the public of my gratitude for its approval than to publish the fourth volume of Medical Police in the midst of most weighty work imposed upon me by the restless calling of teacher of practical medicine and being the head of all medical institutions and hospitals of a very populous province. I hope that this volume will prove no less significant than the previous ones.

But I must ask one thing of my German readers. I am no longer in a position to obtain in good time all the important writings appearing in this remote country and to do justice to every writer as well as using, as I would wish, the various proposals concerning my field. On the other hand, my work should gain much when compared with the first three volumes since I here enjoy every possible freedom to write as I think, and to immerse the brush precisely into that color which I consider most suitable for representing my painting most naturally. Some proofs of this are provided already in the Italian translation of the first volume of Medical Police from which one can be convinced that under Joseph II the rights of mankind also were restored where before nothing prevailed, but the chattering of teeth and whimpering about the sacred Inquisition, and where, in the case of openness in printing, such slavery held sway that only a powerful protective spirit could provide redemption.

Another advantage of this work is that because I was able to carry out a large part of my proposals, I can judge better their consequences and difficulties than most writers are usually able.

My employment provides frequent opportunities for this, and I have already drafted plans for the establishment of a medical college in Austrian Lombardy, for medical studies at the Royal Imperial University in Pavia, for apothecaries, and, finally, for midwifery. These plans have been approved by the Court and there is hope for their execution.

These are numerous pieces ready for Medical Police and as I insert them in the following volume, I shall simultaneously explain everything by giving the reasons required and providing additions which come from experience. Perhaps Providence used my transfer to Italy as a tool for improving the work which I undertook for the benefit of mankind and which, I hope, I shall see through to the end.

The present volume of Medical Police deals with one of the most important subjects of police in general, though it is difficult here to determine what should be judged by a medical tribunal and what is outside the field of state medicine. Everything that threatens the body with disease or injury can be viewed by the physician as cause for disease. If thus viewed, however, the field of my considerations is infinitely large, and subjects will appear which few persons would seek in a work dealing with Medical Police. Yet, just as I pass over many matters that are not in direct relation to Medical Police, I also consider many things worthy of my attention which so far seem to be outside the scope of medical consideration.

I repeat: when a writer himself chooses to treat many subjects, there must necessarily be many deficiencies; but such are always the first attempts at such an extensive work. Those who will run the same course after me by and by can fill in the empty shelves and discard what is superfluous. This is the business of each subsequent century, to which every writer must submit, together with his book.

It remains for me to speak also of saving people who have become lifeless, but the abundance of subjects forced me to defer this important article to the next volume, else this volume would have become too large. Therefore, in the fifth volume of Medical Police I shall add my considerations concerning this matter, and at the same time I shall treat of medical institutes and medical schools, wherein I shall describe my proposals that have already been introduced in the Milan region, and accompany them with the required explanations.

Pavia, 1 August 1788.

INTRODUCTION

On public safety in general

> It was she who turned the animal, the savage, into a
> human; Because of her, instead of freedom, he chose
> the chain!

Public safety as the intrinsic object of all police can be here considered only insofar as it concerns in its narrowest sense the work, life, and health of the citizenry. All else, therefore, is outside the field of Medical Police (Medicinische Polizey) and cannot be placed here.

How can the life and health of the people be ensured against all injuries that are not completely unavoidable?

This is the great question, worthy of a thinking sovereign and in connection with which chiefly the physician should be heard because it can be expected only of him that, in addition to accurate knowledge of the human body, he also knows the relationship of the causes which affect it, and only he is able to discover the manifold springs [of human life] which have many sources, and the drying up of which is not always the unalterable fate of mortals.

It is difficult to answer in a specific order the question that has been posed, and it would be equally justifiable for me to put into this section what I have written hitherto about Medical Police. Even the medical institutions proper, with which I shall deal in the next volume, constitute an important part of the answer to be expected.

However, I am still dealing here with safety measures in the narrow sense, by which I mean measures against accidental and careless, against malicious and malevolent undertakings, against attack by wild animals, etc.

"It is impossible," says von Sonnenfels, "to determine all cases in which citizens may come to grief due to carelessness. The police would have to provide every citizen with a guard. It is possible, therefore, only to give as examples those notable opportunities which can easily be applied to the others."

If it should be said that some such considerations can be put forward by non-physicians, I do not object, except that a physician could, nevertheless, present various interesting points of view when he is aided by his science, and that such subjects may just as well be left to our consideration as are subjects not connected with bleeding or purging, which physicians are given to judge.

If physicians' considerations of the most frequent causes of our injuries should be confined to the different injurious tools, then either every person in authority would have to search for the causes of most accidents and determine their effect in more detail than has been hitherto done, or mankind would have to be left to continue suffering from many avoidable ills, because it would be assumed that physicians should be forbidden to consider such causes of death and injury of citizens which have no proper Materia peccans nor can be purged by rhubarb or aloe.

It is really irresponsible how greatly most authorities sin against the article on general security with respect to life and health of the citizenry. However, if I am not very much mistaken concerning one point, which is only a matter of common sense, I believe that the stronger persons joined together in society, have never submitted to a single weaker person for any other reason than to enjoy the advantages of social life under his energetic protection: secure in both their persons and their property. It is, after all, no mere joke when an entire nation submits to one man, and the nation is entitled in all earnestness to claim from the regent the fulfillment of certain paternal duties which are not confined to protecting his people against the attacks by a greedy neighbor, and for good measure hanging a dozen thieves every year. For the same person in authority, who in his own house puts away knives and forks so that the children cannot lay their hands on them, often lets an entire province suffer an annual loss through the most frequent causes of daily injuries which, taken as a whole, never would be caused by the most terrible foe, whose selfish interest after all always sees to it that the province which he wants to conquer is not completely devastated.

I repeat, therefore, there is no point in making so much fuss about population institutions, which basically are nothing so long as there is no realization of the great advantage realized if the people who are already here are preserved and made happy! . . . In my opinion it would be ridiculous to try to fill a pond before the dams are secured; and to populate a country without protecting and preserving the inhabitants by prudent institutions is tantamount to trying to store water in a sieve. I know a prince who assures everybody that his small country is really overpopulated and that he does not wish it to have more people. Although in this blessed country there are still some uncultivated regions, I nevertheless do not object to the system of a regent who, if he cannot protect his present subjects against all avoidable ills, at least does not desecrate the word population, as is done by so many who seem to enjoy only the spectacle of many people ascending a mountain here and tumbling again into deep ravines over there.

The following sections will convince every philanthropical reader most strongly that it is not of maliciousness that I reproach such authorities who look after the interests of mankind so badly. My criticism is leveled the least at today's great regents; and in the last ten years in some countries such wonderful health measures have been taken that it would be impudent to doubt that one is only now beginning to realize what had been lacking in the past.

* * *

In 1779 in Vienna 167 persons died in consequence of accidents; of them 75 alone were victims of an exploded powder magazine. In 1780 there were 73 accident victims. Specifically 13–16 found dead; 8–4 drowned; 19–11 fallen to their deaths; 9–7 run over.

In Leipzig there were the following accident victims between 1759 and 1774:

Found dead in the house	56
in the street	43
in the water and drowned	50
Fallen to death	28
Run down by mounted horses	5
Run over by vehicles	5
Broken legs	7
Shot to death	6
Executed	10
Murdered	15
Child murder	18
Suicide	12
Hanged	11
Burned and scalded	5
Died of money swallowed	1
Sudden violent hemorrhage	1
Bitten by rabid dog	1
Of poison	1
Frozen to death	1
Self-inflicted wound	1
Crushed by nurse	1
Through various accidents	4
Strangled	1
Suffocated in latrine	1
Total:	284

However, between 1759 and 1774 there were altogether 9255 persons who died in Leipzig. Thus the ratio of those who died by accident to those who died of a natural death was 1 to 81.

In London in consequence of accidents in 30 years there were dead:

Drowned in water	3,189
Found dead	1,191
Those who drank themselves to death	954
Suicides	1,371

Executed	470
Of falls and wounds	1,640
Smothered and suffocated (children)	1,936
Murdered	217
Killed by dagger	20
in the pillory	3
by poison	34
by bites of rabid dogs	29
by bites of rabid cats	2
by bite of a viper	1
by a bear	1
by an ox	1
by a kick from a horse	1
in a duel	3
by wounds received	5
Accidentally shot	21
Blown up by gunpowder	1
Killed by lightning	2
Suffocated by charcoal fumes, etc.	80
in food	3
in fat	14
by a cherry	1
Smothered	70
Strangled	5
Crushed, mangled by carriages	112
Burned	221
Scalded	94
Due to broken arm or leg	182
shoulder blade	42
jaw	10
other limbs	23
amputation of arm or leg	3
breast	1
pulled tooth	1
hunger or cold	17
great shock	23
	————
Total:	11,994

The total of those who had died in London in the course of 30 years was 750,322. Therefore the ratio of those killed in accidents to the total is 16 to 1000, i.e., almost $1:62\frac{1}{2}$; in other words, out of every 62 persons one was killed in an accident. This stable does not contain persons who went to sea and found their death there. That in a city where arms or legs are so easily amputated, only 3 persons died within 30 years after such an operation is as little credible as that only one death should have occurred after amputation of a breast. It seems likely that the surgeons gave the matter another name if the patient did not die directly during the operation, and thus there are many other items lacking which within a period of 30 years must have caused death in such a large city.

According to a table of 1785, 18,119 births occurred in London between 13 December 1785 and 12 December 1786. The number of deaths was 20,454. Of the latter the following were accident victims:

Frozen	8
Wounded and injured	19
Burned	9
Drowned	112
Suicides	22
Poisoned	2
Starved	3
Fallen to death	58
Murdered	7
Fallen into boiling water	1
Suffocated in smoke	4
Total:	245

In the country many causes of the sudden accidents that occur in towns are absent; however, it must be borne in mind how many persons suffocate in clay pits and sand pits, how many are crushed in quarries, that some fall from trees and are killed, or are killed while felling trees, how many children, because of lack of supervision by their parents, who are engaged in work, are burned, scalded, suffocated, drowned, eaten by pigs, fall to death, etc. Thus it seems that the dangers in towns and in the country are almost equal.

These few examples and random thoughts should make it clear that what is involved here is no small matter, but that if accurate calculations were made everywhere, sufficient material for useful cogitation would be gathered.

In times of war I often read accurate reports of persons shot, wounded, captured, and I always thought then: the great men believed that they had to count on only one enemy, and to pay attention only to the losses caused by him. England whose capital lost in 30 years alone 11,994 persons in accidents, would have had to conduct a most unfortunate war if the Empire had lost, relatively speaking, as many persons; and thus it is certain that every country, year in and year out, loses more citizens in accidents than are usually killed within the same time in even the bloodiest war.

I doubt whether there are any of my readers who do not agree that such tables of accidents should be introduced everywhere, and the attention of citizens and princes be alerted thereby.

But what use are the best intentions of a prudent and loving regent if his servants and the nation itself do not realize the necessity of certain improvements, and when they complain of interference with the rights of mankind, when a prince wants to protect the thoughtless people against the influence of deleterious habits and obsolete prejudices. It is therefore well to prepare the nation itself by writing about such beneficial improvements, that force be used to tear away from the eyes of the people the unfortunate blindfold and to let them see the abyss from whose terrifying edge the fatherly hand of the regent wants to guide them away.

* * *

PART ONE

On accidental and careless infringements of public safety

Quid quisque vitet, nunquam homini satis cautum est
in horas.

Horat. Od. XIII.

Accidents and carelessness are the most abundant sources of the troubles besetting mankind, and they certainly account for half the physical ills that gradually destroy the human race. Even if I included the illnesses which are a consequence of our effete way of life, I am afraid that here would have to be taken into account most accidents, which destroy our bodies before their natural end and thus leave to mankind only the distinctive peculiarity that it has to maintain at great cost a special faculty which endeavors to remedy what passions, idleness, and cooks ruin of our health.

However, I do not want to submit here a complete medical treatise, and I choose among the accidental and careless causes of our sufferings only those that are within the domain of Medical Police and which can usually be prevented if the health supervisers make some effort.

It is difficult to put the greatly varied causes of accidental or careless injuries under a few headings, but I tried to put everything in as good an order as possible so that related subjects would remain together unless they had to be separated for good reason, and to make it easy for my readers to find each of them under a general heading.

I class as careless infringements of public safety all acts of people which, without evil intent, are committed out of lack of consideration, experience, or prudence, and which have a direct and very dangerous effect either on the health or on the life itself of the perpetrator or of his fellow citizens.

Under accidental infringements, I class not only that which in the real sense of the word is an accident and deleterious to public health and safety, but also intentional effects, occurring according to certain laws, of causes which may forcibly shorten the natural span of human life.

It goes without saying that since I do not write as a mere physician, I do not speak of diseases which really belong in the domain of medical pathology.

It also goes without saying that here I cannot consider everything that may shorten our life as an accident or in consequence of carelessness; otherwise I would also have to speak of war and evil women, and treat a number of subjects which, no matter how much they harm society, still are not within the jurisdiction of Medical Police.

PART ONE

Section One

On injuries through smothering, collapse of buildings, falls, contusions, running over, etc.

> We accuse nature because of our fate:
> Behold, most was done by man to himself!

§1

Danger in crowds collecting

My considerations concern first of all public celebrations and popular amusements which rarely end without mishap, where the crowds pay far too high a price for pleasure unless a prudent police is able to foresee and prevent the misfortune. In the year 778 after the founding of Rome, when the city enjoyed complete peace, a sudden disaster caused more deaths to the Romans than a bloody defeat by an enemy would have cost. A freedman, Attilius by name, wanted to arrange a gladiator fight at Fidena. Since he undertook this not for glory and honor but for profit, he economized and built his amphitheater on bad foundations. Whoever was able, hurried from Rome to see the fights: the amphitheater, unable to support such a large crowd, collapsed, crushing those in it and at the same time all those standing nearby. The number of dead and wounded came to 50,000. On 28 March 1770 between 1,500 and 1,800 persons were crushed in Paris on the occasion of an unfortunate bonfire on the Square of Louis XV. On 29 June 1780 some 66 parishes were invited for a simultaneous confirmation at the same hour, and among them several were badly mauled by the pressure of the crowds. A woman from Neidhart, six months pregnant, was hit by a guard with his otherwise peaceable musket so hard in the left side of the abdomen that she immediately began bleeding and labor set in, and an abortion occurred a few hours later. The umbilical cord had been torn off the placenta and the brain of the child had been completely crushed although the mother had felt the child to be alive that same morning. Many such examples can be found in many countries where measures for public benefit are either unknown or the people are unwilling to obey them.

Therefore at public spectacles where the populace congregates on special scaffolds or stages, the police must have the scructures examined by building experts most thoroughly and in good time and thus make sure that they are fit to support a certain number of persons.

§2

On building scaffolds

The same applies to scaffoldings which are often put up by bricklayers and joiners with incomprehensible carelessness where high buildings are constructed, much to the detriment of themselves and the passersby. In the Milan region a wooden partition is erected between the building site and the public road, to prevent injury by crumbling of the old brickwork or falling building materials. But, as I have said, even scaffolding cannot always be left to the craftsmen, if it is of considerable size and height, although their own lives depend on it. Often much skill and practical experience are needed for erecting such scaffoldings, around which idle folk gather to gape at those working. There are examples of such scaffolds collapsing, the consequences of which can be easily imagined.

It is necessary, therefore, to ensure not only the proper strength and correct construction of building scaffolds, but also that certain limits are stipulated for the access of the curious mobs. After the aforementioned disaster of the Romans, the Senate decided to have Attilius burnt, and that in the future no gladiator fights should be arranged by anybody who could not produce 50,000 pounds and who had not proved that he had taken every possible precaution. When in Milan in 1787 the many tall and sometimes magnificent statues and pillars, erected with pious intentions long ago in the middle of public roads, were removed upon the government's order because they blocked the roads, the wise precaution was taken to surround the statue to be demolished by a strong barricade at a considerable distance, and to mark a circle which nobody except the craftsmen were permitted to enter.

These are measures which, it would seem, should be dictated by common sense, but common sense must be a rare commodity in many places, because so many indispensable and natural measures are omitted, and the chamber pot is emptied upon the head of the passerby even before the warning cry "Look up" has been uttered.

* * *

Frank then deals with various injuries due to smothering, a few examples of which are in the subsequent paragraphs.

§11

Danger when ramshackle houses are torn down

When old houses are broken up and torn down, when large masses of stones are blown up by gunpowder placed under them, etc., various accidents happen unless the police takes prudent measures. When such work is undertaken, it must be directed by sensible men, and a conspicuous sign must be placed so that passersby and too inquisitive spectators are prevented from entering dangerous places. In Vienna master builders, as well as tilers and slaters, have to announce immediately to a certain supervisor every work they have undertaken so that the supervisor, according to his discretion, can have the street closed off by chains and ropes, and at night have lanterns fixed at both approaches. In the Milan region at night there must also be a lantern lit at such a barrier so that carriages or pedestrians do not run into the unexpected obstacle. In France, all craftsmen working on houses or buildings are obliged to fix on them some kind of sign consisting of two laths which hang on a rope so that every passerby may be warned of the danger, and if these regulations are not obeyed, the person responsible must make good the damage thus caused.

§12

On blowing up rocks

Not every inexperienced stone breaker or laborer should be permitted to blow up rocks with gunpowder, unless the foreman or owner of the quarry is in charge of the work and is responsible for damage that may be caused by this work to people who have not been warned. Public security requires that such work never be permitted close to public highways where strangers, not knowing the warning signs, may be harmed by the horses shying and running away with the carriage, if not hit by the stones blown up. Quarries on steep mountains, which are either built up or where public highways and paths pass at their foot, have to be provided on the side of the downward slope with strong ramparts, so that people or cattle are not injured by unexpectedly loosened stones rolling down the mountain with ever increasing force. Young people in mountainous areas sometimes indulge mischievously in a very dangerous pastime: they throw larger or smaller rocks from steep slopes and enjoy the jumping and crashing of this mass that is left to itself. Once I watched with horror such a dangerous game: a party of thoughtless boys had gone up a very high mountain to amuse themselves in this way. They made certain that there was nothing in danger in the valley, but not seeing a cattle herd feeding on another mountain opposite, they rolled down large rocks which, instead of stopping in the narrow valley, continued for a considerable distance up the opposite slope and dispersed the entire herd, without any of the cattle suffering any damage. If the rocks had taken another, equally accidental direction, half the herd might have been killed. Young people, therefore, must be acquainted with the danger of such games, and similar offenses must be strictly punished. And since other causes, continuous rain, cloudbursts, etc., also detach rocks in mountainous countries, and at the slightest opportunity set them into motion, many accidents may happen without certain measures being taken in such regions by the communities maintaining the roads; a better country police could easily prevent such accidents.

* * *

§ 19

Security of mines

In the case of mines taken over by individual companies, the country police cannot be satisfied that the mines are laid out and supported according to the opinion of each individual. It is true that every miner values his own life but he does not always have enough judgment, and is not always sufficiently acquainted with subterranean building construction, which is necessary for the safety of so many workers congregating at such dangerous places. This is borne out by experience in many regions, where one single error in the layout of the supports sometimes has caused the entire building to collapse and thus become the grave of a number of desperate persons. Later on I shall prove that in any event, the cleansing of the mephitic air in such subterranean caves, which causes many workers to suffocate or to lose their health prematurely, requires various measures which are not sufficiently enforced by all mine managers. The government must therefore obtain detailed knowledge of all mines, etc., in the country, and introduce a kind of mining-police under which mining would have to be managed according to an approved system, compatible with the rules of the building art, and the master builder would be held responsible for all the consequences if he should infringe these rules. It would be very useful if a regulation were issued stating that instead of ordinary wooden props for reinforcing and supporting shafts and other mines, stone walls should be erected. In fact, such round shafts, lined with masonry, can be found in some places of the Harz, e.g., Lauterberg, Strasbourg, in the Stollberg region, also in the Mannsfeld marlpits, etc. Karthäuser* says that by this masonry lining, the country benefits not only by the saving of timber, but being also much more durable than timber lining, which rots and splits and has to be replaced from time to time, masonry lining means considerable savings to the enterprise.

* * *

§ 26

Influence of improved roads on public health

The improved state of the highways in most of our provinces has a much greater influence on the general health of the people and even of their draft animals than one would think at first. For even if we disregard what the working creatures save in strength on better roads, a thousand accidents, dangerous shocks causing hemorrhages in weak people, pregnant women, etc., and broken legs, arms, etc., do not happen any more on straight roads, whereas in some countries these causes are still the source of many endemic injuries (if I may use this term for an evil that is due solely to external force). Since the highways were improved in Lombardy, where they had been neglected for a long time, the number of accident victims has really decreased noticeably, as one becomes aware in hospitals. Thus the improve-

* "Grundsätze der Bergpolizeywissenschaft," p. 82.

ment of highways should not be viewed merely as a matter of convenience and of economic advantage, but really as an object of public health.

§27

Collapse of many overloaded carts

Since we are speaking here of highways and vehicles, another cause of sad happenings occurs to me. In Germany the carters often heap so much on their carts, either out of greed or for some other reason, that if the paving is only slightly bad in towns and villages, the carts either break or, before anybody can take action, lose their balance and tip over. In the former case the cart is often dragged along for some distance, spectators congregate, and in spite of apparent caution, these are sometimes surprised and injured. A few years ago such a defective, enormous freightcar drove through Bruchsal hoping to reach a certain destination; suddenly the car collapsed, overturned, and crushed a child who had been quietly walking next to it.

For the sake of the roads, excessively loaded freightcars are not permitted everywhere, but with a view to public security it would be desirable to allot safer ways for such immense loads than an often narrow road that is always full of people. If the layout of the town is such that similar carloads cannot pass through the crowds, care must be taken that the carters at least are exhorted at the gates to the greatest caution, and especially if the wheels, axles, etc., are defective, they must be made to stop and not continue their journey until the danger is completely eliminated, even if they deny its existence. And while such work is in progress, the owner and the craftsmen who have been called must be under the most stringent responsibility to remove the inquisitive spectators in time [to prevent further accident].

§28

Possibility of a needed improvement of the carts

If our vehicles could be made altogether safer, however, many thousands of persons would be protected from terrible accidents which threaten them on their continuous journeys because of the unsafe construction of the vehicles and the intractability of the draft animals. The attempts of mechanics must therefore be of the greatest importance, here too, and every new invention should be examined without prejudice; even if the ultimate purpose were not achieved, at least the inventor would be encouraged. Wiehem, an art expert, is reported by public journals in 1771 to have invented a very simple machine which can be affixed to all kinds of vehicles; with its aid the horses can be released instantly if they shy. If this invention, as seems quite possible, passed the examinations successfully, its introduction would certainly be of public advantage. But what means are there to stop a vehicle running downhill, even if the shying horses are released?

No matter how great the force of a body put into such violent motion may be, it would show ignorance of the forces of mechanics if one doubted the possibility of prevailing over them. In this matter some artisans have already made their contribution; however, much time passes before such inventions are simplified to such an extent that they become generally applicable. Here there would be a good opportunity for some learned academies of arts and sciences to exchange the frequently occurring prize questions, quite irrelevant to mankind, such as the shape of an old shoe and similar important subjects, for some others for whose solution their medal could well not be too heavy.

* * *

§29
Necessary supervision over public vehicles

That public vehicles, carters' vehicles, and hackney carriages should be subject to police supervision, is indubitably of much concern to the safety institutions. What I have to say on this subject is based on the consideration of the dangers to which the public is exposed because of the carelessness and negligence of those rough people, the carters. If the hackney carriages are ramshackle, their straps and hinges half rotten, the axles and wheels made from bad wood, half cleft or only superficially repaired, the fittings and doors badly, or not at all, maintained, all other precautions are of no use. The police, therefore, must have all the hackney carriages in large cities examined meticulously at the places allotted to them by judicious craftsmen with respect to their durability, and those that are found defective and unsafe, must be forbidden to convey anybody, near or far, and thus expose him to danger. It would only be just that every hackney driver be responsible for injuries and damage to those using his vehicle through his fault, and moreover, if negligence would be proved in this important service to the public, he should also expect an adequate punishment.

§30
The number of persons who are crippled or even killed by careless driving and horse racing in large cities is considerable. It would seem that in a city such as Paris, which is otherwise so well policed, this important part of public safety would not be lacking, and yet here, regardless of all police regulations, any fop, if he can only let himself be driven about in a carriage, may consider himself entitled to grandly run down any creature who is lowly to him who has to use his legs in order to get from one place to another, even if it were a Rousseau! . . . The number of accidents occurring every year due to this cause in that capital is incredibly large and exactly in proportion to the stupid contempt which many affluent persons feel toward the poorer class of their brethren. A hundred poor lose their lives every year under wheels.* In Vienna, on the other hand, despite the considerable traffic of carriages

---

* Tableau de Paris, T. I, p. 37. This number is much larger than that given by a traveling Frenchman whom I shall quote later.

driving to the Prater, there is no disorder due to this. The pedestrians have their special paths on which no driver may drive. The bridge between Leopoldstadt and the Prater, where the crowding is greatest (sometimes as many as 1200 to 1500 carriages [a day]), is divided into four parts. The outer two are reserved for pedestrians, one of the inner parts for carriages entering, and the other for carriages leaving. This order is observed through the forest, and on the thoroughfare, through the suburb, and in the city itself. Several dragoons with bared sabres see to that. On public festivities, no special accidents are known to happen here, and all the accidents and all the harm done here by carriages happen in the daily bustle of the city. Nobody can recall that more than seven persons were killed in one year by being run over, whereas in Paris the number of those killed per year was on the average twenty in the last ten years.*

The police, therefore, must pay attention to this matter and prevent certain malpractices, so that by ceaseless attention dangers caused by careless charge of animals be averted and so as to block that source of public insecurity and maintain the lives of useful citizens.

§31

Most of these accidents happen in cities because people and animals intermingle more closely there and cannot always get out of the way quickly enough when crowded. In a large city, where the streets are daily as full of people as occurs in small towns only on the occasion of the annual fair, there is no end of a din. A pedestrian, regardless of the calls of cold-blooded drivers, is in constant danger of being run down and broken alive by the wheels of the hundred hurriedly passing carriages. The police, therefore, does well, as has already been introduced in several cities, especially in Italy, to raise and pave a footpath for the people walking up and down, so that riding and driving in the lower and wider road can safely take place.

* * *

§32

Because of fast driving and horseback riding, the strictest order must be maintained. In London one hardly sees phaetons, cabriolets and similar vehicles which fly like a bullet most dangerously along a road. Only carriages drawn by two, three or four horses are usual. In Paris the police sentenced Antoine Janton, who by fast riding had struck down a man and a woman and thus had injured them, to be publicly put in the pillory and a notice put on his chest on which his offense should be written; on 5 December 1731 this sentence was confirmed by order of the parliament [principal judicial court]. However, this example did not have a great effect.** In the meantime,

---

* Letters by a Traveling Frenchman in Germany, V. I, p. 383.
** Louis XV once said: "If I were head of police in Paris, I would forbid the cabriolets altogether . . ."
Tableau de Paris," T. I. p. 37.

according to public notice in 1783, this dangerous use of cabriolets has been prohibited in Paris, and only merchants are permitted to use them, but these must be marked by numbers.* In Vienna, the matter was brought to the notice of the police in 1772 by an accident to the Hungarian Bishop of the House of Steilfurt, who was crushed to death by a dainty carriage. The young driver of the carriage wanted to make honorable amends for his fault by making out an annuity to the sisters of the unfortunate prelate. Joseph II was not quite satisfied with this compensation, and ordered the improvident man to pay another 2,000 ducats to the hospital in Prague, remain at home until further orders and never drive a vehicle in the Austrian states. At the same time it was ordered "that nobody, no matter of which class, be permitted to ride or drive in towns except at walking pace, under heavy penalty."**As late as April 1777 an old man in Vienna was run over and killed by an Italian count who gave his shortsightedness as an excuse. Recently, according to public notice, a regulation concerning fast driving has been issued in Munich. It says that when the master and his family are in the carriage, it should be driven only at medium trot; but if the carriage is empty, the horses should constantly only pace. Carriages drawn by four horses, whether with the master or without him, should be permitted to drive at a walk only. The drivers must be strictly exhorted to call pedestrians in time so that they can give way, or stop altogether if they are old persons or children. Infringement is punishable by arrest and corporal punishment; moreover, the master is also responsible for damage done.† In and near the residential city of Dresden, fast driving and riding in the streets, through the gates, and past the guards is forbidden to everybody, no matter to which class he belongs. On the other hand, the pedestrians are also advised that as soon as they see and hear carriages and riders approach, especially if someone calls to them, they should go to the side of the road and not deliberately stop immediately, especially when the carriages turn.†† However, the drivers usually give as their excuse that they have called and it seems that this additional stipulation only causes confusion. Furthermore, many persons are hard of hearing or the noise is so great that one cannot distinguish the voice of the caller.

Drivers in large cities stake their honor on passing close to each other's carriage without touching, or taking corners with outstanding dexterity. If moreover the deleterious habit has been introduced that when four horses draw a carriage, the leading horses are harnessed far from the wheelers, the carriage often takes up a large stretch of the road, or the leading horses are already in another street before

---

* "Ffrter. Reichszeit," 1783. 46.
** "Journal encyclopédique," Janvier 1772. Since then, nevertheless, I have seen that carriages in Vienna drive about as fast as elsewhere, and I am surprised that not more people suffer injuries than actually do.
† "Erfurter Reichspostamtszeit.," 1780, No. 112.
†† Pal. of 17 April 1728, 17 August 1731, 4 August 1742, 12 April 1770.

the driver comes around the corner and is able to distinguish that people or children are thus being crowded. It would be desirable, therefore, that the drivers be advised to drive at a slow pace, especially at street corners, not to overtake another driver, and in general carriages drawn by four, not to harness the horses further from each other than necessary to prevent the lead horses from injuring the wheelers by kicking. Altogether, strict order must be introduced in regard to the carriages making way in towns and on highways, for lacking this, it often leads to great disputes and accidents. This subject for long has been given attention. The Saxon provincial law says: "The empty carriage shall give way to the full, the least loaded vehicle to the heavy one. The rider shall give way to the carriage and the pedestrian to the rider. But if they are on a narrow path or on a bridge. and a rider or a pedestrian are chased, the carriage shall stop until they have passed. The carriage that entered the bridge first shall pass it first, be it empty or loaded."* Instruction for drivers and carters couched in clear terms and explained to everybody are very necessary in every country.

* * *

---

* Lib. II. Art. 59. The laws and regulations belonging here can be found in Feltmann," Diss. Acad. de vehiculis obviis," Struv. in "Jurisprud. forens. Roman. German," L. II, T. 3, §8.—Ferd. Harprecht, "Tractat, jurid. de Jure Aurigarum," 1739.—Urban. Levin. Gabriel.—Luedecke, "S.R.I. Princeps, Politiam circa commercia & studia civium fuorum rite adornans," Goett. 1746. §17. p. 102.

PART ONE
Section Two

On injuries through accidents by water and fire, etc.

* * *

§5

Of floods and the aid necessary during them

As every year so many persons and animals are the victims of floods and are carried away by waves that unexpectedly sweep over inhabited places and drown in the most pitiful manner, the country police cannot choose any worthier subject of their attention than the prevention of these terrible occurrences in the threatened regions.

On the other hand, what can be done is proved by Holland which is built so-to-say beneath the seacoast. There, warned by the terrible flooding of a large stretch of land, all human ingenuity and immense sums are expended constantly for the maintenance of firm dams and bulwarks the damaging of which carries even the death penalty, and at the slightest indication of danger from the water entire provinces are mobilized to prevent the imminent disaster.

The regions most exposed to the danger of flooding are those which, either like Holland, are lying on low ground, close to the sea, or which have large rivers, streams, creeks, close by rising on snowy mountains, or which are in narrow valleys surrounded by mountains over which the water plunges down when the snow melts, or after cloudbursts, without having immediately sufficient space for discharge. The many dykes which are maintained in a valley region either break during such floods, or the badly maintained dams are breached and abandon the lower-lying villages to the waters.

Measures must be taken in good time against all these causes. Of course, a country that is almost alone in possession of a large river can do more than when the river is flanked by several principalities. It is terrible to see the devastation caused by the otherwise tranquil Rhine at a time when the snow begins thawing rapidly in the Swiss Alps in some years, and what immense sums of money and how much labor are wasted, only because all the Rhine regions have such different rulers, and their measures are so contradictory that some reasonable defense against the common enemy can never take place. Instead, every rampart erected on one side is regarded on the other bank as an attack, and as such it is destroyed by the more powerful neighbor, and moreover, the communities in addition to the loss of property, are embroiled in bloody fighting as well. If there were greater unity and readiness for agreements, millions could be saved and the lives and fortunes of righteous citizens preserved.

Without dealing here with the rules that the hydraulic experts may be expected to promulgate, according to which dams and the banks of dangerous lakes and rivers have to be protected, I only want to point out the necessity of cleaning the river beds and lake bottoms and to excavate them. The bottoms of flowing waters must be prevented from being clogged and filled up by rubbish thrown into the water. Ice accumulating in roads and houses near the water has to be hacked away in time. At different places, especially in towns and low-lying apartments, which are more exposed to danger, several sufficiently large drainage ditches have to be dug. Locks have to be constantly kept in good repair. Mills, bridges, and steps above such waters have always to be laid out with a view to preserving the freedom of flow of the river. The number of dykes in the valleys has to be reduced, and even when the first human habitations are planned, there the dangers of the water must not be left out of account.

In addition to that, neighboring villages exposed to the danger of flooding should cooperate and arrange certain signs with which to announce present or immiment danger. As soon as these signs are made, they should lend assistance to each other without delay. Prizes should be set out for the saving of weak and pregnant women, children, old men, sick persons, etc. At certain places a number of boats and barges should be kept with which assistance could come to people and cattle overtaken by water, etc.

* * *

§7

Saving of people when fire breaks out

Inasmuch as I considered sufficiently the dangers of water, as far as seems indicated, I must also examine the dangers which threaten human society in regard to life and health through fire. I do not speak here of the necessity of good fire brigades the founding of which in our days is the primary task of the police, and which has considerably reduced the number of those unfortunate ones whom this element has robbed of their fortunes, but it seems that in the important endeavor of saving buildings from complete destruction, too little effort has been expended on saving the persons exposed to the fire.

As fire often breaks out in the interior of buildings and causes havoc before persons, either asleep or living in the upper stories, are aware of the danger, they are often prevented from saving themselves because the stairs are on fire, or they have to jump with their families through the flames or through high windows into the paved street, which is almost as dangerous to them as the fire. Very often timidity and fear, sometimes illness, too great or too young age, stupefaction due to terror or suffocating smoke, etc., make the unfortunate unable to avail himself even of this means of saving himself. Desperation grips the abandoned whose whimpering and cries of fear are largely smothered by the crackling of the flames, the collapse of the burning beams, and the noise made by the populace rushing to put out the fire.

It seems to me to be very desirable to appoint everywhere certain persons whose only task with the fire brigade would be the saving of trapped persons. Without this arrangement one either relies too much on the other or too many persons, under the reigning disorder, expose themselves to danger and leave their other posts. But if some citizens are specially appointed who have no other task in case of a conflagration except extricating persons, and when these are saved, also to look after domestic animals, the remaining congregated persons can busy themselves with extinguishing the fire, and the police may be relieved that this important part of the care necessary in such cases has not been neglected.

These special rescuers should be selected from a suitable craft, if possible from the guild of the joiners or bricklayers, etc. They should be provided with distinguishing markings so as not to be hindered by anybody in the execution of their duty and they should be provided by the police with all the tools necessary for the rescue of persons . . . Very simple and light clothing that could resist the fire for some time would enable the rescue-men to brave the flames even more. And, moreover, if an award would be given for the rescue of a person from such dangers, one could certainly hope for immense benefit from such an appointment.

* * *

§11

Dangers of hunts

At great public hunts, which are still current in Germany and to which the populace comes from faraway places and in crowds out of curiosity, many spectators often take up a position where they are exposed to the bullets of the marksmen, and from such improvidence they are often injured or even killed by them. Thus, here too, the eye of the police is indispensable, and the great act irresponsibly if they either do not prevent the idle crowd from attending these pursuits of animals altogether, since they are anything but edifying, or if they do not stipulate and stake out a certain place for the spectators whose transgression would be punished on the spot by guards; and they must instruct the marksmen not to shoot in the direction of the spectators.

The same precautions should be taken during military manoeuvers or during routine shooting exercises of the garrisons in spring. These always attract large crowds, and especially foolhardy boys who, in order to get hold of unburnt cartridges, come far too close to the firing, or who by heedless pushing forward, are often gravely injured when the corps carries out unexpected turns.

May I, in the name of the poor people, beg of the masters of forests and hunts, to better protect their lives during the driving of game or in the so-called battues? The brutality of the hunters and their carelessness in employing negligent marksmen has cost many a poor peasant, the provider of a dependent family, his life. Is it not enough, then, that these unfortunate persons must leave their work in the fields for weeks on end, in order to drudge for the pleasure of their fellow men while subsisting on nothing more than bread and water? . . . Is it then necessary that an unfortunate act of negligence and gross disdain of this useful class endanger their lives so often! I knew a canon who was an ardent marksman and who lauded his shotgun so much that when a peasant had been shot in a battue, without the perpetrator being known, he gave himself out as the one who must have shot the peasant since none of the other shotguns present could have hit at such a long distance. This he did merely to save the honor of his firelock!—If this was a means of generously indemnifying the unfortunate or his family, and to contest the right of others to this merit, it was a way of somewhat alleviating a very bad thing. But on the whole, when a few peasants at hunts are shot, there is at some German courts still such unconcern to this which does not all redound to the honor of mankind.

* * *

§13

Dangers of chemical laboratories

Laboratories of chemists, alchemists, apothecaries, materialists [grocers] and others may be dangerous to passersby and to the entire vicinity if experiments are made in a certain careless manner. It has happened several times that such workers were gravely injured or even killed upon unexpected explosions, and that part of the laboratory was blown up over quite a distance as if by a mine. The dangers in connection with the spoiling of the atmosphere, and the increased danger of fire, I have mentioned elsewhere, and as regards poisonous preparations which are often made ready by such laboratory workers, measures are necessary of which I shall speak in another article. The police thus determines the disposition and position of such laboratories. It sees to it that their owners choose a place far from the highway, where it must have free access of air. It orders the greatest possible cleanliness. The walls and chimneys must be fireproof. And the workers must be instructed to carry out their experiment carefully and to be responsible for damage which they might cause through negligence.

* * *

PART ONE
Section Three

Of injuries by dangerous games, of sleepwalkers, insane persons, etc.

§1

Disadvantage of too serious a police administration

In the third volume of this work, I demonstrated how necessary it is that the police should make it its business to provide human society with every opportunity of innocent entertainments and amusements, and that one would have a very bad opinion of this supervisor of the citizens if one imagined that the police, always with irons in hand, banning all the natural freedom of man, had to seek its honor by lording it over slaves. This strange opinion of the duties of the police administrators has the regrettable consequence that the public, instead of feeling grateful to the fatherly care of its protector, expresses the greatest aversion to everything that is called police, and considers as nothing all the good that the police provides for him against the tyranny of his impetuous judgments. Like those stubborn parents who rule their children with an iron rod and thus extinguish in them every spark of natural love for them, the obstinacy of the police superintendent, under the pretense of good order, draws upon himself the hatred of the entire nation which finds itself ill-treated by a few men chosen from among its midst. A father who is too strict does not bring up good children, and a sultanic government may be certain that the public, which trembles at the sound of its chains, will at the first opportunity permit themselves more than the most untamed rabble of a free country. Just look at the wise government of the Romans, a nation which as regards might and prudence did not have its equal on earth! How careful was the government to make every citizen forget that he lived under strict laws! How many kinds of feasts, plays, and other public spectacles were not only permitted to the people, but even arranged at the expense of the republic! . . . And now, how gloomy do the people look at the most philanthropic governments. How hypochondriacally do entire nations drag themselves under the huge number of unattractive, but oh, salutary laws!

§2

Yet no matter how necessary pleasure and amusement are for persons living in society, none of these should be deleterious to public morals and peace, and a prudent

222

police must be able everywhere to promote calm and moderation. Good morals especially must have the greatest influence on popular amusements, and the enlightenment of the citizens must be obvious from their pleasures. All plays, all pastimes which entail dangers to the actors or to the spectators cannot have much attraction for a cultured people, and if still here and there too strong a shadow, and a hankering for cruel amusements shows in the features of a society, it is the duty of the police to quietly erase this shortcoming in the mentality of a nation and to substitute more humane amusements.

§3

Of animal fights

A pastime which would be more worthy of animals than men is the bullfight, and animal fights altogether. I am not at all surprised that such spectacles which so dishonor mankind still meet with the approval of the Spaniards. Who can quietly snooze during an auto-da-fé, may of course listen unperturbed and without compassion while his fellow creatures around him howl with pain. But it has always been incomprehensible to me that the gentle Viennese still lack all human feelings to such an extent that they storm in crowds to animal chases in order to enjoy the bloodbath of innocent creatures. And just as incomprehensible to me is it that the wise police can close their eyes to this. I know, the Roman principle was to imbue the people with a martial spirit by such spectacles. It is not unknown to me that a Roman lady at a real fight between human beings which was usual in Rome, was offended that a dying gladiator gave up his ghost in too effeminate a position. However, did the heroism of the Romans ever gain anything from such inhuman games? I must be permitted to doubt this. Constantine, at least, did not share this opinion, and this probably does more honor to the Christian faith than to the heart of this emperor, who would not really shrink back from a human bloodbath . . . However, it was not so easy for Constantine to put an end to the spectacle of the gladiators in Rome. Even the imperial guards and a class of soldiers hired themselves out for these inhuman games. Finally in 361 Constantine forbade them this dishonorable trade with their own blood. He decreed a penalty of 6 pounds of gold for persuading and luring someone to such a fight, but whoever freely offered himself for such a purpose was to be put in chains. In Tuscany, at Pisa, there were up to our times less bloody fights which, nevertheless, never passed off without injuries. The citizens were divided into two parties, and half the town went to fight the other half, both armed according to old custom. Long before the event, both sides enlisted friends and helpers. Even the nobility took part in the honor of being permitted to break their necks mutually, although there was no lack of police laws prohibiting most strictly all use of cutting and pointed weapons. In time the matter became so serious that one Pisan looked at another with such disdain and attacked so ferociously in the fight as he would hardly do against a real enemy in our time. Provided with helmets and weapons they took up positions, party against party, at the very beautiful marble bridge over the Arno. Each man chose his adversary, and then each fought the other as well as he could, until one of them was defeated and had to capitulate to the other. But this often did not happen until substantial, and sometimes lethal, injuries prevented further fighting; then the defeated party under frequent humiliations had to recognize his victor publicly and extol his triumph.

One can imagine that this arrogant behavior of the victors had to incite the defeated to revenge. In fact quarrels which were more ferocious than the fighting games themselves often followed among the citizens. Even the women of the two parties had their crosses to bear, since their parents, brothers, and brothers-in-law often had served with the opposite party, and belonged either to the proud victors or to the base crowd of the worst half of the town, and consequently were despised or hated, and reproaches were heaped on them. Elsewhere fighting games were held on the water, and these also had the saddest consequences. Finally, much to their chagrin, the present grand duke forbade the Pisans this wild fighting game, which had such unfortunate consequences and bred continuous enmity among the burghers of one and the same town and lost many of them their lives. That is also why Fabroni wrote against this cruel custom with all his fire. Only in 1785, when the King of Naples arrived, did the grand duke permit this ancient fighting game to be again enacted once, but with all due moderation.

All such games, even if they do not entail bodily injury, and even animal fights, leave in the minds of the spectators an impression which is not to the good of mankind. He who can coldbloodedly watch the sufferings of an animal and fellow creature, without having more to expect than delight from its death, need make only one more step to remain unfeeling to even the wailing of his fellow men, and society should take good care to repair such an attitude as much as possible. Therefore Apollonius Tyanensis already heaped the gravest reproaches on the people of Alexandria for their great passion for horseracing, at which it often occurred that the participants threw stones at each other or fought each other with swords, and thus, for the sake of idle pastime, shed human blood.*

* * *

§8

Nocturnal noise

Altogether, quiet for the public should be respected at night more than is done at present, and roaming idlers should be forbidden to make any noise which robs the citizens, who return tired from work, of the necessary sleep, and the poor sick who so longingly seek an hour of quiet or have already found it, and who are without any regard, being disturbed or startled. In Italy nocturnal commotion can perhaps be more easily forgiven, because there people only go visiting late in the evening

* Fleury, "Hist. Ecclesiast.," T. I. Lib. 2, p. 238.

and because in summer the fierce heat altogether forces people to turn night into day. However, it is not the going hither and thither of the people or the rumble of the carriages which annoys the people who are used to this way of life; in most streets there is often such noise at night as would not be permitted in daytime. In the Milan region also this was settled a short time ago, although at night some guns are still being fired, which in Germany would bring together half the town. The robbers, therefore, make a play of it, for nobody takes heed of a call for help, since people may indulge in this for their pleasure.

* * *

In Section Four Frank deals in great detail with accidents caused by violent weather (lightning) and earthquakes, as well as with protective measures which may be taken.

PART ONE
Section Five

On injuries caused by enraged, harmful animals

* * *

After §1 in which Frank has dealt in general with man's attitude toward animals, he gives examples of how dangerous some animals (pigs, rats, vipers, and wolves) can be, and discusses the measures taken by people in various countries to protect themselves against these dangers. In this matter, he also touches upon hunting, and addresses the following impressive appeal to the great:

§7

Appeal to the great

The establishment of great hunts in Germany, of which I have already spoken in another connection, deserves to be mentioned again. How dearly has mankind to pay for the pleasure of its gracious sovereigns who have their poor subjects forced by merciless hunters, at the threat of a thousand permitted abuses, to expose their lives to the fury of stags and wild boars that are to be locked up. It happens very often that the poor defenseless peasant who is doing the beating, after having had to leave his field for weeks, is impaled or cut down. When will the great finally get to know and respect the rights of mankind! . . . But perhaps we come closer to the happy time when several regents follow the example of the German Emperor, who by limiting the harmful game, endeavors to secure, in addition to economic advantage, the safety of the diligent peasant. I have never, when in the Palatinate, in the Zweybrücken, the Saarbrücken, the Darmstadt, Speyer and other regions, and formerly (for the philanthropic Margrave of Baden has long since abolished this nuisance) in Baden-Baden, watched without aching compassion in the fall, when the harvest began to ripen, the tired subjects who watched all night and cried to each other; in that way they endeavored to keep the harmful animals in their forests. Here the poor peasant, the abandoned one, who had to work hard on hot days, perhaps because he had to do homage to his sovereign, and was bathed in sweat, now on cool autumn nights, lies at the fire which is to help him keep the game away, clothed in a thin, torn, linen smock, and in order to preserve a little grain for his children, often exposes himself to catching a cold which may be the cause of his death, or, and I know of examples of this, he is attacked by stags, or especially wild boars, which he has to chase from his field without any weapons, in order to preserve his painfully acquired property, and often miserably loses his life, or is at least maimed. . . . My God! . . . Why does the subject pay all this money to the lord if not to secure his property and life under the protection of his sovereign? . . . One should not believe that the nocturnal watches of peasants against the all-destroying game are only a minor cause of all the rheumatic, bilious, putrid dysenteries and bad autumn diseases among them!—No, these watches last for weeks on end, at a time that is most critical for health, and it affects so many people that in many villages which lie near forests, often everybody must turn out to watch at night, and thus a considerable number of subjects may be sacrificed for the sake of the pleasure of merely a few great persons. In the Austrian Emperor's hereditary countries the philanthropic decree, dating from Emperor Joseph II, was recently renewed. According to it, noblemen have to keep their wild boars in enclosures, and the peasants are permitted to kill these animals if they encounter them on their land.

* * *

PART TWO

Of deliberate infringements of public security in general

In nature every living creature takes care, according to laws hidden in its mechanism, to provide for its own preservation. Temper and eagerness to defend themselves are allotted to many animals in order to protect them in case they are endangered by others, and to fortify their well-being.

Usually the mutual anger ceases when either the ultimate purpose has been achieved or, conversely, there seems no hope of achieving it. The most important causes of animal disputes are hunger, thirst, a pleasant dwelling place, and love. Every living creature seeks to assert its right of satiating its instincts, even if this seems to entail general harm.

In human beings, these otherwise inevitable passions have become more dangerous for the race since the epoch of civilization. Now man no longer fights a short battle for a river bank rich in fish, for forests where the hunting is good, fights in which the weaker, without the potent stimulant of a feeling of honor, gave up as soon as he recognized the victor, still retaining the hope of enforcing his own will elsewhere against even weaker ones than himself. Just as in the first days of spring, when the happy herds leave and their bulls fight each other with terrifying violence for the prerogative of love, and then, when the fight is over, concede the victor rank and choice for the rest of the year, likewise the weak among human beings, first with grief, later willingly, gave in to the stronger, and looked round for another maiden when the stronger had cast his victorious glance at his maiden.

Now a special constitution and the most unfortunate concepts of honor have changed everything and have armed one half of mankind against the other half. Poison, dagger, and fire have now to be in readiness, at the beck and call of imagination when the human heart's exaggerated sensitivity creates for itself injuries, and when one word causes entire provinces to be destroyed and dyed by streams of human blood. I have said it earlier: even the ennobling of love between the sexes, which in other animals does not go beyond the physical, resulted in a greater degree of morality, through the sociable life at the time of the first people. But it could not but increase considerably the inner disquiet of their minds and the quarrelsomeness of those yearning for the fair ones, and thus greatly reduce the security of the weakest suitor, etc.

But, when I consider in general the injury to health or life which one human being inflicts deliberately on another or on himself, I find that poisoning of various kinds, fist fights, stabbings and shootings, suicide, secret removal of one's enemies, damage to them through superstititon and prejudices deleterious to health, deserve the greatest attention of the police. Elsewhere I have already dealt with deliberate faults in the use of foodstuffs, with means of abortion which so often degenerate into tools of murder, and with the weakness of despairing unmarried mothers which induces them to murder their own fetuses.

PART TWO

Section One

Of injuries by applied poison

§1

On poisoning in general

Of unintentional poisoning I spoke in another part; here I want to deal with the intentional endeavor of eliminating one's enemy quietly with the aid of deadly poisons. Poisoning or executing a person by the quiet administration of some small dose of a very dangerous agent, hidden under others, is so easy and requires so little courage of the murderer that any vile and malicious soul must be all the more ready to use it, the more difficult it is to detect the culprit and to convict him of his evil deed.

§2

They used to be more frequent

There was a time when poisonings were one of the main occupations of courtiers, and history teaches that these decreased only when the Asiatic way of life on the part of the regents was replaced by a manly feeling of their rights to mankind and of the forces, allowed by mankind itself, to support their pre-eminence, and also when the sciences began moderating the darkness and wildness which befogged the minds of powerlusting subjects and those who obeyed them, who could still imagine that they served the state or religion when, with the cup of poison in their hand they murdered princes who had the misfortune not to judge the world according to their own light. It is known that among ancient nations, just as is done by some of the Americans, hunters used poisoned arrows to kill wild animals. Many permitted themselves to use poisoned weapons even against their human enemies, whereupon death was certain to follow. The cup of poison was the usual punishment for those who displeased the prince, and all of history is full of the frequent use of poisoning in ancient times. As long as Rome adhered to its innocent customs, little was heard of poisonings; but closer acquaintance with its depraved neighbor introduced this evil, too, as can already be attested to in the laws of the Twelve Tables, introduced 304 years after the foundation of the town. Not until 20 years later, under Valerius Flaccus and M. Claudius Marcellus, did a society of noble women for the first time engage in mixing poison; a large number of unexpected and unusual deaths among all classes of the inhabitants occurred which filled the city with terror. A female slave who knew of the secret revealed it. The poisoners wanted to pass off their concoctions as medicines; twenty of them were forced by the authorities to try them out themselves and to devour their concoctions themselves. They all died of their experiment; their assistants, 170 in number, were immediately arrested and received their deserved punishment. About 200 years after this terrible occurrence the Republic again had cause to take action against spreading poisonings. Then Lucius Cornelius Sulla drafted the well-known law (L. Cornelia "De Veneficis") according to which poisoning met with the same punishment as other murder. The Council even decided to punish by banishment from the country those who, though not intending to kill, gave a woman with lethal effect medicines to speed up birth. Immediately afterward the punishment according to Cornelius' law was also extended to those who, under the guise of a cleansing or purgative drug, advised the taking of suspect medicines or herbs. On the other hand, the 8th law stipulated that governors should condemn to banishment also those women who took similar drugs in order to abort their children prematurely.

It can be seen from these laws that poisoning in ancient Rome was nothing rare. This may well be the same in the history of most nations which gave up their original innocent way of life for alien vices, and combined ignorance with cruelty, two popular properties that are usually connected with each other.

§3

Decrease

Enlightenment among people, a better concept of religion, and natural duties banished to a certain extent this vice from the world. But it was not abolished completely, so that a more thorough examination of the various poisoners' skills, which came down to us from dark centuries, could be dangerous. Krünitz maintains that knowledge of poisons is of variable use to the entire state, especially to the peasant. He says: "Instead of unjustly accusing the physicians, who spread the knowledge of poisons among people, of irresponsibility, their philanthropic hearts should be appreciated. They should be thanked for their efforts, by which so many righteous citizens are saved for the state, and the health and lives of others are maintained. They should be commended and the state should endeavor to promote the successful progress of their work by powerful support and joint participation in it. Would it not be worth the effort if the authorities, who have to provide for the good of the state, even if they do not deal with the entirety, at least made provisions that every citizen of the state be acquainted with either all poisonous products of his country or with all the poisonous plants, since these are similar to foodstuffs and thus may cause the greatest calamities? How many accidents could have been prevented by such a measure, and how many could still be prevented in future! Besides, knowledge of poisons is also useful to the state in order to unmask the long-hidden wickedness of its unworthy members, which rages in the dark, and, on the other hand, to save the accused and oppressed innocence and absolve it, to eradicate deleterious and shamefully ingrained prejudices and to stop up their source."* Mr. Krünitz also endeavors to prove his sentence by the provision that peasants may derive much advantage from the knowledge of poisons, with regard to their animals, or the extermination of harmful predators, insects, etc.

Though these are weighty reasons, nevertheless, I do not concur in this opinion without reservations. Of course, once the generally known main poisons, such as arsenic and caustic quicksilver, are accurately known as to their effects and properties, not so much that is worse can be learned, and perhaps no deadlier substance may be expected. However, I believe that one should proceed with the utmost caution in the practical solution of such important problems. If in the accurate description of poisons and all their properties we would not have to admit publicly so often that one or the other among them does not leave any discernible trace of its effect and may kill quite unnoticed; if we would not have to say so often that against this or that poison there is no known remedy; if the generally known poisons would be sufficient to satisfy completely all economic and agricultural purposes; if it were possible by closer acquaintance with all poisonous plants to achieve their destruction on a large scale, etc., I would not hesitate to agree without restriction. Since the opposite is true, however, I believe much caution is still indicated, at least in countries where murder is still in fashion, and I wish that works dealing in detail with the subject should be written in scientific language rather than in the people's language, as long as the police is not confident that it can prevent all misuse that can easily be foreseen. I am of the absolute opinion that it is good to warn the people against the ordinary poisons, and to describe them to impart the necessary knowledge. There is no doubt that many persons and animals can be saved if the surest way of combating poisoning is added. Yet a detailed treatise on poisons in popular language still seems to me to be a very questionable matter. Mere popular books on medicine have already caused so much harm that I shudder at the thought of a book on the art of preparing poisons written in popular language.

§4

Continuation of poisoning

I will therefore confine myself here to general considerations of this subject and not enter upon that which concerns the best antidotes which must be known not only to the police but also to physicians, and which should not be a secret to them because of the many writings on this subject.

In large and populous cities, where the most violent passions are more at home

* "Oeconom. Encyklop.," XVIII. p. 452–454.

than elsewhere, some persons die in a manner which leaves grave doubts as to the cause of their sudden death. It is said that in Paris some years ago poisoning, it seemed, became the fashion, and a number of physicians and surgeons were charged at the expense of the Court to examine all those who had died suddenly and without a physician being called, and to testify to the illness, and to report on it to the government.* In Italy, where poisoning is said to have been formerly more current,** one now hears little of it, whereas every year so many thousand persons die of dagger and knife wounds. Perhaps this is so because poisons are more the murder tools of noble people who, as far as I know, do not cherish murder more in Italy than in other countries. Yet perhaps some deeds are still committed on the quiet, and this is all the less reported, since even stabbing does not arouse attention among the people.

* * *

§5

Difficulty of preventive means

If it were possible to prevent the sale of all poisonous substances, poisonings would become much rarer, but as I said before, closer acquaintance with poisonous plants growing in each region may thwart caution with regard to sales of poison. In pharmacies and in ships selling spices, arsenic, caustic quicksilver, some quicksilver precipitates, and other chemical preparations are the most hazardous poisons. Unfortunately, some of these dangerous products are indispensable to some trades and arts; their sale, therefore, cannot be completely prevented. The police, therefore, can only draft in regard to these substances some cautionary measures concerning the buyers and sellers. As regards poisonous plants which grow wild near human abodes, special measures need to be taken.

§6

Restrictions on poison merchants

If anything is to be achieved in this important matter, the number of sellers of poisonous substances must be greatly reduced, so that it will be easier for the police to assume supervision. The sale of poison should therefore be entrusted to a few duty-bound men who are well acquainted with its effects, and it should be strictly forbidden to all middlemen, no matter how good their reputation. And since, in addition to physicians and apothecaries, other persons in the community deal with the chemical treatment of natural substances, the police must gather information on this too, record their names, situation, and way of life, so as to find the source immediately in case of calamity. Certainly, since the study of chemistry has become the favorite or fashionable activity of a large number of individual citizens, this science has made

* Ffrter. Zeit., 1777. No. 89.
** Renatae, "In Italia artes Veneficae, familiarius exercebantur."—Hahn, "Oratio de usu Venenorum in Medicina," p. 69.

giant strides because of the contributions of so many collaborators, and this zeal deserves to be encouraged by the authorities. But it must be admitted that in Europe this refinement of the taste for practical sciences caused an increase in the number of those who may and do without constraint busy themselves with the preparation of poisonous substances. It may be rightly said, therefore, that now there is a large number of poison factories which were previously unknown since such products were tolerated only in the hands of certain sellers. Of course, every citizen who feels a natural urge to such scientific activity and pursues it at his own expense, may be supposed to be honest and conscientious, but if it occurred to a malevolent citizen to carry out such work with evil intentions, and to concoct poisons for secretly selling them under the guise of learned investigations, what means would there be of distinguishing him from other and harmless workers? . . . One need have no knowledge of people not to allow for such a presumption. But assuming that the devotee of chemistry did not misuse his products, who guarantees the coarser persons, who often assist him in his work, or who guarantees us that even the most conscientious chemist is also a careful man who never permits himself some rashness or forgetfulness in the storage of his poisonous products, which would make it easy for some rogue to seize them to the detriment of society? Are not our apothecaries and druggists also honest and upright men, so that laws are needed only against them and not against others who engage in the same trade?

It can thus be seen that so far the police in many regions has not paid sufficient attention to an important subject, and that even in a noble occupation of the citizens, the police may find a significant subject of its care for public safety. Nobody in the republic, therefore, should be prevented from busying himself with the important field of chemistry, which is so useful; but nobody should be permitted to engage in chemical work without previous knowledge of the police and its permission, based on the known integrity and honest disposition of the devotee. On the other hand, the police should have an accurate list of all chemists of its region, their laboratories, the use to which their products are put, etc., and all precautions should be taken in regard to this class of people also, since there are such weighty reasons to apply these precautions to apothecaries and druggists.

* * *

PART TWO
Section Two

Of injuries in brawls, assassination, duels, suicide, etc.

§1

It was rightly stated that religion and education will contribute most if brotherly love and unity among mankind are to be enhanced. However, until these important shortcomings of so many persons are remedied, it is the duty of the police to think of other means to control the evil. I believe that I have already given very good advice for reducing the number of brawls that are often lethal, by proposing that the immoderate consumption of wine and brandy should be restrained, that neighboring villages should become better acquainted with each other, and that young men should become accustomed to not considering it an attack on their honor if a strange young man courts a maiden from their village. In the country, these are two of the most important causes of brawls, and even some manslaughter has not had any more important motive. In Italy, in addition to the very cheap wine, it is the passion for gambling, which among the peasantry and the rabble is incredibly great—especially in the Piedmont region, which is close to us—which causes a large number of deadly conflicts. However, here I want to mention various other things which may not seem to belong exactly to the field of Medical Police to those who have too limited an idea of this science.

* * *

After discussing the custom of carrying swords and firearms and the attendant dangers, Frank deals very completely with students' duels and the aggression which was prevalent in Italy at that time.

§5

Murders in Italy

It is a terrible truth that by daggers alone Italy loses every year more persons than France and Germany combined in perhaps ten years. Thanks to prudent measures by the government, this madness has decreased considerably in Austrian Lombardy, but there is still a long way to go before this will be completely eliminated, as I have learned from the many persons wounded by daggers and similar weapons who are admitted to the hospital in Pavia every year. On the other hand, the only nearby region, which is now under Sardinian rule, Lomellina, but still has the right to send its sick, like the province of Pavia, to the hospital here, supplies more wounded than perhaps all other regions which use this hospital. As late as 20 April 1788, the respected Count of Crema was murdered in the Venice region by a pistol shot in broad daylight, on a public highway, close to the city, while sitting next to two ladies with whom he had gone for a drive. The presumably hired assassin retired after he had done his deed, without robbing anybody or without asking for anything but the death of the victim. In Lucha, a very small free state, about 60 persons are murdered annually. In the nearby Genoa and Piedmont regions, things are unfortunately similar, and one cannot but regret that such a nation is still so close to barbaric times in this respect. When in 1787, I was in Turin for some time, I had the opportunity of revealing to His Majesty the King how many of his subjects from Lomellina were annually admitted to the hospital in Pavia of which I was in charge with murderous stab wounds. Although an alien, I considered it my duty to bring to mind these atrocities, since I had such a desirable opportunity. To His Majesty, the situation of his subjects was not unknown; this good-natured prince, who was even so affable toward foreigners, had long since issued the best laws. However, so far, they had not been able to prevent the irascible people from committing annually 500 to 600 murders in all the royal states together. Even in Rome some time ago forty murders of this kind were committed in a mere 9 months, and what things look like in the Naples region is known from Archenholz, although his tales, here as everywhere else, should be taken with a grain of salt. In a single Neapolitan province with 447,465 inhabitants there are annually 500 murder victims.* In the Venetian states, the mischief is no less, and in the Papal state one cannot expect any better order either.** In Germany, there is quite a number of accidents due to brawls; however, the first move of an enraged peasant is to put away the knife which he may have had in his hand, and to tear off a chair leg or seize a bottle in order to attack his forewarned adversary, who is thus better able to defend himself. In this country, upon the slightest flaring up of the rabble, the first move is to grip the knife, which everybody carries on him in his trouser pocket, taking care that it is as pointed and as sharp as possible; and a mere controversy may be the cause of fatal injuries. Children 8 to

---

* Bartel's "Letters about Calabria and Sicily," Part I.
** Archenholz, on the other hand, says that knife wounds now are much rarer in the Papal state than in Genoa, Naples and Sicily. In Rome these murderous deeds are now mostly prevented by the strictness and watchfulness of the present governor of the city, Spinelli. As soon as it gets dark, the Sbirri have to patrol the streets, and they have the right to search the pockets of every commoner. If a knife is found, punishment by galley work is inevitable, even if the man in question, due to his class and character, is beyond suspicion. L.c. Section 7, Part. 4.

10 years old already feel this unfortunate impulse, and not so long ago, a wounded man was brought to the hospital in Pavia, who, upon exhortation by his father who was present, raised the murder knife against his adversary, but was felled by him before he could put his intention into effect.

It would be wrong to believe that this raving of the Italian people extends to all commoners. At least, I know of no instance where people of rank and education caused such scenes; it would be wrong, therefore, to impute this vice to the entire nation. In my opinion, the main reason is the incomprehensible ignorance in which the Italian country folk are brought up. Greater vivacity may of course have its share, but if such a common cause were the only reason, the evil would not be confined to certain countries and classes of people. The Italian rabble has no religion, no morals, and I believe that the main reason lies with the clergy who think too little of moral impressions, and sacrifice all instruction of this kind to idle dallying with religion. Moreover, the laws are usually too lax: as soon as a murder has been committed, the murderer escapes across the border. In many regions, the matter is only superficially investigated, and after a year or two, the culprit returns after he has lost part of his fortune, and then he lives quietly as before. Thus in some regions, murder represents part of the judges' income, and it is known that it is difficult to abolish such perquisites. But Austrian Lombardy, where there is now much less trouble than in the past, is proof that the frequent murders can be stopped in Italy just as well as in Germany. Even more conclusive proof is provided by the region of Brescia, however, of which there will be mention later on.

* * *

There follow examples of ordinances issued by various towns and countries against the carrying of arms.

Prevention of brawls   §6

Although it may be very dangerous sometimes to act as intermediary in serious quarrels, nevertheless it is the duty of every good citizen to prevent a very great evil, even if there is danger to himself, and to prevent murder or manslaughter. Even the Kalmuks have a law for this: "When people quarrel," it says, "and one is killed, all those who acted as idle onlookers are to pay a fine of one horse."*

It seems to me that in few places do the police safeguard those who are engaged in prevention. I know regions in the country where communities are so incensed against each other, that they only wait for a good opportunity such as parish fairs, holidays, etc., in order to choke the life out of each other. A person who would dare enter such company without having any authority, could easily be killed himself.

* Pallas, "Russian Journey," Vol. I. p. 264.

I know of a very honest and peace-loving peasant under Baden rule whose room was full of people who fought tooth and nail, with murder and death threatening. When the peasant realized that it was impossible to separate peacefully so many raging peasants, he decided to throw into the room and among the fighting men one of the beehives that were standing outside the window; these insects acted excellently in place of the most courageous policemen, and in less than five minutes all the peasants had fled through windows and door, and had also forgotten their grudge. However, without such presence of mind, what can one do with such raging combatants?

* * *

What is there to prevent the police from delegating on the spot their authority and power in all cases to the person who is first at dangerouus quarrels, or that a general law be enacted according to which any citizen is to be regarded as a member of the police in such situations, and that even the smallest disobedience, any resistance against or attack on him, would be punished in the same way as if they had taken place against the authority itself which could not always be called quickly enough? For why should not the authority of the not omnipresent police be delegated to any honest citizen in case of necessity?

* * *

§8
Of suicide

As regards suicide, there is little I want to call to mind: a disease cannot be punished, least of all on the dead, and the police cannot order anybody to be healthy unless it abolishes the causes which lead to this kind of insanity. I call it insane to endeavor to end one's days by force; however, great philosophers found a more beautiful name for it, and they collected all kinds of reasons in order to prove that one can reasonably put an end to all reason. I need not resolve this dispute, I side with those who value their lives, who know how to use life in every situation, and who are convinced that it is always worse to be a quitter knowing that one lives in the certainty of one's parting. Be that as it may, the police cannot but view suicide as an act that is very detrimental to the community, and even if the philosophers were right (of which I can convince myself as little as of their philosophy itself), the laws cannot possibly favor those who disdainfully tear up the bonds of society, and who may teach by their example that one may boldly challenge creation and curse one's existence, as soon as a violent passion, unpleasant sentiments, or mere boredom makes the post allotted to us by nature somewhat burdensome.

There were nations which excused suicide under certain circumstances, and which granted every citizen who was displeased with his situation in this world the release he demanded. In Marseilles, the authorities themselves kept a poison prepared from hemlock, which was given free of charge to those who had previously disclosed their motives to the Council of the Six Hundred.* When Sextus Pompeius left for Asia, he found on the island of Cea that a noble 90-year old lady, after having submitted to her fellow citizens the reasons for her having wearied of life, prepared for her violent death, and asked him to solemnize it by his presence. Many nations applied all possible leniency toward old and feeble persons who had wearied of life; however, there were also clever heads that realized that physical pain is not a reasonable cause for choosing death.

In view of all this, the ancient Romans did not punish suicide committed after some misfortune or out of weariness of life, and only the possessions of those were confiscated by the treasury who having committed some grave vice and fearing punishment, resorted to suicide after their crime had been taken to court. On the other hand, whoever did not carry out the suicide he had decided on and was prevented in it by others, was punished by death because he had judged himself.

Christian morality has gradually supplanted the abhorrent teaching of the Stoic sect, which the teaching of the wise Plato was unable to dislodge in Rome. Later it was established that suicides were to be deprived of a public funeral and were to be buried like cattle. This was called the burial of an ass (sepultura asinina), and since people were used to taking everything from the Scriptures, they referred to the prophet who said of King Jehoiakim: "They shall not lament for him, saying, Ah my brother! or, Ah my sister! They shall not lament for him, saying, Ah Lord! or, Ah his glory! He shall be buried with the burial of an ass, drawn and cast forth beyond the gates of Jerusalem."** As is known, Jehoiakim was still living then, and there was no question of suicide in his utterance. Thus, what the prophet threatened the depraved regent with was meted out to suicides. In Saxony, and in several other German provinces, suicides were not even removed by their domestic animals so that they could be buried: instead, they were lowered through the window.† In France, the suicide is deprived of burial, and if he should have already been buried, he is again exhumed; the corpse is dragged with a noose by the feet and taken to the knacker's yard. If the suicide is not found, at least his memory is branded.

Thus it can be seen at least according to our traditional notions, the relatives are punished rather than the dead; therefore, in some regions this custom was gradually abolished, and rightly so; possibly, as the Catholics do, the body was quietly buried at a separate (nonconsecrated) place. The worst was that the abhorrence of this crime went so far that nobody dared to cut loose such an unfortunate person as had hanged himself but still showed signs of life and to use on him the means which people had already learned to use on other accident victims (and if he had been saved, as was often possible, he may have repented his evil deed). People hoped that by such

* Mich. Montaigne, "Essai," Liv. II, p. 256.
** Jerem. XXII. 18, 19.
† J Casp. Bocrisius, "Dissert. de eo quod justum est circa sepulturam Propricidarum," Alttorf. 1760.

harshness of the laws, the living would take an example and be deterred from similar acts.

However, when a large number of the maidens of Miletus began to hang themselves, the inhabitants stopped this nonsense solely by burying the suicidal girls in the nude, with only the rope round their necks.* Long experience has shown, nevertheless, that only the beauties of Miletus, who probably suffered from some hysterical frenzy, were deterred by such a sentence after death and desisted from similar undertakings, and thus if the natural love of life does not prevent suicide, no lesser cause can ever prevent it. It is only right, therefore, that the police desist from such indecent punishment for these unfortunate beings who already paid dearly enough for their madness. The authorities should take all the more care, as far as it depends on them, to counter the causes of suicide. It is well known that in England suicide is very widespread, this being the consequence of an unfortunate state of mind which often affects the brightest heads of this enlightened country. It has even been noted that the passion for doing away with oneself is on the increase there. Whereas among 10,000 dead there were fewer than 10 suicides around 1690, around 1756 there were 19, i.e., almost 2 out of 1,000 and one out of 500 dead.** Under the more auspicious Italian sky, suicide is something very rare, just as duels are. This is proof that the ancient Romans committed suicide more because of a moral doctrine rather than because of physical reasons that affected their minds, and that these combined offenses are usually based on different concepts of the so-called strength of mind and of bravura. In France in recent times there has been a much larger number of suicides than one would expect among such a merry nation, which, by the way, so affects anglomaniacs that they copy the original exactly in this characteristic trait also. Germany, too, has its Werthers and unfortunately in our time suicide has become much more widespread. In Berlin in the course of 17 years, beginning in 1758, there were 45 such miserable ones among 81,133 dead, i.e., one out of 1,803. In Leipzig between 1759 and 1763 there were two suicides among 9.255 dead; and in the course of 11 years, from 1764 to 1774 there were 12 among 13,220 dead.†

Various causes were ascribed to this observation. If suicide were really a heroic act, it would prove that we Europeans come ever closer to such philosophy, and thus suicide would be a new scale on which our forces of reason would stand at an advantageous height compared with those of our fathers. But as long as the other proofs do not testify equally to our wisdom, a new argument could be derived from it, namely that all suicide is based more on a weakness of the mind and philosophical walking on stilts rather than true determination of a soul not bound to worldly things.

Closer examination of the causes disposing toward suicide may prove this sentence

* Aul. Gellius, "Noctes attic.," Lib. XV, c.X. Plutarchus, "De virtute Mulierum."
** Süsmilch, "Divine Order," Part I, p. 549.
† S. Baumann, in the new edition of Süsmilch's work on the Divine Order, Vol. 3, p. 246.

even more. I read a terrible letter written by a talented young man whom I knew, which he had written half an hour before he killed himself with a pistol shot. He recognized the horror of his impending deed, foresaw his virtuous father's desperation, deplored his fate which he was unable to resist, named the originator of his misfortune the source to which he referred being the cesspool of masturbation, and his teacher in this vice having already gone on that same path of desperation. Tissot described the state of mind of the lovers of self-abuse so masterfully that I need not explain why I ascribe a large part of the blame for the unbridled dissoluteness of youth and the increasing number of suicides to this spreading vice. I have already demonstrated elsewhere that most of the suicides are persons who live in celibacy. The chastity of this large class of people is so much exposed to suspicion that I do not want to ascribe to it such a terrible effect. Therefore, it follows that the celibate perhaps has an indirect effect on the suicides, enhanced by the additional effect of secret vices. This theory is strongly supported by data supplied through a true history of monasteries and convents.*

The gradual spreading of suicide was also ascribed to dramatic performances of the suicide as a hero. Of course, it may excite the imagination of excitable spectators, and one should be careful with such misrepresentations and not submit for applause examples of an act the imitation of which is so terrible. The eyes of the mass of weak people daily become better acquainted with the picture of suicide, full of admiration for a deed which makes an otherwise insignificant man appear important; now, they search for a similarity of their own suffering, and even at the slightest provocation, their sick souls easily fall prey to a quiet insanity which may cause in the most cowardly weakling a paroxysm of convulsive determination. However, the main causes of such confusion probably most often are the spreading vices which undermine health, gnaw at the conscience, and entail sadness and desperation. Irreligiousness, debauchery, and idleness, lavishness and its attendant unaccustomed misery, but especially the reading of poisonous novels are the most common causes of suicide, and if we disregard the cases of real illness, perhaps the only ones.

If the police wants to put a stop to this spreading taste for arbitrary shortening of life, it must, in addition to the effect, also fight the causes of this evil and uproot them. It has been usual so far to have the corpses of suicides dissected by physicians in order to hear from them whether or not an illness was the cause of the crime. But this ceremony is of little use as long as it is uncertain whether the dead was really his own murderer; in that case, it is necessary to examine whether his injury was

* That exaggerated monastic virtues may have the same effect is proved by the history of the Carthusian order in Rome, where some years ago many became melancholic, and some even mad. Archenholz says that from this ensued deliberate murders, they murdered each other without insult and without any cause whatsoever. These occurrences caused the monks forcefully and against their will to restrict their senseless over-piousness and to be more sociable. "England and Italy: Part V."

really lethal so that if another perpetrator perhaps is found, the right judgment can be made about the direct influence of the mistreatment on the victim's life. If, on the other hand, suicide is proved, the physicians' opinion concerning whether the presence or absence of a physical cause for his act is not very reliable, as was already shown by Schönmetzel in one of his treatises.* The causes of insanity are not always as tangible as one may imagine. The whole body may be full of blockages, without the head being affected in any way. Conversely, the main fault may lie in the organization of the brain or the nervous system, without anything unnatural being found in the spleen, which for so long has been wrongly accused, or in other viscera. The faults of the Sensorium commune are often not amenable to manifest representation, as has been taught by so many dissections of insane persons where not the slightest deviation from the normal state has been found. On the other hand, the strangest damage in the brain structure has been discovered without the mental functions having been in the slightest way affected by this, as I confirmed from my own experience in the treatise referred to. Thus, very often, accidental deviations have been taken advantage of in order to excuse a suicide, while on the other hand really insane persons were declared physically healthy, which they were not, and consequently through the physicians' fault they were unjustly condemned after their violent death, to the disgrace of their entire family. Of course, attempts were made in such cases to judge also according to the Vita ante acta, but this is not always the most reliable touchstone for making such an important decision. Insanity may be the work of an unfortunate instant, and it does not always require the usual precursors. It may prevail in only one object, whereas the criminal can judge everything else in the proper light. The Taedium Vitae, or the spleen of the English, leaves everybody the freest and often most extensive use of his mental powers, and only one single string of the spiritual instrument is too highly strung. Whoever does not play on it, deems the whole harmonic; but the chaffing, or the dissonance lies in another chord on which only the sick plays his song of grief, and there he finds harmony whereas healthy ears are insulted. And which anatomist will seek this so finely spun string in the instrument that is out of tune, and reliably state the degree of its excess tension, or its causes?

Who, then, does not realize that in judging suicide, one cannot set much store by the dissection report, and that in most cases there are assumptions that such an unnatural act has a merely physical cause which does not leave the judge much room for accusations? Therefore the community should ensure better education and better morals; debauchery should be curbed; ruinous gambling, which leads to desperation, should be restricted; the praise of suicide should be banned from the stage, and novels praising suicide also should be banned; the state of celibacy, and monasteries, where desperation and insanity are bred, should be reduced; gymnastic games and other

---

* "Quaestio Medico-Legalis, an sectio anatomica in Cadaveribus de Autochiria suspectis?" Heidelberg. 1766. I had this treatise reprinted with some additions in my "Delectus Opuscul.," Vol. I, p. 65 ff.

popular amusements that keep the body healthy should be promoted*; the misery of the poorest class should be alleviated; finally, care should be taken that melancholic persons and persons suspect of quiet insanity obtain help from their relatives in time and are brought to safe places, etc.; then the number of suicides will soon drop, and by combatting the accidental causes, more will be done than the strictest laws can achieve, which anyway cannot ever catch up with the deceased.

* * *

* Zimmerman says that even peasants become hypochondriacs due to too much sitting; this is perhaps as little known as the observation that in Switzerland there is a large, beautiful and rich village in which there is not a single house in which somebody has not hanged himself or committed suicide in some other way. "Of Experience," Part II, Vol. IV, c. 8.

PART TWO
Section Three

Of injuries through prejudices of sorcery, devilries, and miraculous cures

§1

Intention

I flatter myself that to many of my readers the present section must seem superfluous, for they imagine that I fight against the empty shadow of a subject that does not exist anymore. I wish that this reproach were well founded, and that all accusations of gullibility applied only to the dear past; however

> Tell us, sagacious women! . . . Interpreters of signs! . . .
> Gypsies! . . . Tell us, are we cleverer? . . .*

Enlightenment among people is, in many regions, like the illumination of a spacious temple by a few bright candles during Holy Week. The light is all the more effective, the darker the place is; however, nobody can read by that light unless he stands very close to the altar, and at the end the candles at each reading are extinguished one by one by persons employed for that purpose, until at last, when they are all extinguished, the old destruction begins which to us Catholics is known by the name of rumble-matins (Rumpelmette).

Unfortunately for mankind and the sciences, it is often men of otherwise recognized merit who, through prejudices acquired in their early education, use the esteem which they have acquired in the community for either defending or reviving precisely those absurdities which many righteous persons fight at the price of their happiness and peace, only to free mankind from the slave chain to which it had been fettered by the coarse, stone-blind ignorance of centuries.

Sennert** and a fairly long time after him, von Haen,† two of the first general practitioners in Europe, the former after the most courageous attacks on superstition by Wierus, who deserved more gratitude, the latter after so many successful works by the best heads from all branches of science, as physicians came to defend the

---

* Uz, "Lyrical Poems," Vol. I, p. 58.
** "Tract. Medic.," L. VI, p. 376.
† "De Magia," Liber. Venet. 1775.

reality of sorcery only at an advanced age. Even later, very distinguished scientists from all faculties (and even Protestant schools) had to let themselves be deceived by the appearance of the miraculous in a way that exposed our Germany to the danger of being thrown back, at least for a considerable time, into the old quagmire which had been its saddest age!

It seems necessary to me, therefore, to dare here an investigation in which many a well known matter must be mentioned merely to remind the Germans of the horrors under which their fathers, more than other nations at that time, suffered for centuries, and, as a physician, to show them on a hitherto little trodden path, the devastations that the prejudice of sorcery caused and still continues to cause their health and the lives of their fellow citizens in a more or less remote manner.

§2

That a large part of human sufferings is the work of a certain class of persons who through close association with an evil being from the rank of higher and more powerful creatures who have the gift to destroy the health, fortune, and fruits of their fellow creatures' diligence by murmuring certain mysterious words, wishes, benedictions, songs, etc., to change themselves or others into all kinds of animals, to travel through the air, etc., all this is a general, popular belief, and a thing of whose reality our forebears were as convinced as they could have ever been of the principal dogmas.

§3

It would be quite pointless to give here the entire history of sorcery, but I shall, as a physician, supply the skeleton from which it can be seen, as regards its influence on the life and health of people, how important it is for the police of a country to counter the monster of the most awful superstition, which under the mask of religion and piety, makes a large number of persons at least suspicious to the state and an even larger number completely useless, and lulls the simple country folk into security as regards their most important requirements.

The history of all nations teaches that, just as in his first years of life, man accepts as certainties everything true and untrue without further investigation. All nations in their childhood also believe confidently in the craziest fairy tales. When a nation has staggered about for a long time in this state of childhood, and if the deceit has lasted longer, the time must come when the nation grows up toward greater enlightenment. The coarse man is more receptive to prejudice than to anything else, for ignorance in all things is the vehicle by which every crazy tale is greedily swallowed, and the child who has been instructed by his governess to such an extent that he does not dare go outside the house as soon as it is dark, listens much more avidly to the tale of the terrifying appearance of specters than he listens to anybody who would want to tear him away from his delusion.

When completely uncivilized nations are today the victims of some misfortune, they cannot seek the cause in anything else but what happened around them approximately during the last week. To such nations, the idea that all man's misfortune is due to some malicious, powerful, invisible being does not seem so far-fetched. It was very natural to a nation that is steeped up to its ears in prejudice and is bereft of all sentiment for the works of the Creator, that under such a system of religion, the fear of this malicious being considerably reduced confidence in the strength of the charitable but weakly recognized god to the extent that the sum of misfortunes on earth prevailed over the number of good deeds it enjoyed. That is why the blood-thirsty idol has an incomparably larger number of worshippers in all parts of the world than does the god of peace and benevolence toward men, and why less than one third of the sacrifices offered to the diety are due to gratitude. All the others are enforced gifts in order to ransom ourselves from all the evils which we believe are ordained for us. The first prayer of most primitive peoples to the barely recognized deity may very well have been exactly like the one that is still said by the Tatars very devoutly every morning with faces turned to the sun:

Do not kill me! . . .

Where the idolator is permitted to bury the sacrificial knife with sacred fervor in the breast of the fellow citizen he has chosen as the placating sacrifice, and where he is the undoubted interpreter of the most secret hints of his blood-thirsty deity, his reign is much more unrestricted than that of the mild mediator between an infinitely indulgent being and the penitent or grateful man. It was more profitable, therefore, for the large class of persons on whom all enlightenment solely depended anyway, to serve the bloody rather than the rose-covered altar.

Even in the first Christian centuries, one usually had no other notion of a spirit than that it was a special being, consisting of an extremely fine and transparent body. With such a premise, it was difficult to understand the omnipresence of the good, and then of the bad being, and as with human legislators, certain subordinate beings provided with full power (demons, both good and evil) eventually had to take their place. These two kinds of beings of semigodlike nature, like their supreme commanders, had to act in constant antagonism, and were engaged mostly in loud controversy because of the object of their mission: the important point was always who was able to win most adherents. Just as people among themselves gradually lost faith and belief, the evil suspicious being was not satisfied with what its party promised it merely verbally; nay, it demanded signature, and with blood of its allies at that. Now this being was much more certain of its victory, and the effective influence of the good being was necessary to prevent this; however, this influence was not so general, and eventually the largest part devolved upon the evil spirit.

* * *

In order to be able to distinguish his own better, the Evil One, as our very wise jurists were able to discover, imprinted his seal in the form of certain stigmata, as if scratched by hare's paw, under which, as executioners and equally discerning physicians in later years asserted, no drop of blood circulated and no nerve yielded any perception. Part of the hellish power was thus implanted in the recruit, and it now depended on his will to make the dear neighbor's leg disappear, to make his wife completely lame upon her next confinement (where the devil received from God greater power over the fertile mothers anyway! . . .), and to play a trick upon his daughter on her wedding day, whereby her husband, against all former mutual experience or at least high hopes was unmanned into a very useless tool, against all temptations of the flesh. To prevent a rich harvest, and through induced lightning and hail, turn into a desert the most beautiful land, with whose blessings the Beneficent Being rewarded the diligence of industrious citizens, etc., was the favorite activity of these selected friends of the malevolent demon, and with their almightiness to do evil, they could never make such use of it that there would not be room in addition, for further reproach.

It was easy for them [these evil ones] to make themselves or good friends invulnerable or impregnable, so that, as Frommann asserts and many people still consider completely certain, neither fire nor sharp weapons, nor even bullets from a firearm could penetrate their skin.*

* * *

Generally speaking, this is approximately the nature of the system of belief in sorcerers and witches whose origin we must seek in the pitch darkness of heathendom. Without many changes, however, but with noticeable additions, we then see it transplanted into Christendom.

The history of the oldest nations shows that they usually put all their trust in soothsayers and fortune-tellers and magicians in general, and that these altogether boasted of a special intimacy with the demons through whose assistance they obtained all their extraordinary excellence. Whoever among the Teleuts [Tartars] had once been ordained to be a Ram (priest), could already practice sorcery. Of such a Ram, they said that sometimes he sat for several nights in the field in order to find out what he should order his believers to do. Such a priest can neither read nor write; and the signs by which he proves his suitability for this office consist in contortions of the body, such as our insane usually make.** To this day, among the Kalmuks, all the unfortunate occurrences are ascribed to evil-doing spirits of the air which, however, are subject to the power of certain Tangut prayers and exorcisms and have to yield.†

Astrology and medical practice were necessary arts to gain trust and admiration

---

* "De fascinatione," lib. III. P. IV. p. 595.
** Gmelin, l.c.
† Pallas, "Russian Travels," Vol. I, p. 282.

among the people. Among the ancient Germans, women who did not seem to be suitable for such honorary office, were more disposed than they were among any other nations to deal with demons. Among them and the ancient Celts, the women did not have much more to do than to observe the course of the moon, collect herbs, and extract signs from certain occurrences indicating whether some undertaking or other of the nation would take a fortunate course. In each province, these aged women were subordinated to some overlord; in others, they were ruled by a respected mistress of the order. These women were also called soothsayers (Allrunnen) who had knowledge of secret things, witches, i.e., prudent, wise women.* By singing special songs, they exorcised ghosts, released them, forced them to reveal certain secrets, and they worshipped Freya, Wotan's wife, etc. On certain nights, especially Walpurgis Night, sacrifices were made to this deity on mountain peaks. Occasionally people were sacrificed and eaten there by the Celts to propitiate [their god] Dys; and of these, too, various tales were current of men being turned into wolves and women into owls, cats, etc.**

* * *

§4
Necessity of understanding the witch doctrine
   The main actions of witches and sorcerers deserve to be examined here in some detail, although for reasonable persons the completely foolish system will soon be changed into the previous naught from which stupidity and self-seeking created it. Thus, if means applied by the authorities will not help, this aberration will yet have among the people (nobility, bourgeois, and beggars) much unfortunate influence on public well-being, and under these circumstances repetitions, spiced with the memories of one physician working for the police, do not seem superfluous.†

§5
The most striking function of the witches was the making of the weather, and so few persons doubted its reality, that prayers were said about it, even at a sacred site.

* * *

Frank lists examples of alleged changes in weather, caused by witches.

---

* A. Rieger, "Instit. Jurisprudent. Ecclesiast.," Pars IV, p. 276.
** See especially in Krünitz, "Oeconom. Encykloped., etc."—Hexe (witch).
† Meanwhile what has happened in France and Germany since Cagliostro's appearance proves well that we have not yet advanced sufficiently in commonsense; otherwise, it would be unnecessary to say a word about these matters.

§6

In addition to the art of ordering thunder and lightning, sorcerers had another singular ability, namely to cause other persons the strangest diseases by otherwise ineffective, or at least harmless, means.

* * *

There follow examples of illnesses caused by witches.

Women, wet nurses and maidservants, says Chrysostomus, dip their fingers into a kind of sludge which has been deposited on the bottom of baths; then, they press their fingers against the forehead of the child in order, they say, to remove the evil eye of envy from it. The Romans hung certain amulets around the necks of children; they had the shape of Priapus or a phallus;* and this figure, which does not seem very edifying to our eyes seemed so inoffensive to Roman eyes that even the vestal virgins sacrificed this fascinas to their god. Thomas Bartholinus supplied a drawing of this amulet. The drawing, which had been made known by Pignorius before him, represents only a clenched fist with the thumb protruding between the index and the middle fingers. Delrio and others maintained that the use of such clenched fists, made of silver or ivory, was still customary in Spain, they were worn by children around their necks, and Spanish women would force those they feared put a spell on their children to touch this clenched fist.**

Even among the Jews in former times there was a spirit, known by the name of Lilith, which killed or dragged away the boys who were to be circumcized.† As early as in the eighth century Queen Fredegund had Count Mummolus tortured most cruelly because some Paris women had said that in order to prolong his life, they had taken their prince's life by witchcraft.††

Next to the children it was mainly women in confinement over whom the devil had great power, as I have said elsewhere. Altogether nothing was easier for the witches than to conjure old nails, pieces of glass, potsherds, hairs, live animals, especially toads, lizards, and similar loathsome creatures, into persons who were odious to them, as can be seen from a large number of writings, even by physicians (who, however, were not themselves sorcerers) which make very edifying reading.‡

* * *

---

* Plinius, "Hist. nat.," lib. XXVIII. c. 4.

** Frommann, "De fascinatione," p. 66. "Mémoires du Chevalier d'Arvieux," Tome III, p. 249.

† Samuel Strikius, "De jure spectrorum," §3. Frommann, l.c. p. 7. c. 2. §2.

†† Gregor. Turon. L. VI. c. 35.

‡ See Sprengerus, "In malleo maleficarum."—Bodinus, "De demonomania."—Remigius, "De demono-latria sagarum."—Sennertus, "Prax. med." T. VI.

§11

Although many evils had been perpetrated by sorcery, the fiends on the other hand had a special skill in making up for some misfortune that had afflicted someone or other. In this art, they had less experience, but there were persons who boasted of having found the secret of how to force the witches to end their witchcraft and to replace unimpaired the health they had robbed. This, of course, was more than the hexing itself; for since in the means to this purpose again there was no, or relatively no, medicinal power, again supernatural forces, and of a higher order at that, were required to make the devil retract. It is strange that here the mere invocation of the good being by creatures who served under his flag usually did not suffice, and that prayers and the strict observance of his orders were of little avail unless one tried to use mysterious means of coercion and certain words of incomprehensibly high meaning.

A purer notion of religion forced the prudent ancient theologians to simply forbid the people such curative methods although Constantine justified by a special law the use of magicians against hoar frost, hail and storm, and some ranking canons agreed with this silly opinion. The executioners and physicians who were used at the rack, where the fiends were to confess their deeds, partly paid great heed to the testimony of the wise women, or they at least tried to make the world believe that they themselves knew their tricks from this source. That way these gentlemen secured for themselves special confidence in all cases at the root of which there was some witchcraft. Barbara Dore confessed that she was able to help those whom she had previously hexed by placing on their stomachs a dove split in half (with the words: "In the name of God the Father, the Son, and the Holy Ghost, of St. Anthony and the sacred Archangel Michael, be in good health again!") and by having Mass read in the parish church for nine days running. This prescription, of course, indicates that this was a pious witch. A thousand such magical medical tricks, whose history is told approximately in the same manner, was a mysterious heirloom of entire families of torturers whose predecessors are still remembered with trepidation by all fiends. The more ignorant a nation is, the smaller is the number of the natural evils, but the larger is the number of unnatural evils that befall it. It is the same with medicines. The Kalmuks hardly know any other medicine except prayers, certain formulas, and figures which are worn as amulets. In a nation which ascribes almost all its ills to witches, bases its great confidence in executioners on tradition, a person who is eager to utilize the common practice as much as possible among the country folk, must be in possession of a rich collection of such mysterious prescriptions in most regions, or must be prepared to be put to shame at the first opportunity by any old hag, as Zacutus Lusitacius admitted in regard to himself. A maiden who, because of her cruelty, had been cast in wax by her lover and bewitched by obliging women, suffered from terrible convulsions and vomited the strangest animals, etc. He [Z.L.] and several other physicians were unable to restore her, but a sorcerer who had been called immediately, provided relief for her for considerable remuneration. During an attack he shaved the maiden's head, put a sheet of white paper with the two letters T.M. and a half-burned donkey's hoof on her head, and whispered in her ear.

That is why our so very wise village physicians provide themselves with the most powerful sayings against bleeding, against inflammation, and against the four-day fever. Thus, the upright Wierus, himself, was called to a dying man to whom shortly before such a quack had given three pieces of some root against the fever, into each of which the patient had to bite once and say at the first, "I wish Christ had never been born;" at the second, "I wish he had not died;" at the third, "I wish he had never been resurrected"; but after all these endeavors he died of a breast abscess.*
I remember that in my early youth as a student, I came to my superior who, as a monastic man, also acted as physician. There was the question of a hexed child; I heard the highly enlightened man prescribe that of the three pieces of a root, which he gave to the messenger, one was to be placed in the cradle, the second under the threshold, and the third was to be buried in some place which I have forgotten. My respect for the extraordinarily sagacious man increased, and I am very proud to have had such a superior. In the Principality of Speyer, I had to examine a country surgeon; he did not know a single answer, and when I rejected him, he believed that his honor had been insulted and told me that he had achieved some great cures. I asked him about them in order to talk them over with him; it was bleedings which he pretended to have cured. I wanted to know how he had approached the matter . . . these are secrets, he replied; but in order to earn your benevolence, I shall reveal them. I begin, he said, by secretly blessing the wound, then I say the most sacred three names, God the Father, Son, and Holy Ghost, and in this and in the name of St. Anthony, etc., etc., I order, etc., whereupon the bleeding must cease. But since the good peasants, whom this surgeon should have cured, live in a consecrated country, anyway, where there is an abundance of blessing, I did not consider it wise to permit the dispenser of benedictions to practice his science in the future.

§12

Hexing of domestic animals

It is certain that the peasant fears the effect of witches less on himself than on his domestic animals. According to the notions taught the people, the pathology or the study of cattle diseases is very brief. Most of the things that happen are the doing of a fiend who vents its fury on the poor dumb creatures, who without Balaam's miracle, can never reveal the perpetrator of the evil, unless some extra wise monks eventually learn the language of the cattle and discover the cause of the evil. Since the peasant does not easily seek the fiend outside his own or the nearest village, he saves himself even more exertion in the search for his witch if the number of old ugly hags in his community is small. He is also expectedly spared unnecessary expenditures

* Jo. Wierus Gravianus, "de praestigiis Daemonum." Basil, 1564. Lib IV, p. 422.

which he would have otherwise incurred in purchasing some physical remedy against a physical disease by the verdict of the mendicant friar. The many wax images of all kinds of domestic animals that are sacrificed on every pilgrimage explain sufficiently the peasant's complete theory concerning the illnesses of his animal companions, and consequently of the power of the Evil Being to cause him and his family damage at will. This belief holds that even a virtuous life, devoted to professional work and arranged entirely according to the Creator's wish, is unable to prevent the health and fortune of an honest man, acquired through hard work, being completely dependent on the caprice of the adherents of the Evil Being.*

* The frequent journeys into the country by the court of S. after a famous pilgrimage to W. enabled me to amass an excellent collection of important parts of animal and even of human pathology. There is probably not a single limb of the body which did not appear, cast in wax, on this pilgrimage; and I am very much surprised that it took such a long time before people went over from these sacred attempts to the profane but excellent anatomical wax casts which do Bologna and Florence so much honor. There I saw so many waxen wombs and female breasts heaped up at every Mass, that the good fathers should have been sickened by such objects. When Gassner worked his many miracles at Ellwangen, there were also many in the Rhenic regions who endeavored to imitate or even surpass this famous man. An interesting story that happened on my well-attended pilgrimage deserves here to be rescued from oblivion. A young man from W. confided to me that he had undertaken to cure a girl of 12, whom neither I with my physics nor Gassner with his spiritual means, had been able to restore. The Father was so gracious as to excuse my failing, and assured me that the devil had a hand in the matter. I replied modestly that even if this were not so, my inability might still be excusable.—Since this candid man did not know how to flatter, he admitted this, too, without noticing that it made me blush slightly... But Gassner was not let off so easily, and despite the miracles he had worked, he was charged with ignorance. The girl concerned was suffering from spasms, and had taken the medicines prescribed by me without effect. She also had traveled to Ellwangen, and came back no better than before. The monk assured me that the illness, nevertheless, was of devilish origin, and he wanted me to cure the remnants (as they put it in this region) or the physical remainders of the illness, in my own way once the cause of the illness was removed. Although I was disinclined to work after a monk, nevertheless I asked whether he was certain that spiritual remedies were necessary here. He said yes. The proofs are (and here he pulled out a Ritual from under his arm) that I [sic, i.e., he] 1) had already carried out the Exorcismum probatorium with the girl, and had obtained all the signs of my assumption; 2) I had made her climb into a bath in which I had had boiled various blessed herbs, as is prescribed in my book; 3) and that the girl had vomited cats' hairs and evacuated pebbles with her stool.

I promised to investigate the matter the following day in the presence of the mother and the girl. The mother, full of confidence in spiritual help, confirmed the Father's statements and told me that since he had given his assistance, her daughter, who was present, was much better. I enquired about her aversion to the bath, but was unable to discover anything except that the girl had been afraid of the water and had refused to climb into the bath. The third point in question was more interesting to me. "Did the girl really vomit cats' hairs? Yes.—Were there many of them?... No, about ten or twelve.—Where did the vomiting take place? At the monastery at W.—At what place? In the cell of the witch-Father (I knew that no woman was admitted to such a place, and from this I concluded that the law did not apply to young bewitched girls).—Did the patient vomit onto the floor or into a vessel? Into an earthenware dish.—How did the Father come to have this dish? It was standing outside a cell.—Did the vomiting occur without any previous inclination or loathing? Yes, my daughter had only just taken a little of some white powder which the witch-Father had given her for the purpose,

§13

This is approximately what the whole witch system is like; I had to provide in advance a notion of it before I could explain its influence on the public well-being.

No matter how willing people always are to let themselves be hoodwinked by the miraculous, such a miserable system must arouse opposition sooner or later from good heads of which there is always a larger or smaller number among all nations.

* * *

The belief in witchcraft was never more dangerous than when persons began burning those who had been accused of it. Conversely, those are most deserving of mankind who, at a time when it was so dark and consequently so dangerous to face almost alone the onrushing prejudices, risked their happiness and lives in order to defend loudly the innocence of the accused, to censure publicly the injustice of such court proceedings, without fear of the tyrannical inquisitors, and to describe as an abomination the complete hitherto existent witch system. In respect to human reason, one must believe that many learned men in former times well realized the weakness of the belief in witches; but either for well-founded fear, or because they did not deem it advisable to enlighten the common people, they left the foolish people to their fate. Their names, therefore, remain unknown to posterity, for they lived only for themselves and put their own well-being before the salvation of thousands.

* * *

Frank then lists the names of men who fought against the belief in witchcraft: Johannes de Poncinibus, Joannes Wierus, Hermann Wittekind, Francis Bacon von Verulam, and Friedrich Spe.

§14

Symptoms of bewitching

For the most part, general prejudice [of the public] maintained the symptoms and statements of guilty women accused by the Inquisition, whose leaders said, in order

---

when soon afterwards the vomiting occurred." Now it was fairly clear to me how the first miracle had occurred, but the second one seemed to me to be just as deserving of closer investigation. "Did your daughter really discharge pebbles with the stool? Yes.—How many? Three.—Were they large? No, not very large, like large beans and of unequal size.—And where or at what place was this? In the garden behind my house." Since I knew the soil in this region well, which is sandy and contains so many small pebbles that if the 12,000 virgins of St. Ursula had sat down there in a row, they could have left a similar Sedimentum behind, I did not deem it necessary to investigate the matter any further. —Poor good country folk! How you are deceived because of your gullibility by idiotic or fraudulent persons, and how dearly do you often have to pay with your lives and the lives of your useful animal assistants! . . . I insert this story here as proof that I speak not without reason of witchcraft as a police matter, and that the whole article will still be amenable to some application up to the very end of the eighteenth century.

to give their cause a veneer of piety that God would necessarily teach them how to distinguish an innocent person from others who had been arrested.* This was really a stupid continuation of the nonsensical statement, approved in the past by secular and spiritual authorities, that God had to work a miracle all the time in order to prevent foolish people from continuous mischief and breaking each other's necks. For those suspect of witchcraft, the so-called water test was the method mostly used. Hands and feet were crossed and bound, and a rope was bound round the middle. Then when the bound body was thrown into the water and swam on the surface, people were convinced that they were dealing with a witch; if the body sank, innocence was established.

* * *

Once someone was seized, there was not much hope of his release, even if the rack had not forced a confession, for it redounded to the judge's dishonor for having been too rash with the arrest.** When Voigt looked through the files on witches at the Royal Prussian Prefecture at Quedlinburg, he was amazed to read a record of 11 June 1569 regarding some suspicious beggars who were eventually convicted of arson and witch-craft. The records were kept fairly neatly and completely. As long as the other crimes were being investigated, the judge proceeded correctly: he did not accept every charge as true, but examined it thoroughly. As soon as sorcery and witchcraft were involved, however, he immediately, and without proper charge, began with the rack. If one of the arrested bore witness against another, it sufficed, even if the accused denied it, to bring him to the rack, too, after all hairs on his body had been shaved off (so that the devil could not play his game with them). Since the executioner usually removed the hair from all parts of the body at a remote place, says Spe, this offered him opportunities for some amusement; also, being convinced that such a person must already have had intercourse with the devil, an occasional rape or defloration also prefaced the proceedings. But the testimony of the arrested against others had to be given on the rack; there, persons who were otherwise considered dishonest, were accepted as valid witnesses. Tanner taught that no matter how many accomplices there were, they could never give valid testimony; but Delrio and others of his ilk stipulated their number to be three or four. Thus, each examination of witches became the preparation for much more widespread investigations, whereby entire villages were gradually stripped of all mothers and daughters.

* * *

There follow examples of cross-examination of witches.

---

* To this Spe said: "Mox! . . . . scilicet, cum in cineres jam involuti sunt!" l.c. [Cautio Criminalis, seu de processibus contra sagas liber. Ad Magistratus Germaniae.] p. 50.
** Spe, l.c. dub. XXII, p. 146.

§15

Decline in the belief in witchcraft

Finally the efforts of the meritorious Balthasar Becker and the unforgettable Christian Thomasius succeeded in this matter being viewed differently, even in most court houses. And the polemic by the latter, published in Halle in 1712* completed the great work of changing the hitherto so barbaric criminal laws which Spe had begun. Gradually it was realized that some persons did not shed any tears on the rack because violent pain usually dries out this source, completely interrupts the excretion of moisture, and makes crying impossible, until finally the pain becomes more bearable, whereupon often a violent flow of tears follows and usually provides some relief for the sufferers. Ariosto expressed this state beautifully:

> L'impetuosa doglia entro rimase,
> Che volea tutta uscir con troppa fretta,
> Cosi veggiam restar l'acqua nel vase,
> Che largo il ventre, e la bocca abbia stretta:
> Che nel volta, che si fa in su, la base,
> L'Umor, che vorria uscir, tanto s'affretta.
> Enell' Augusta via tanto, s'intrica,
> Ch'a goccia a goccia fuore esce a fatica.**

People now realized that what in the unfortunate creatures on the rack was called laughing was, really, as Spe had already said, a terrible distortion of the twitching facial muscles with the jaws firmly locked, so that every needle prick was not felt so much and always caused bleeding to death, for one sees mischievous boys who put pins deep into their calves without complaining and because a very violent mental state may smother both the lesser pain and the coursing of the blood through the tender vessels in the skin. People now know, too, that a scar on any part of the body may be the play of nature or the consequence of a skin injury after which sensitivity is usually diminished;† that the fact that some persons, when thrown into the water, remain on the surface may be due to a paunch distended by flatulence or by fat, or to other causes;†† furthermore, it has been realized that it was unconsciousness which

---

* "De origine ac progressu processus inquisitorii contra fagas." Also by the same author, "Theses de crimine magiae," Halle Magdeb. 1731.

** "Orlando furioso," canto XXIII.

† With slight talent for witchcraft which, I am sorry to say, I observe in myself, I would have in the past been considered by any honorable grand inquisitor a very worthy subject for the rack because on my Christian crown of the head along the top suture there is hidden a scar about three inches long, which was caused neither by human hand nor by illness. In one of the previous centuries I would have been well advised to trust only my wig with this secret.

†† When in 1767–68 I was in charge of the warm baths at Baden, in the County of Baden, I observed several patients who did not go under in them or sink to the bottom, but, like blown-up frogs, swam on the surface, which is not very unusual in hypochondriacal and hysterical persons. At Baden it was thought that the warm healing water did not accept certain patients, but this would show too much

made the unfortunate victims stretched out on the rack seem to be asleep, or that the extreme exertion of the nervous system through the insufferability of the pain affected the brain in such a way that parts of the body were paralyzed briefly and conscious-ness and voluntary movements were suppressed, that the admission of the cited evil deeds was the fruit of desperation because of the pain and of the firm preference for certain death to the pain, that the accusations against others were either due to the fact that the torture continued until the victim had named a certain number of accomplices; or because persons tortured to distraction, often still suffering from old ills, thought that a larger company of unfortunate ones could provide some consolation or a kind of satisfaction. The aforenamed Tonnissin who was burned for witchcraft, was according to the record "admonished to confess further, revoked all, saying she had said anything because of the pains, and in order to be spared these pains, confessed. She was therefore tortured again in puncto revocationis, and at half past nine in the morning Tormento Vigilae was applied, but she persevered in her revocation. Post meridiem circa septimam she confessed that what she had said before was the right truth as known to her."—On the other hand, poor women endeavored to have their revenge on richer women: "Yes," said the Muscher woman, "if they would burn the Wenecker woman and let the rich ones go, the devil should take them."*

§16

The physicians, of whom it could have been expected that they would endeavor to demonstrate physically how foolish this superstition is, tried rather, as mentioned before, to mislead theologians and jurists in their judgment of natural occurrences. It was really their task to open the eyes of a deceived world to the causes of illnesses and natural occurrences. Yet, they were often the first who in their duty-bound, expert opinions carried the torch ahead in order that they could light the unfortunate pile on which the unfortunate women had to be burned alive, those women whom they could not heal and would not excuse. Thus theologians and judges were long led about in darkness by the physicians and fobbed off with principles that could not bring any sound consequences in their train. In vain did Wierus demonstrate to them that the so-famous witch salves consisted entirely of things that robbed the persons to whom they were applied of their reason and made them somnolent, dreamy, and insane. In vain did they see similar effects of similar causes daily with their own eyes. They remained too indolent to make comparisons and distinguish the true from the false.

---

sense in warm water. Stranger is the observation by my friend Doctor Frambaglia, a skillful physician at Voghera near Pavia, of a girl suffering from tetanus. When suffering from an attack of this illness, she swam on the surface in the bath, but when the attack passed she sank in the water. Bielfinger made the same observation about tetanus; I never encountered this. Several years ago an abbé died in Naples who could walk in the sea without sinking in further than to his loins. He tried this several times, and publicly at that. See also Haller's "Element. Physiol.," T. VIII, addenda p. 152.

* "Materials for the Statistics," l.c. p. 343. 46.

But then it was such a beautiful thing, in view of the immense number of senseless hypotheses on which practice was then based, always to find an ever ready excuse in the belief in the devilish origin of illnesses when healing did not make proper progress . . . Instead of laboriously broadening the frontiers of science, they preferred to state certain sentences according to which devilish illnesses could be judged, and stipulated symptoms according to which they could be distinguished from natural ills. Among them was one of the most prominent: if several skillful physicians could neither diagnose nor heal the ill, or if the illness, without a known cause, suddenly reached a peak, it was certain that it had a supernatural cause. Instead of thoroughly answering the many questions that are usually asked of physicians in regard to natural occurrences, or admitting their ignorance freely in a way which they deemed humiliating, they ascribed all extraordinary, seemingly miraculous events to a supernatural power, and thus, thought to have sufficiently saved their own honor and the honor of medical science.

It is quite incomprehensible how carelessly men of otherwise good knowledge went to work in this most important matter, and how they let themselves be bamboozled by the most ignorant and unreliable persons into taking fairy tales for facts, which they then raised to principles. Mercurialis says that thinness and emaciation in children, of which one cannot say that the cause is their condition or the condition of their nurses, is ascribed to bewitching. And this settled simply the question of explaining most of the lengthy children's diseases.

* * *

There follow examples of the gullibility of physicians.

§18

Thanks to the common interest of philosophical physicians, many deceits, and superstitious, murderous prejudices have so far disappeared. These efforts relieve me of the need now to disprove formally and at great length the madness of belief in witchcraft, especially since the distinguished physician in ordinary so thoroughly treated the subject of witchcraft as the supposed cause of illnesses. First of all, it had to be proved that all the signs from which conclusions were drawn as to the presence of supernatural causes of natural occurrences are anything but conclusive evidence. The incurability and wonder of various illnesses no longer served, as in Sennert's time, as the touchstone of natural ills. The boundaries of the art were determined more accurately and it was admitted, without that ridiculous pride of omniscience, that there was still much in medicine that was dark and that our knowledge still had many weaknesses. As we became better acquainted with nature, we began to trust its force more in usual occurrences and upon daily exertions and stimuli than we once did, and we began to withdraw even from the views of a Willis, who still supposed a supernatural force and a devilish origin caused spasms which were so violent that a healthy person could not imitate them. A convulsively moved muscle compared with a muscle moved by mere will, or the usual mechanism, is in the same relationship as the force of the entire body in the healthy state is to the power of the little finger. A man of medium strength, when a violent fever makes him obstinate towards his attendants, becomes a giant, and in him all the former relationship between mass and motive power disappears. Thus one no longer needs a devil in order to explain the super-human strength of a weak girl gripped by convulsions or all her unnatural contortions for it became known that what electric power was able to do in nature on a large scale, could be achieved in man on a small scale by what the physicians called dis-ordered nervous strength.

Among the frequent examples of hysterical convulsions, which I found in sus-ceptible persons, I encountered such notions that would have seemed to any unpre-pared person as more than natural. In Bruchsal I saw a girl, aged seventeen, whose superstitious father, guided by even more fanciful clergymen, proclaimed her to be possessed, and therefore requested written permission from the bishop to have his daughter exorcised. The sick girl was just attacked by a violent spasm while I and her 80-year old father were alone with her. I have a strong body, yet I was far too weak to keep her in order. She sprang with a few steps toward the vertical wall; her other-wise relatively thin neck swelled within a few moments so much that it was almost equal to the chin; she threw her head about so rapidly that it almost seemed to be impossible to believe anything but that her head turned in a complete circle on her neck as the axis, both her breasts swelled up, became hard as stones and were larger by half. Since the supplicant father was, for good reasons, not permitted the shameful exorcising of his marriageable daughter, it was not surprising that the gullible old man took it upon himself to rid his daughter of the accursed devil. Of course, the manner in which he went to work to do it was droll and characteristic of this old man: Exi! . . . he called very loudly, Exi immunde Spiritus! etc., while nobody except he and I were with the girl! . . . I remarked on this at once in order to upset his exercising earnestness. However, the good old man (who was at the same time Doctor juris) continued maneuvering against the devil until the girl was exhausted by her attack and fell asleep.

* * *

How little common sense is needed to discover all the great secrets of the devilish causes of illnesses, or at least to realize that no matter how obscure the matter is, no devil need be presupposed to make the correct indication. People who are used to drawing conclusions quickly, even physicians, may easily commit some foolishness which one forgives. I want to give a small example. It is known that Gassner some-times ordered the pulse to cease in the name of Jesus and that the physicians who were present really could not then feel any pulse in certain persons. Gassner extended the order to this or that arm, as, in the meantime, the artery in the other arm beat properly. To tell the truth, I do not believe this story. My friend, the Privy Councilor and Professor May from Mannheim visited me unexpectedly when I still lived at Bruchsal and asked me what I thought of Gassner's talent. I replied: Just as little as you, Councilor, whose disbelief in such things I know. And yet, he said, I want to prove to you that this phenomenon is true . . . feel my pulse! It beats as in a healthy man, I said. Well, replied May, but I order in the name of Jesus that it should not beat any more. Ha, I thought, I want to see that. I did not feel any pulse in his right arm while the pulse in his left arm continued to beat as before. This is strange, I said . . .* Of course, very strange, but now I order that the pulse in the left arm cease and in the right arm be felt again. This really happened, and I was at a complete loss. My friend laughed and thought I would now believe in Gassner's deeds.—And who among my dear readers would have refused this for long under such circumstances?—No, my friend, I said, I do not draw any conclusion from what I felt and did not feel, except that it depends on you to make the artery in your arm jump according to your own will, though I must admit that I feel as if I did not have a doctor's degree at all. May took pity on me and my surprise, although I had not been misled and only my attention had been aroused. You see, he said, since I, like other people, have only one artery in the arm, I arrange things in such a way that under the armpit I induce pressure, which can be easily done when the camisole is somewhat tight and I press the arm firmly against the chest; this immediately stops the pulse or at least makes it weaker.—I should have thought of this, I said, and I tried to imitate it, without, however, being able to master my artery completely. Privy Councilor Zimmermann from Brunswick, who honored me with his visit in Pavia in October 1787 on his journey through Italy, had hardly heard this little story from me when he immediately repeated the miracle and gave me his arm in which no pulse could be felt.

Sometimes phenomena may occur, as Eberhard demonstrated especially in his important treatise on magic, which may disconcert even physicians; however, a reasonable man will not conclude that there are supernatural causes involved, only

---

* Of course I knew that certain people can stop certain vital motions according to their will for a certain time. Cheyne gave various examples of people who made such experiments on themselves and lay for some time completely stiffly and without pulse. The example is known of the Englishman who was able with his hand to stop the motions of his heart as often as he wanted to. He earned much money with it, but in the end he died from this trade for he was unable to make his heart move again (Haller "Meth. stud. med.," T. I). Monti, in a letter to Herr von Haller, collected a number of similar cases and added an example from his own country of a man who pretended to be dead and for long was believed to be dead. He held his breath, and an enormous number of flies already descended on his body. A skilled physician found no pulse, no heartbeat, a burning candle held in front of his mouth did not move, the cruellest experiments were in vain. The peasant, who was thought to be a spy, got up and went away when he was left alone with a clergyman. (Ignazio Monti, "Dettati medici," Volume I. pp. 30–36.) The clergyman of Cealius Rhodiginus was able to pretend to be dead when he wanted to; he could be stabbed, pinched, and even burned, without anything moving on him. ("Lection. antiqu.," lib. 20. C. 14.)

because he cannot immediately solve the riddle. No, first he investigates, and if he cannot find the key to the secret, he confesses to his ignorance rather than take refuge in explanations that contradict common sense.

* * *

There follow remarks concerning the speaking in foreign languages, and impotence.

The inducement of illnesses which were attributed to witchcraft was based either on real poisoning and the administration of noxious substances, or on the imagination of those who considered themselves bewitched, or finally on more hidden but natural causes of rare but conspicuous cases (mostly nervous ones). The ignorance and the pride of the physicians who, being unable to cure the ill, preferred to put all the blame on the devil rather than admit the inadequacy of their art, contributed in no small measure to the rapid spread of such Hottentotic notions of the causes of diseases. But it was especially our crafty and unutterably ignorant monks who endeavored with all their might to maintain and increase the inclination of the simple folk to the miraculous, which was the source of their income. Besides, the profit to be derived from the performance of sessions with the devil, or from rare accidental cases, had always been one of the strongest mainsprings for marshaling all one's powers to perform such an important role to perfection. Sometimes it was merely a stupid idea of not-quite-so-stupid clergymen, who wanted to prop up religion by such stories, even though they themselves were convinced of how feeble their proofs were. Sometimes there was also sanctimoniousness and the wish to be deemed an important person or a saintly man, and people gladly sacrificed all comforts of life and even the satisfaction of their most urgent desires in order to acquire the reputation of a miracle worker, soothsayer, or the victim of the fury of evil spirits and sorcerers. Of course, the so-called witches had no such prospects, and one would have thought that the fear of the stake would have made every human being recoil from the mere assumption of belonging to such a class of people. However, experience shows that an extreme inclination to carnal lust and a sick imagination can overcome all punishments meted out by a terrible, albeit still uncertain, fate. In reality, many of the women who were burned as witches were not completely innocent victims of a slanderous accusation; there were such among them who indicted themselves and voluntarily admitted the worst misdeeds. Most of these, however, disregarding poisonings and the satisfaction of carnal lust with disguised men, were mostly a product of the crazed imagination. The salves of stupefying, soporific herbs, of henbane, thorn apple, poppy juice and other things, accompanied by violent visions and imagination, induced dreams that made everything seem very real, and were able to deceive the sick soul in such a manner that upon awakening, the impression remained and left the conviction that everything had been real.

Here I do not want to disprove the Devil's power over people: who cannot be convinced by the mere telling of the nonsense prevalent in such things, will not listen to proofs stemming from reasoning either. I do not want to spell out what the Devil can and cannot do, for that is not my business. I do not state that in the past the Devil did not make diseases of which the physicians who only have to treat the presently fashionable ills know little. In short, without detracting from the former Devils' domains I only want to state here, that in our days there is no reason any more to believe such stories, and that all the possessed, no matter what name they have, and all the sorcerers, must be considered either the cheats or the cheated. The stories of old visitations by the Devil are of such a nature that we no longer have any data today to examine them, or they are open to a more reasonable interpretation than our theologians are willing to apply.

* * *

§20

I abstain from any further mention concerning this abundant matter, so that this treatise does not develop into an entire book. But what I have mentioned so far may suffice to make the police take more notice than they have hitherto done of the influence of superstition on the physical well-being of the people. The police must forbid with much severity all superstitious remedies for illnesses, and call their originators to account. The police must also strictly punish simulation of various illnesses and dissimulation meant to arouse general compassion or to indicate miraculous cures.

* * *

PART TWO
Section Four

Of the maltreatment of dying persons

> What does Your Reverence call temptation on the deathbed?
> The Philosophical Physician, Part I, p. 196

§1

Contemplation of our natural end has a certain usefulness in improving the moral state of man, and this influence was already realized long ago by non-Christian philosophers. But this contemplation can even help promote our physical well-being if we do not undertake only monkish meditations on this subject and endeavor to forget the fate of the living while we busy ourselves with the world of the ghosts.

§2

So far, the police has given very little attention to dying citizens, partly because one dislikes dealing with the image of death, partly because at this instant, when all should be considered as lost, everything else is inevitable, whereby all nature has to take only a passive part.

§3

But I believe that, because of their care for the living, the police should not completely forget the dying, and that people will be grateful if the police will at least concoct a soothing balm for this sensitive portion of our lives rather than try to control less general ills.

However, what can be done for person when he is in the process of ceasing to be? The physicians admit the powerlessness of their art; in desperation our relatives kiss the cold hand for the last time or wish us an early blessed end—and then the clergyman takes over his spiritual object without giving much consideration to the physical body. Even this instant is supposed to add shadow and light to the picture that remains after we are gone; and natural convulsions and contortions of the facial muscles, easily explained fright of the wise man's ruined machine emitting a death

262

rattle, have been viewed by respected theologians as decisive signs of the dying men's desperation. Nor could they always completely disguise the inclination to detect at least spots in the setting sun, and thus deprived the dying of even the last consolation of knowing that posterity would judge him more justly.

§4

And why does civilized man die with such an appearance of dreadful terror, whereas all of remaining nature, most so-called wild nations—disregarding a few muscle contortions which spoil the entire course of life for us—await calmly enough the last heartbeat and do not permit any added artificial torment to natural dissolution? . . . Is it a merit for the enlightened human race that misunderstood religious notions stuff us with images of death, so that we lose our health and the calm of all our life, and that the religious man's last moments compared with those of the animal-like human creature appear in the worst possible relation? . . . That certain persons spend part of their lives in depicting death in the most terrifying way to their brethren, because, according to the most lenient interpretation, they are too indolent to submit better reasons to the healthy. As if we still lived in the dark days where such bogies were intended to put the believers into the right frame of mind to the temporal advantage of the church!

I wish very much, indeed, that the reproach by non-Christian philosophers be removed, namely that Christian morals paralyzed the old courage of manly nations by increased fear of death, and the Christian was the first to teach to tremble those who sang the pagan German death song with a smiling face, and who believed themselves to be dying the death of their fathers amid the loud calls of the bards, without awaiting on their knees a future battle . . . But reproaches often leveled against the Christian religion applied to only a few of its teachers, and the prudent Christian finds causes unknown to the dying pagan for calming down in his last moments.

§5

Why not seriously counter this reproach in a matter which has such a great influence on our lives; why thus expose the large class of suffering persons to an unnecessary deterioration of their fate, without thinking of means of banishing from the sickbed an unfounded fear of death, which is so often the cause of earlier breakdown, or at least a terror that is deleterious in every respect?

In the past I have found many examples of the most ill-advised treatment of the sick, which would not have occurred if the clergymen were better acquainted with the duties of the healthy and of the dying. That is why I noticed a pronounced fear of such visits in many sick, and this may not always be based on the prejudice that once the priest has been called one has soon to die. In France physicians are obliged under pain of being deprived of their office to warn the patient or to have him warned to make his confession immediately on the second day after they have been called to a patient whose condition seems to be dangerous. If the sick and his relatives are not inclined to do so, the physician himself has to report to the priest and ask him for a written testimonial that he had fulfilled his duty. Now, if neither the priest nor his chaplain attest in writing that the sick man either actually made his confession, or was at least visited by the clergyman in order to be prepared for receiving the sacraments, the physician is forbidden to visit his patient on the third day and to give him medical treatment. I refrain from expressing my thoughts concerning this ordinance, in which Cardinal Rohan, in view of his special system, is supposed to have taken a leading part, and the carrying out of which is hardly likely to be strictly enforced now.

But do not such ordinances prove that even the believing often shrink from spiritual succor? . . . What are the causes of this? . . . Are they generally to be found in the aforementioned prejudice? . . . And if so, are they not perhaps based on the sometimes just complaints which dying persons have against the ill-advised help of an inexperienced clergyman? . . . Or what is really the true source of the frequent disturbances around the deathbeds of so many persons?

* * *

§10

Turmoil at the deathbed

Once and for all, why such turmoil at the deathbed of believing Christians? . . . And why should they alone be deprived of the privilege of being able to die in peace? . . . I have often heard commended that the best moral would be to see a man die . . . This may be true for a few persons but why should one be forced, to his great torment, to hold moral lectures when just about to die! . . . And then, it is known for certain that it is not rare that a member of a gang of robbers secretly mingles among the people at the execution of one of his fellow robbers; yet, the next day, if the opportunity arises, he plies his old craft sometimes with even more confidence, for he has just seen how edifyingly his brother ended his life, and how he gave up his ghost in the certainty of a blessed end, no matter how great his misdeeds had been throughout his life.

* * *

PART TWO
Section Five

Of the danger of being buried alive, and of belated funerals

§1

I must better acquaint my philanthropic readers with the close relationship between life and death than I did in the previous section dealing with mistakes committed on dying persons, in order that they are prepared for extremely important investigations. This article will make everyone shudder because of the large number of human victims killed through ignorance and rashness. And I hope that I will incite in all reasonable persons the fervent wish, by earnest application to the police, to prevent the terrible fate that everywhere threatens our closest friends and relatives, and perhaps even ourselves.

§2

The excellent Unzer made observations on the life and death of people which may not have the value of complete novelty, but which certainly have the merit of truth and great lucidity. "The sum total of the parts and forces of a body," says this man of merit, "make up its nature. Since the human body is not by its nature substantially different from all other bodies, I call this nature the physical nature.—The capacity, the ability and the forces for human economy I call the mechanical nature. The new forces by which this able machine, which without them is dead, moves, feels, thinks, differs from the mechanical laws of an ordinary, artificial, or a dead natural plant machine, I call the animal nature.

"The nature of the human body is thus the sum total of its physical, mechanical, and animal nature.

"The continuance of the nature of a thing is called its life. The end of the nature, however, is its death.

"The human body is therefore capable of threefold life and threefold death."*

From this concept it can be easily understood that man is not immediately dead

* "The Physician," Part II, Chapter 36.

265

but mostly dies partly, gradually. Unconsciousness is an example of how this usually happens: he who is overcome by it, almost always feels how he loses hearing and sight beforehand; then, the muscles fail him and leave the body to its own gravity and the position in which he is, the pulse becomes completely imperceptible, the skin, especially in the face, becomes deathly pale and ice-cold, the eyes close, and when they are opened by force, the soul does not perceive anything of the image which external objects project upon the retina. Occasionally the sick person, without his knowledge, excretes urine and feces; in other words, the sphincters of the urinary bladder and rectum are subject to some kind of paralysis. Thus all parts that now refuse to function are separated from real death only by little more than the power of the heart, which should it be lost and not restore circulation for some considerable time, all is lost. Meanwhile, life in the unconscious person, albeit very weak, is restricted to a few parts, the heart moves or it remains at least in possession of its sensitivity; by imperceptible breathing, the lungs distend sufficently to let through the little blood sent to them by the heart.—Those animals which spend the winter without a sign of life, without food, without evacuation, are in every way like dead animals of their species, so that nobody can immediately and easily state a difference which consists only in the very slight circulation, confined to the innermost parts, and the constant ability to be awakened by returning warmth. Thus, real death differs from these and similar cases only in degree, and this difference has at first simply no certain symptoms at all, when the entire animal machine, so-to-say, lies wrecked in front of us. I know of only a few parts without whose activity the human clockwork cannot run on for some time, and it is known that even the noblest parts sometimes are destroyed in the most incredible manner without death occurring immediately. The writings of physicians are full of such important observations, and the physiologists are often at a loss to explain the continued functioning of the whole when the most important springs have already burst and the leading driving cogs are as if crushed.

One must precisely differentiate between the invisible life of an animal and the visible life, therefore, and take it as a constant principle that the latter may have disappeared for a considerable time without the former ceasing, and without this hidden spark, fanned into flame by some stimulus, being unable to reproduce the general life of all the bodily parts. Malouin rightly says: One knows death only as opposed to life, as the clock is distinguished from its movements. At first a corpse differs from a live body only in regard to movement. The organs are able to begin functioning again for some time, until putrefaction, which occurs sooner or later, severs the cohesion of its parts, and the machine becomes forever incapable of movement. Thus one can assume two stages of death. In the first, man is only incompletely dead, still amenable to help, and amenable as long as his vital organs are no more than inactive but capable of being put into motion again. Complete death follows after that, and consists in an earlier physical or mechanical destruction of the vital organs, and consequently of all possibility of being put into motion again.*

* * *

Frank subsequently deals with signs of death and the ordinances issued in various countries to protect the apparently dead.

---

* "Dictionnaire encyclopédique," Edit. de Genève. Tome XXII, p. 272. 73.

A SYSTEM OF COMPLETE MEDICAL POLICE

Volume Five

Safety Measures as Far as Public Health is
Concerned and the Interment of the Dead

PREFACE

Opening the fifth volume of my Medical Police (Medicinische Polizey) with a treatise on apparent death, I must admit that those of my readers who, to the credit of the grateful author, complained about the long interruption in this work, were really entitled to conclude that the interruption of 24 years was due to the real death of the author. But the resurrection of this work of mine indicates that if its apparent demise has been ascribed to a real demise, at least it cannot be said that in the long intervening period I did not give any sign of life regarding state medicine and thus gave no grounds for doubting my resurrection. It is known that in the ten years I was in Italy, and my equally long employment in the Austrian capital, my four-year service in Lithuania and in St. Petersburg, in addition to the many tasks of a public teacher of practical medicine, and the publication of several treatises on this subject, I was constantly busy as ordered, organizing the study of medicine, equipping a physicians' higher college, improving the administration of pharmacies, regularly managing many hospitals, preventing or stamping out various epidemics, and in general carrying out the duties of a medical expert and having an extensive practice. If the continuation of the present work was necessarily delayed, nevertheless its further elaboration, in view of the applicability of the proposals it should contain, may have gained more than it lost.

After the long time that has passed between the publication of the fourth and the present volumes of my work, it is to be expected that if I used part of my remaining days for other matters, there probably would not be enough time to complete my work. I therefore decided as early as 1808, after I had been visited by several illnesses, and my otherwise sound forces were unable to resist the northern climate, to renounce not only it but also all medical activities and to devote all my remaining time of life to the completion of the books promised to the public, and possibly to the publication of my most important observations concerning practical medicine. In 1809 I chose the gentle Rhine regions, and among them the Breisgau, which was particularly favored by nature, as the place of my future sojourn. However, a fate whose description would make my unhealed wounds bleed again, led me after barely a year and a half into the arms of my steady friend Vienna, which had become gray together with me, and to the apartment that remained there to me. In the midst of powerful storms I have repaid part of my literary debts; if I will be granted the necessary lifetime, and according to my strength, I will repay the rest, of course only in old— in our so highly learned times not so popular—but at least not in counterfeit coin.

In the first volume of this extensive work I dealt with healthy procreation and desired reproduction, in the second with extramarital procreation, and the physical education of newborn infants into adult citizens, in the third with their nutrition, clothing, maintenance and dwelling, and in the fourth and fifth, finally with the security institutions required for the protection of the population. Since the number of subjects to be dealt with was so large, I was unable to merge these last two volumes into one.

Thus I have, as far as my strength permitted, described everything from procreation to death and the funeral of mortals, in relation to public health administration, and concluded almost all subjects that do not belong to medical institutions and hospitals proper.

It remains for me to deal with these last, which require no less than two volumes. Of the supplements to Medical Police (Medicinische Polizey), the first volume is to appear at the next Easter Fair, and the second is to follow soon. For them I have already put in order the most important chapters which relate to health matters and hospitals, and which on various occasions I already elaborated in the past. Thus, if I should become prematurely unable to write any more, or if death should thwart my well-meant intentions, it will at least be clear how I thought and acted in regard to subjects contained in the promised volumes of this work.

Vienna in Austria, 19 March 1812.

PART TWO
Section Six

On apparent death and preventive measures required in general

* * *

§2

What is apparent death?

Most forms of apparent death could be rightly considered some kind of suffocation, and thus treated under a single heading; however, the variety of remedies justifies a more accurate distinction of the subjects treated here. Under them, I shall consider various subcategories of apparent death, but I shall always stipulate the method of treating the victim with hope of success in every case, no matter how remote this may sometimes seem.

Apparent death is in reality vital capacity hidden under the image of death and expressing itself neither by constant body heat nor by breathing, neither by heartbeat nor by pulse, neither by perception nor consciousness, nor by any movement. Therefore inactive ability of resuscitation I call apparent death; and this ability may be found for a longer or shorter time in any animal, without any of the usual signs of life. Life, as it is used in common language, is merely an expression of life rather than life itself, which may be present without there being any sign for others to perceive. Man, formed by the activity of his vital organs to give proof of his continued existence, is sometimes, regardless of the season, put into a state in which he, like the bat, the swallow, the marmot in winter ceases, not to live, but to give proof of his living. In the previous volume, I have explained the difficulties of distinguishing this state from real death, but I must now recall the fact that the causes which usually end our lives most rapidly are those which most often under the same terrifying aspect destroy all vitality, but not always as rapidly as they usually suffocate all visible signs of life. The most violent of these causes which suddenly robs our vital organs of their apparent activity affects the breathing usually. I shall, therefore, examine mainly the effects of air that is unsuitable to be breathed in; then, I shall proceed to the remaining causes of sudden apparent death. In that fashion on the basis of experience and reason I shall point out the most suitable countermeasures to be taken.

* * *

Frank then deals with the various kinds of apparent death. He provides a short history of the rescue service and sheds light on the insufficiency of the measures taken hitherto, giving individual examples, whereupon, in §9, he lists three generally obligatory guidelines.

§9

General measures

In every well regulated state, therefore, must the following three conditions be emphatically provided for saving accident victims and apparently dead persons:

1) That everybody without exception be obliged to help, as quickly as possible as far as can be done without jeopardizing his own safety, a person who is in obvious danger or who is apparently dead, if he lacks any other assistance.

2) That nobody may plead as an excuse ignorance of the remedies to be applied before the arrival of a physician or surgeon.

3) That everywhere, but especially at dangerous places, physicians, surgeons, supervisors, and rescuers be appointed and the tools and medicines necessary for rescue be purchased and stored, and constantly maintained in a good state, at places where they can be easily found.

As regards the first point, I need not prove perhaps the justice of such a law, which is based on Christian morals, and I hope for the sake of mankind's honor that nowhere will the judicial authorities place a deplorable, not to say ridiculous, obstacle in the way of faster rescue of accident victims.

A revised and enlarged mandate of the Council meeting in Hamburg of 11 February 1793 says: "First everybody is repeatedly reminded and exhorted that in any case it is the duty of every man and Christian to provide for the rescue and recovery of victims of accidents, and that everybody should obey the following regulations and contribute all in his power, and not be deterred by the unfounded prejudice that it is forbidden or disgraceful to voluntarily touch, pull out, or give shelter to somebody who fell into the water, is being strangled or otherwise suffocating, especially if such a person wanted to take his own life, as if one could thereby get into trouble or incur expenditures. Also, the prejudice that there is no help possible for a body that is already stiff or seems dead. The authorities assure everybody who receives such a body into his house that he will receive the speediest protection against any crowd, that if the body cannot be revived it will be taken away as soon as possible, that no expenditures will be incurred; on the contrary, all damage and costs due to the reception, or the providing of beds, blankets and other implements, and the relative share of subsequent rewards are guaranteed by the authorities."—"On the other hand, those who impede or prevent the rescue, or prevent others who want to aid the victim, as well as those who, by their intrusion or otherwise, obstruct the rescue attempts, will be held responsible and if found guilty, be subject to severe punishment."

* * *

There follow examples of further ordinances in different countries, these explaining the first point.

Universal education

In regard to the second point, my opinion is this: 1) in all elementary schools the duties, so closely connected with religion, toward persons who have had accidents should be thoroughly explained, and young people should be acquainted in time with both the causes of such sad accidents and the main means of rescue. This has already been ordered in Hamburg. It is still a remainder of our former cruelty that in elementary schools the necessary religious dogma is taught, but little of the rules of self-preservation and the primary duties toward oneself, one's fellow citizens and his domestic animals. If our first catechisms had been drafted by not only zealous theologians, but together with them, prudent statesmen, economists, and physicians, it is certain that useful education of the people would have progressed much more. Although the catechism and the popular calender have no place in our book collections, they are in my opinion the most important books for mankind, provided they are what they should be. And the priest and the schoolteacher, even if they were only half as learned, only taught in addition to the principles of the faith, all the good they could, they would be the most eminent and (not only according to time) the first professors in the State. In my opinion it would not be beneath an academy of sciences, no matter how famous, either to itself prepare the non-theological part of a catechism or to set out a considerable reward for the best draft. German physicians have already supplied important contributions to such a useful undertaking, especially in regard to physical accidents and apparent death; I may flatter myself that in my work on Medical Police, too, some useful hints for such work are contained.

* * *

Personnel and equipment for rescue

The third condition for appointing experts, superiors and assistants first requires that at the countries' universities there should be thorough instructions as to how physicians and surgeons should proceed with accident victims and the apparently dead, and public examinations should establish strictly the extent to which the instruction was fruitful. Physicians who learned their science at universities abroad should give proof of the knowledge they acquired in this field before being appointed, especially to civil service. The medical districts of the country should be stipulated in such a way that they would not lack physicians and surgeons, especially in communities where there are river or lake ferries, bathing establishments and pools. It goes without saying that physicians and surgeons who do not draw a salary from the state, if called to save people who have suffered accidents or who are apparently dead, are also obliged to aid them as quickly as possible. When the cities of Lyons and Rouen, following the example of the capital, made arrangements for the rescue of drowning persons, the local physicians and surgeons decided that the first of them who would be called in such a case should immediately proceed to the indicated place.

It goes equally without saying that each mayor, upon the first report of an accident, should immediately take the prescribed measures: providing both the persons from his community required to give aid and the tools and means necessary for the rescue, and by his authority, he should maintain good order during all the actions that have to be taken.

* * *

PART TWO

Section Seven

On apparent death due to the lack of good air for breathing

* * *

In the first subsections, Frank explains what is meant by "atmospheric air," "mephitic exhalations," and "carbonic" and "flammable air." He then speaks about fermentation, carbonic vapor, fountain air, exhalations above latrines, and their dangers for human beings, as well as the protective measures to be taken. Of these latter, the following subsections emphasize direct reanimation measures.

§9

When the accident victim has been pulled out of the mephitic fumes and transferred into fresh air, it is important to note whether he suffers only from strong numbness, or whether he has already passed into the state of apparent death. In the former case he usually recovers soon if he is placed in a somewhat upright position or half sitting, while somebody holds his head straight, neither forward nor back, if he is quickly undressed and brought into fresh air, into the open in summer, possibly under a tree, into a spacious room where windows and doors are open in winter, if he is sprinkled with cold water or if his face, head and neck, as well as the rear part of the ears, are washed with cold vinegar. Care must be taken, however, that the oral and nasal cavities are not filled with water which might prevent breathing, which begins later. Also blowing into the face with clean bellows is useful. The head is to be swathed in folded cloths that have been immersed in clean water. When the suffocated person regains consciousness, he should be dried and placed in a half sitting position in a cool bed and covered with a light blanket. At the same time the suffocated is to be given an enema of equal parts of vinegar and water neither of which must be applied warm. Poultices of cold water are to be placed on the chest and the pit of the stomach, as well as in the armpits.

* * *

§12

Restoration of breathing

If no signs of life follow upon these ministrations, the activity of breathing should mainly be sought, for the motions of the heart, the circulation of juices, the body heat, and its sensibility depend on it.

By breathing in air from mouth to mouth

It is strange that only as late as 1744 the first attempt was made in England to restore breathing by artificial inflation of the lungs, and this was done with an adult. This attempt was made by William Tossack, surgeon at Allon, on a man who had suffocated and had not given a sign of life for 3/4 of an hour. The attempt was successful and was first described in "Medical Essays," Edinburgh.* However, Borellus had already reported that a servant saved his suffocated master by breathing air into his mouth.** Such blowing in of air was effected either by the volunteering philanthropist putting his mouth upon the mouth of the apparently dead person, compressing his nose, and then blowing his breath into the lungs of the victim, or a tube was inserted in one nostril of the apparently dead person while the other was held shut, and thus breath was blown into the lungs of the unfortunate. Vogel rightly admonishes that when air is blown in, the head of the windpipe should be gently pressed backward because the way to the gullet which lies to the left behind the windpipe, and to the stomach is thus blocked to the air.† However, in apparently dead adult persons in whom rigor has already set in, the head of the windpipe cannot be pushed back so easily without using violence. It is always necessary when breathing or blowing air into a drowned person, to lay him on the side, preferably the left, and to hold the body firmly in this position. In a publication which appeared as early as 1740 at Strasbourg, the German translator says: "It happened to me that three young chicks got into freshly slaked lime and suffocated in it. They may have been in it for an hour and did not show any signs of life. I had them placed into a fairly deep dish but in such a way that the necks and heads were above the edge of the dish, and had water poured in, at first quite lukewarm, later somewhat warmer, so that their bodies were cleansed of the adhering lime and were warmed at the same time. Then I had them warmed and dried at a fire while held in hands and swathed in cloth, and at the same time breath was blown into their throats; two of them soon recovered so that after a few hours they were able to follow the hen." Thureton made experiments with fowl, and Muralt with dogs, blowing air through the oral opening. John Fothergill†† spread the news of the rescue of a suffocated person by Tossack,

* Vol. V, part II, p. 605.
** Centur. III. obs. LVIII, p. 241.
 † Thoughts and Remarks on the Rescue of Drowned Persons.
†† "Medical and Philosophical Works," London 1781.

who blew air into the person's mouth and who even further exhaled his own breath into the victim, from mouth to mouth and after closing up the suffocated person's nostrils. Fothergill states that he approves completely of this procedure. "I have been told by some of my acquaintances," declares this enlightened physician, "that bellows would be better for blowing air through the mouth into the lungs of an accident victim, but if there is a philanthropist present who is ready to carry out this charitable act, it seems to me that it is better to have him breathe out the air. Firstly, there are not always such bellows available; secondly, the human lungs can supply exactly as much air as those of another person can inhale without damage, and this is a thing that is not so easy to determine with bellows; thirdly, the moist, warm breath, which a living person breathes into the suffocated one is much more suitable to restore circulation than could be expected of cold air that is pressed into the lungs by bellows."*

* * *

§15

Respiration of vital air

After experiments showed that an animal lives seven times longer in oxygen gas than in atmospheric air, and that it is precisely this kind of gas which makes up the breathable part of the air, Chaussier, and in particular van Marum** advised respiration of vital air into the lungs of suffocated persons.† As is known, this kind of gas is obtained most cheaply from manganese dioxide and purified saltpeter. This vital air can be gathered in several bottles and properly stored. When it is needed, it is conducted into bladders, and these, after having been filled, are connected with Gorcy's bellows, and the oxygen is driven through them into the lungs. "After oral and nasal cavities have been freed as much as possible of mud," says Holst, "we blow air into the lungs through Gorcy's bellows by means of a bent pipe which is led past the root of the tongue to the upper opening of the larynx. Until traces of the restored respiration become apparent, we use oxygen gas as the most concentrated and natural vital stimulus for the lungs; when spontaneous breathing returns, we use the atmospheric air. We never used a mixture of hydrochloric acid with atmospheric air because this gas seemed to deviate completely from the recognized vital stimulants, and even in mixture it seemed to have only a corroding effect on the tender structure of cells and vessels.†† The van Marum syringe is also suitable for

* * *

* L.c. p. 118.
** "Observations and Experiments with the Means of Rescue of Drowned Persons," p. 106. 19.
† See also Daniel Hill's "Observations and Experiments on the Curing Powers of Oxygen Gas or Vital Air," P. 21. 19.
†† Günther, l.c., pp. 100, 101.

this purpose. According to Ackermann, in rescuing even apparently dead persons, one should rely exclusively on oxygen gas while avoiding all attempts at stimulating the nervous system, and the gas should be conducted to the blood of the seemingly dead, and mixed with it in suitable form.*

* * *

Part Two, Section Ten deals with undertaking establishments, funerals, and cemeteries. It is typical of the enlightened and at the same time economic attitude of Frank that in §40 he sympathizes with the ordinance issued by Joseph II, viz., that the dead are not to buried in coffins but only in sacks.

---

* "Apparent Death and the Rescue Procedure, a Chymiatric Attempt," Frankfurt, 1804. See also Poppe, l.c., pp. 499, 199.

A SYSTEM OF COMPLETE MEDICAL POLICE

Volume Six

Medical Affairs

1

Medical Science and Medical Educational Institutions in General

PREFACE

In such a work, encompassing so many and varied subjects concerning public health, which is so comprehensive and so cumbersome that, as in the present case, only five volumes were published in the course of 37 years in very long and irregular intervals, and though this delay has its good reasons,* nevertheless, each volume requires its preface as a due by the author to his honored public.

In our times hairsplitting is an everyday occurrence, especially in Germany. Daniel was the first to introduce the name "State Medicine" (Staatsarzneykunde) and he raised it to the dignity of a genus to which two very different branches of study, medical police and forensic medicine, were to be subordinated as species. Later writers called the medical police simply health police (Gesundheits-Polizey), sanitary police (Sanitäts-Polizey), public health police (öffentliche Gesundheits-Polizey), and even life security police (Lebenssicherheitspolizey). J. B. Eberhard likes the name medical legislation (medicinische Gesetzgebung), and to this he subordinates medical police and police of medicine as species. Gruner views both this classification and the names, "natural science for legislation—dietetics of the state" (Naturkunde für die Rechtspflege—Diätetik des Staates) as wrong and therefore unusable. Not because of Daniel, but out of deference for the learned men who approved Daniel's expression, I myself used in my work now and again the expression "State Medicine," and for the sake of myself and my contemporaries, who are in no mood for daily change, I remain faithful to the old name, though not out of ridiculous predilection for the name of a child of which I am neither the parent nor the godfather, but which I only adopted and, no matter how immature and small-limbed I found it, raised it within ten years to considerable size, and almost without outside assistance, at that.

In the preceding five volumes of this work I contemplated man living in society, in all the situations involving threatening danger and requiring assistance from the Medical Police. The assumption might now arise that with this my work has reached the end; but whoever remembers the preliminary announcement of my work, or even my promise given on its title page, namely the promise of completeness,

* Preface to the fifth volume of "Medical Police."

will easily notice the gaps which I deliberately left and which to fill where it seems fitting, I shall now devote the few days that are left to me.

I do not think that I have to apologize to knowledgeable people for the length of my work so far. Folio volumes have been written about the art of curing mankind's illnesses, and some have been received with thanks. Why should my work be considered too long-winded, therefore, as it is destined to eliminate from human society a host of physical ills and is much more certain of success in so doing? Without wanting to disparage practicing medicine which has risen so high in our time, I am prepared boldly to wager that if two empires were in everything equal except that one were sufficiently provided with the most skillful practitioners, but were deprived of all the advantages that are to be expected from a good Medical Police, while the other, conversely, would have no physicians at all, but except for this shortcoming would enjoy the most suitable health institutions, I say that of these two empires the latter would undoubtedly have the advantage of the former, both in regard to the number of inhabitants and their health and longevity. Although this statement may sound too harsh to some, to prove it I need only mention the ravages caused in Europe by the plague, yellow fever, leprosy, and smallpox because of the lack of strict police supervision.

No matter how much I have been rewarded for my work by the approbation of the public, I am not so vain that I cannot bear criticism by some, and in view of my mentality, which makes me never in a mood for learned disputes, the "fac melius" (except of the defense forced upon me) is all that I permit myself to reply to my critics. With such a large number of subjects treated by me, how could I have failed to offer an opening to the quarrelsome?

It was said of my work that "with all its recognized value, according to experience so far gathered, the beneficient consequences, which the citizen of the world expected of it, have not been observed."* If this were really true, the blame should be ascribed not to me, but to the ill-fated times of war, which paralyze all humanitarian institutions that require some expenditure, and also to the well known recklessness of the people, who usually receive the warnings of the physicians with the greatest indifference so long as they are in good health. In the meantime, some salutary health ordinances have appeared upon my indirect instigation, even if my name did not appear in them, and if the seed of the good does not sprout as quickly as the seed of calamity, why blame the indefatigable plowman? Stoll says that the cause of failure is that I, "firstly, stipulated the concepts of constitution and administration of the state, and thus also of medical matters, as a partial intent of realizing the aim of medical policy, not distinguishing one from the other"; nay, that I "even assumed

---

* Dr. J. Stolls "Staatswissenschaftliche Untersuchungen und Erfahrungen über das Medicinalwesen," Zürich 1812. I. Theil. S. 156–158.

the organization of medicine as given, and immediately stipulated only the very objects of administration."

To this I can but reply that my intention was not to draft the metaphysics of Medical Police, that I am still of the opinion that we physicians should deal less with the business of administering the state than is the custom nowadays, that medical matters should be organized more according to the state than the state according to them, and finally, that I should not be judged according to what I have omitted in my work before I have concluded it.

* * *

Another reason for the imperfection of [my] work," says Stoll, "as far as it has already appeared, lies in the lack of a perfectly determined concept of the Police, and that even the criteria of the system are not given, i.e., which subjects really belong to Medical Police. Therefore many subjects are included in it which really do not belong to it: e.g., on the prevention of various accidental dangers."

To tell the truth, I was never inclined to stir up the wasps' nest of scholastic definitions and thus to take part in the time-wasting quarrels which were conducted also because of the word "Police." It suffices, therefore, so far as I am concerned, that immediately on the first leaf of the first volume of my work, I informed the reader of my concept of the general police, which I share with v. Sonnenfels, and of my concept of Medical Police. Scherf says rightly: "According to the judgment by Herr v. Berg and after sifting of the definitions of the general police given by the writers, or of the concepts of police given altogether, it seems certain that the jurists still lack a philosophical concept of the police which would reduce the variety of it to a common principle from which this variety could again be explained and deduced, its nature or its essence determined, and its limits defined. If such a concept were either given from experience or, independently of it, were given a priori, the physicians could subsume under it the concept of Medical or Health Police, and they would have to modify its duties, rights, and limits accordingly; it would then be very easy to determine from it the nature or the peculiarity of Medical Police, which is only a department or branch of the general police. But since jurisprudence and political science lacks such a certain and circumscribed concept, the physicians should be forgiven for not defining in their textbooks the concept of Medical Police accurately, and succinctly, but only superficially and briefly."

Could it not be said that the general police is appointed by the state as the supervisor and administrator of order and mutual security, which does not in the least encroach upon domestic peace, and Medical Police is the same guardian administering public health of the people and their cattle living in a society according to the same liberal principles.

Just as the physicians, though they do not know what life is, have nevertheless described with sufficient accuracy its functions and the means of its maintenance, the same also applies to the general and Medical Police: only that there is room for argument whether this or that belongs within its jurisdiction. Thus, I was also reproached for having included in the latter subjects that do not belong to it; but I believe I have long ago satisfactorily disposed of this objection and I, therefore, refer to my public declaration.* In a culturally and in many other respects inferior nation, many subjects must at first be ordered by law, but once introduced, many laws within no more than a lifetime are observed voluntarily, as mere customs, without mentioning the law anymore.

* * *

Of the present volume of my work, there is little I want to say by way of preface. The great number of subjects to be dealt with made it necessary to divide them up. In the second part, which I have to deliver for printing still in this year, I spoke in particular of the public teaching of medicine. Since I have taught at five famous medical schools as public teacher, and since I myself worked out and implemented the curriculum at some of them, I did not approach this important task unprepared.

All the more, I know the obstacles that often are in the way of such an endeavor. It is the same in planning a scientific edifice in a certain field that has already been built on, as with building a new and regular city at a place where houses and streets, founded without plan, are to be preserved: only complete razing to the ground can provide free flight for the builder. However, most universities in France were as good as calcined owing to the long revolution, but in Germany, and in most other European states, they were shaken almost to overthrow, and thus the present building plan offered by me may be in good time, no matter how strenuously the owners of a few houses that are not completely dilapidated resist. I would show unforgivable conceit if I declared that the draft study contained in this volume is a plan, corresponding perfectly to the requirements not only of the present but also of much later times.

Vienna, 19 March 1816.

---

* "Med. Police," Vol. II. Preface.

PART ONE
Section One

On medical practice in general and on its influence on the well-being of the state

* * *

Frank gives a survey of the development of medicine since antiquity, and then deals with those arguments against it as expressed by Rousseau and other critics of medicine. He counters these arguments with his view of the utility of medicine set forth in subsection 7: A special subsection (§9) deals with the duties of the physician, from which we present the main parts.

§7

[On the utility of medicine]

Considering that the objections to the possibility, the reality of medicine, are based only on shallow scoffing or on idle sophistry (§6), I want to speak here of the benefit which this art has already partly provided for mankind, and could in future provide to a much larger extent if the obstacles from which it suffers were removed. For the sake of better order of this brief examination it is necessary to stipulate first preventive medicine, second curative, third the merely palliative, and fourth and finally forensic medicine.

Assuming that the offensive plans of the physicians do not come up to the expectations of suffering mankind where the sworn enemy is already in possession of the prey, nevertheless, the thoroughness and force of the defensive system of medicine cannot reasonably be doubted by anybody. Even those who despise medicine, pay homage to that part of it which teaches how to maintain health and prevent illnesses. Muratori says: "Is it beneficial to society to have physicians or not? There is quite a number of people who believe that they are dispensable or even deleterious; the large mass of people is of the opinion that the physicians bring the state much profit. Regardless of this variety in judgments, the most enlightened men consider medicine an honorable and valuable science. To tell the truth, it is less because of their luck in treating human illnesses but because of the useful warnings and instruc-

289

tions which skilled physicians usually give for the sake of maintaining health and preventing disease."*

It is either the physician alone, or upon his request the state itself who prevents the possible or very likely impending physical ills that concern private or public health. In the former case it is medical, in the latter case it is public prevention which includes most of the subjects that are considered part of public health. Since it is infinitely easier to prevent physical ills than to remedy them once they have arrived, preventive medicine is the most important part of medicine although it has been neglected for a longer time than any other part. Yet Hippocrates was the first who developed the laws of a healthy way of life and taught according to eternally true principles the prevention of the most frequent diseases occurring in each geographical region. Half the people's illnesses, especially the catching ones, are certainly due to neglected preventive measures. Physicians properly distributed in a country are the most natural guardians of public health. Only through them can the governments be informed of the diseases that are endemic in various provinces, of the incidence, the spreading, and the consequences of each epidemic affecting both human beings and their cattle, its communication, as well as of the surest preventive means. He is no physician who, in the case of spreading epidemics, even before being called upon by the authorities, does not endeavor with all his strength and by suitable advice and active intervention to prevent the spreading of the new ill in towns, villages, and families entrusted to his care. How far have we advanced in the art of eliminating the dangers of infection of malignant hospital, jail and ship fevers since the great chemist Guyton de Morveau, called upon by the French government in 1773 to cleanse the atmosphere of the cathedral of Dijon which had been poisoned by the disinterment of bodies, taught how useful was hydrochloric gas,** and later James Carmichael Smyth introduced the widespread use of nitric vapors† in crowded hospital rooms, jails and ships! Just look at the many excellent portions of treatises which the physicians published and endeavored to disseminate in the most selfless way, for the sake of abolishing habits deleterious to health, and of having a healthy offspring, and for completely preventing pernicious epidemic diseases from whose treatment they might expect a rich livelihood. It must be admitted that few other classes of people ever made such an endeavor to make themselves less

---

* Cf. excerpt of the treatise by Muratori, "Della felicità publica," in Robinet's "Dictionnaire Universel des Sciences Morale, Économique, Politique, et Diplomatique," Londres 1779. Vol. IX–410, p. 40.

** Cf. Instruction sur les moyens d'entretenir la salubrité et de purifier l'air des salles dans les Hôpitaux militaires. Guyton de Morveau, "Discours préliminaire au traité des moyens de désinfecter l'air," published by the Medical Council of Paris under the 5th Ventose of the 2nd year of the French Republic.

† A description of the Jail Distemper, etc. Description de la fièvre des prisons, telle qu'elle se manifesta parmi les prisonniers Espagnols détenus à Winchester, en 1780, ainsi que les moyens, qui furent employés pour la guérir et pour détruir la contagion qui y avoit donné lieu. London 1795. S. Odier, bibliothèque Britannique; science et arts Vol. XVI, pp. 250, 335. Vol. XVII, p. 27.

necessary to the state. I still feel gratefully the great value of the weighty words with which Emperor Joseph II deigned to address to me at my first introduction in Vienna, 1785: "You are not orthodox," he said, "you taught the regents how to maintain their subjects in good health, and thereby you did not spare the interests of the physicians!" Yes, I am much more proud of my endeavor to prevent the ills threatening mankind from all sides than of the successful healing of many patients no matter that I have grounds to appreciate their loud gratefulness in various countries. And how many of my brethren in office have entered the path, where I had the good fortune to lay the trail, to the greatest advantage of mankind! Was it not the physicians or their writings which brought about the many excellent ordinances of enlightened governments that concerned public health and achieved such signal successes? Did not some of them for years, despite all the shouting of the people,* now and again even despite the shouting from the pulpit,** and to set a convincing example, inoculate their own children first† before this procedure was approved, protected, and finally ordered by regents? The result was that whereas previously out of a million people suffering from smallpox at least a hundred thousand succumbed, after inoculation only one thousand eight hundred lost their lives, consequently ninety-eight thousand two hundred people were saved for the state by the art. When through the immortal Doctor Jenner, cowpox vaccination and its usefulness first became known, it was again the physicians through whose unfailing diligence and zeal this great discovery was spread everywhere and used, despite all the objections. Now it depends only on the reasonableness of the authorities whether by the general use of this invention they want to save the twelfth part of all the inhabitants of the earth who up to now have fallen victim every year (which smallpox alone used to carry off, i.e., several million people annually), whether they will achieve more beautiful, less disfigured and healthier offspring, and finally, whether they want to eliminate this pestilential disease completely from the surface of the earth and thus make the use of this medical discovery itself superfluous. If we now find ourselves so rarely attacked by the plague, as compared with the previous

* The Royal Prussian physician-in-ordinary, Dr. Eller, one of the first physicians in Germany (1721 or 1722) who inoculated with smallpox, says that this useful undertaking would have found an earlier reception in Berlin if the people would not have adhered so firmly to the prejudice of predestination with regard to illnesses and death. "De cognoscendis et curandis morbis," pp. 152, 153.

** The preacher, Massey, stated in England from the pulpit that inoculation of smallpox was an invention of the devil who had applied it already to Job.

† In 1748 Doctor Tronchin inoculated his son with smallpox for the first time; thereby, he introduced this operation in Holland, and in 1750 he prevailed on his native town, Geneva, to accept it. In that same year when a murderous smallpox epidemic caused destruction at the borders of Tuscany and in the Papal state, Dr. Peverini from Citerna inoculated first his daughter with smallpox matter drawn from lethal smallpox, the purpose being the same [prevention of contracting the virulent disease]. In regard to this, see Hensler's letters on smallpox inoculation (Henslers Briefe über das Blatterpelzen). Altona 1765.

centuries, or if it does insinuate itself somewhere, we are able to choke it off quickly, is this not the effect of our better measures of public health policy on the water and on land against this source of the greatest human misery? And are not these measures the fruit of medical admonitions and writings on its feasibility, based on the accurate knowledge of the mode of propagation and the main vehicles of the contagious matter? Is it already forgotten how readily the physicians everywhere, when there was an attack of plague, proceeded right into the center of the disaster, and how often they found there, foreseen by them but disregarded out of fierce philanthropy and unbounded zeal for service, their own end but not a consoler for the family that was left behind, often without means?* How often does the physician succeed, when he is consulted within the first few days, in cases of venereal contagious matter, which appears first locally, in destroying this matter quickly, and consequently in preventing its spread, and thus the spread of general venereal disease, including its sad consequences, which often affect an entire innocent family? The philanthropic physician often earns urgently when he first notices signs of the contagious ill, which to the infected person often seem quite harmless, to desist completely from intercourse with the opposite sex, or, if he already suffers from venereal disease but flatters himself rashly that it has been completely healed, and therefore intends to marry prematurely, the physician entreats him that this already in the first weeks of married life would disturb all his domestic happiness and would threaten his ability for healthy procreation, and that he should therefore desist for a time from his intention and wait conscientiously for his complete recovery. Does not the physician often succeed in combating rabies, by a quick destruction of the surface of a wound caused by the bite of a rabid animal and covered or penetrated by the venom, and does this not prevent most opportunely the certain outbreak of this, the most terrible of all human diseases? Did not a similar skillful process creatively save hundreds of people who, wounded by poisoned arrows or bites of vipers, were certain to die? How many thousands of hopeful young men, who had already caught the vice of masturbation and were thus lost to the state, have been saved by physicians rather than by the most eloquent moralists, by the fatherly exhortation, a shocking representation of the terrible consequences of this unnatural offence, and have thus been transformed into useful members of human society! The extermination of the coarsest prejudices, which were deleterious to the health and life of the people, is mostly the work of the physicians who more than others are gifted with understanding of

---

* "Who else but the physicians were in those times of contagion the sheet-anchor which the dismayed leaders of the state tossed out when outraged nature threatened the citizens of the state with destruction! Here it was where all human knowledge, even the most thorough, was inferior to medical knowledge. The time had to come to show to our state authorities how great was the disadvantage which follows neglected medical constitution and the consequent lack of a public health policy." D. Ant. Fried. Fischer's "Darstellung der Medicinalverfassung Sachsens nebst Vorschlägen zu ihrer Verbesserung," Leipzig 1814. 8. pp. 35, 36.

natural science.* Whoever thinks that this service is not so very valuable, should read what I wrote elsewhere in this work about many diseases which were formerly, neglecting all reasonable antidotes, ascribed merely to evil nature and witches.** The physician-in-ordinary of the Duchy of Juelich and Clere, Doctor Wyerus (Wyer) was one of the first who emphatically attacked the belief in witches and sorcerers, and in view of the opinions then prevalent both in clerical and in secular courts, this entailed the great danger for him of being burned at the stake.† How great is the difference between this mentality and that of Charlemagne who decreed as early as the eighth century that "nobody, no matter who he is, be burned under the pretext of witchcraft, but that the sorcerers should be donated as serfs to the church."†† The blind belief in vampires, with its sad consequences, which was so completely destroyed by van Swieten, is still fresh in memory. Such applications in the interest of mankind always caused the physicians to be reproached with unbelief, a reproach that is as dangerous as it is undeserved, and we unfortunately know how dearly some of them had to pay when this reputation attached to them. Never were the warnings heeded, about dangers entailed for the inhabitants of human abodes too close to swamps, about the heedless clearing of woods which prevented the poisonous exhalations from the swamps reaching the houses exposed to them, especially in hot regions, until finally the great papal physician-in-ordinary, Lancisius,‡ opened the eyes of both his colleagues in office and the authorities, and supplied convincing proof that the draining and reclamation of swampy lowlands and the preservation of high woods are urgently needed, both for economic reasons and mainly with regard to public health, and the eradication of the frequent and murderous and variegated intermittent fever (febres intermittentes perniciosae), endemic dropsy, scurvey, and other, often lethal ills. Thus history teaches that one of the most famous

* "Pendant longtemps les hommes adonnés à l'étude de l'art de guérir ont été les seuls qui ont professé les diverses parties de la vaste science de la Nature. C'est aux médecins en général qu'on doit les progrès de la Physique générale, de la Zoologie, de l'Anatomie, de la Botanique, de la Chemie, de la Minéralogie: Ce sont eux qui ont d'abord peuplé les académies de l'Europe, qui ont même institué plusieures d'entre elles, ou qui en ont posé les premiers fondements." Fourcroy, "La médecine éclairée par les sciences physiques, Vol. I. pp. 3, 4.
** "Medical Police," Volume VI, Part II, Section 3, §3, pp. 533 ff. §§6–12. As late as under Gustaf Adolf's rule, witch trials were very frequent in Sweden. The most cruel means were used to make people suspected of sorcery confess: the hangman tore out all their hair, subjected them to the water trial, etc. The daughter of the great Gustaf, Christina, seems to have risen above the superstition of the age and to have curbed this terrible misuse of justice. At least she ordered a court in her German states "to desist from all further Inquisition and trials concerning witchcraft because it is obvious that the longer one deals with these things, the more one gets into an inescapable labyrinth." D. Friedr. Ruehs, "Geschichte Schwedens," Part IV. Halle 1810, p. 459.
† Jo. Wyerus, Gravianus, "de praestigiis Daemonum et incantationibus ac Veneficiis," Basileae 1564.
†† Ad. Ecclesiae servitium donentur. Saxon. Capitul. art. 21. It is recommended to read Gaillard, "Histoire de Charlemagne," Vol. II, p. 245.
‡ "De noxiis paludum effluviis."

philosophers of the Pythagorean school, Empedocles of Agrigent, became immortal and acquired the name of the tamer of the wind because he plugged the gap between two mountain peaks and thus cut off the path of the midday wind which destroyed everything and caused malignant diseases. This philosopher is also reported to have put an end to malignant diseases when the inhabitants of Selinunt suffered from the plague because the nearby river Hypsas contained stagnant and putrid water, and Empedocles brought other running water into the swamp whose exhalations had caused these diseases.* The beneficial distance between burials and churches and human abodes is no less the work of frequently repeated remonstrations by physicians against this abuse. The physical well-being of a large class of useful citizens, the artists and craftsmen, was enormously endangered daily by improvident procedures in their professions, and only a few physicians knew the source of the diseases which were restricted to these people, until the excellent Ramazzini finally discovered it and at the same time taught with great success to drain their noxious effluents.** Barely two centuries ago the specific nature of the so-called lead colic was only half known (although this disease must have afflicted a large number of people in the past millenia, in lead mines, in sundry work by painters, in tin and lead foundries, among potters, typefounders and printers, goldsmiths, apothecaries, chemists, confectioners, and in the long-established adulteration of wine) until it was described by Citesius†: nowadays, when help is sought in time, and the best cure†† is immediately applied, thousands are successfully healed and the sad consequences of this illness, which is so frequent especially in large towns, are averted. Croup, which nowadays seems to be more frequent than ever and still causes the death of a great many children, is now successfully cured much more frequently than before, if an experienced physician is called in good time. Previously the business of physical rearing of children was badly neglected and this neglect, based on gross ignorance and prejudices, had many fatal consequences, but in our time this has been ended, at least in the nurseries of enlightened parents informed by and actively using written warnings from physicians! Since children afflicted with contagious diseases, or only half cured of them, met in public schools, a constantly glimmering fuse was contained therein that could easily ignite a spreading fire, until finally the loud calls of concerned physicians caused several governments to stop this offence, etc.

If the usefulness, in the narrower sense of the word, of the physician to the citizen is to be assessed properly, the physician's art, although it is an entity, has to be

---

† S. Sprengel ["Versuch einer pragmatischen Geschichte der Arzneykunde."] Halle, 1800, Part I, pp. 312–314.

** "De morbis artificum," Genevae 1717.

† "Diatribe de novo et populari apud Pictones dolore colico," Parisiis 1639.

†† Among the many writings on lead colic published up to our time, the "Traité de la Colique métallique, vulgairement appellée colique des peintres, des plombiers etc.," deuxième édition, Paris 1812, 8, by F. V. Mérat is most worthy of being recommended here.

resolved into its main components, and each of these has to be examined separately. Innumerable diseases attack the entire system of the human body or predominantly some parts of it, and though they often also develop externally, they are called internal diseases in view of the origin of the incidence which is hidden to the senses. Other injuries are merely external, and they do not presuppose a fault of the whole, e.g., contusions, wounds, sprains, broken legs, etc. For several centuries the treatment of both these kinds of ill was left to one and the same physician, regardless of the name; and it is as impossible as it is unnecessary to determine whether he should deal first with internal or with external ills. Since in ancient Egypt each part of medicine had its own artist,* it stands to reason to assume that even then the external and internal ills each had their physicians. According to what history teaches, however, it was not until the times of Erasistratus and Herophilus that individual parts of the art were practiced by different physicians, and the entire science was divided into dietetics, pharmacology, and surgery.** It is impossible here to work out what advantages or damage the imperfect medicine of those most ancient times wrought. Apparently a large part of the successes must be ascribed not to the art itself but to the highly strained imagination of the sick, a result of the application of the Temple method. But when Homer says: "A healing man is worth esteem like many others, who cuts out the arrow and bandages with soothing ointment," this commendation refers mainly to the surgeon; and in reality, no matter how limited surgery was, it must have surpassed greatly the healing ability of the physicians in real utility. Yet if we draw conclusions from the considerable wealth of experience, for which we are indebted to Hippocrates in regard to the reserve from which he drew, it seems to me that what this great man gave to us permits us to conclude that in his few writings that are held to be genuine the mass of experience of a thousand previous years, scattered in various temples and families, is far from being exhausted. There are various experiences whose correctness presupposes many others, even if this is not explicitly stated. Just as the few fragments of Chaldean astronomy passed on to us permit the conclusion that these were based on far broader knowledge and even on mathematical operations which later times are thought to have invented, in the same way some Hippocratic sentences reveal a mass of otherwise lost experiences (which a single man, or even his whole family, devoted to medicine, could never have made alone). Just as in the outer mantle of the globe, which has been subject to so many upheavals since time immemorial and is turned over by fiery abysses of the interior, when it is dug up at some distance, frequently superposed layers of lava are found, and between them other layers which could have been formed from the fertile surface soil only in the course of centuries, likewise, under

* Herodotus, Li. II. According to Maillet, this practice still exists in Egypt. "Description de l'Egypte," pp. 264, 265. Likewise the fairly skilled physicians in Coromandel are distinguished according to the diseases which each of them treats. Grundler, "Med. Malabar."
** Celsus, "De Medicina," Praefatio.

the sand and rubble, partly because of original ignorance, and the crassest prejudices of prehistory, partly because of repeated ideas of barbarians, which during lengthy and bloody wars, with pestilence, hunger and misery, again collapsed and were rebuilt again, but later again repeatedly collapsed, scientific edifices contain some rich seams the property of which can convince us of the frequent almost periodic disappearance of human discoveries and experiences, before the power of the perpetuating printing art fixed them on earth.

If we judged only from the existing writings originating in the first centuries after Hippocrates, it would appear very doubtful that in those early times mankind had more good from medicine than harm. However, in later times and certainly even now, no matter how hypothetical and contradictory their publicly expressed opinions are, at the sickbed the physicians tread the way indicated by experience rather than by their theory; likewise the medical practice of the ancient Egyptians cannot with certainty be deduced only from their writings.* But we know that for a considerable time after Hippocrates the physicians imitating him had in many ways an advantage over many of our contemporary physicians: they emphasized more the observance of a regimen appropriate to the illnesses than did later physicians, they used the expectation method more, and they used gymnastics more, both for prevention and for curing chronic cases. But this must be noted here: as soon as the class of the priests had lost its influence, the authorities used the amassed medical knowledge very little or not at all for legislation, policy, or in the administration of justice. While medicine dealt only with treating diseases, it was unable to provide for mankind all the good that it could have provided. Of course, now that medicine is not practiced any more exclusively by people who derive their respect and income from prejudices deleterious to public health, it should be easier to combat and finally destroy completely these prejudices. For centuries, however, people were governed even in regard to the most ordinary natural processes by Egyptian darkness which laymen had diligently maintained in the past: it was a grave crime, hardly to be punished even by the people itself, which had been deceived so long, to obtain knowledge from human corpses of the construction of the body and of its injuries due to illness, knowledge that was so important to the physician. It was equally forbidden to doubt the immediate influence of the gods or the evil spirits on the origin of many illnesses,

---

* We can see that under the Hindus, even very long ago, the physicians did not act so blindly in treating their patients; this is indicated by the dramatist Kalidasa, who more than 1900 years ago (in his "Sakuntala or The Decisive Ring," p. 251) let Anasuya say to her: "We cannot possibly know, Sakuntala, what goes on in your bosom; yet it seems to us that you feel as we often hear it told in love tales. Tell us outright what causes your illness. The physician cannot begin ordering remedies before he has found out the cause of the illness." Third act, pp. 47, 48. Sir William Jones maintains that the Indian physicians are often more learned than the Brahmins, without being so haughty, and they are the most charming and most virtuous among this people. The Sudera study their medicine from books which are called "Waidya," and it seems to follow from the explanations of Kalidasa that they must have contained some good principles.

especially widespread ones. We see from the narratives by St. Jerome himself, that in his times several ills, especially convulsive ones, were considered the effects óf devilish sorcery*; and the endless wars were a hindrance to progress in all sciences, and thus also in medicine.

Although it was in the fifteenth century that medical art woke from its sleep that had lasted more than a thousand years, and despite all the obstacles, important progress was made in the treatment of even the gravest diseases. More than any other, venereal disease, which never disappears without medical intervention, proves incontrovertibly how badly the mockers and doubters treated medicine the benefits of which they sometimes had reaped themselves. It suffices to bear in mind the history of the appearance of [venereal] disease in Europe: there millions of people were attacked by this terrible disease because then no physician was able to prevent it, and they were desperate, and see how far these days the art alone and not good nature (as is usual to say when patients recover from some other ill) has progressed! "Previously," says Zimmermann, "mortality among sailors was so great that on the short journey from Holland to the East Indies, often only to the Cape of Good Hope, or even before the Equator had been reached, it was assumed that every tenth man would be dead. This is especially borne out in [reports] of the older Dutch journeys at the beginning of the seventeenth century, e.g., by Houtmann, Sebald de Weest, van der Hagen, Rogge, Weens, etc. Now on his second journey around the world, Cook lost in 3 years and 18 days only four men out of 139; three were killed by accident, the fourth by a disease which he had already brought from England. In his third journey around the world, both ships in the course of 4 years and 2 months had only five dead out of 192 men. Of these again three had left their country already ill; therefore the journey again accounted only for one man sick. La Pérouse found upon arrival in Botany Bay in New Holland after a journey of two years, only one single sick man among 199 persons. Mortality among 100 people in the prime of life on dry land is three dead in two years. Our methods of sailing the seas therefore has so-to-say defeated nature. One travels around the earth in order to ensure a longer life."** And of what do these methods consist except the most meticulous observance of the medical precepts, given in view of diet and other reasonable treatment of the sailors, the highest cleanliness of the ship's air, etc., and drawing on long experience? "It was deemed impossible," says von Krusenstern, "to prevent scurvy on sea journeys, and at the expense of great wordiness it was proved, e.g., by the historian of Lord Anson's journey, that the greatest precaution against it cannot

---

* "Auriga Gazensis, in curru percussus a Daemone, totus obriguit, ita, nec manus agitare, nec cervicem posset flectere. Delatus ergo in lecto, cum solam linguam moveret ad preces, non prius posse sanari, quam crederet in Jesum, et se sponderet arti pristinae renunciaturum. Credidit, spopondit; sanatus est." "Vita Hilarionis," in opp. omn., T. I. p. 325.

** E. A. W. von Zimmermann, "Die Erde und ihre Bewohner nach den neuesten Entdeckungen," Part I, pp. 17, 19.

help because this illness has its origin in sea air. In spite of that, this terrible disease seems to be all but stamped out or not to pose any great danger at sea because on the longest sea journeys people were able to prevent it completely."* Even curing scurvey that has already progressed far is more successful now than it used to be, unless the required remedies are lacking. Before the nature of malignant intermittent fever was known to physicians, at least ninety-five out of a hundred patients lost their lives, whereas today the same number of people are saved unless the first or second attack, by its quick fatal effect, forestalls all help by the physician. "Among the declining diseases," says Süsmilch, "are colic, diseases of the head and caused by disordered conformation of the skull of children, women in childbed who died of king's evil or goiter; equally the number of those declined who were born too early or were injured at birth. Deaths by colic decreased from 170 to 7 per thousand. Illnesses of the glands decreased from 19 to 4, deaths in childbed decreased from 14 to 8. Does this not permit us to conclude that the cause of this decrease lies in the progress of medical and surgical science? Cannot such proof save the honor of medicine against its detractors, against the witty mockery of a shallow La Mettrie in his "Pénelope," and those who throw out the child with the bath water because medicine is not omnipotent, because the physician alone cannot help, especially when people have worked for too many years helping along the ruin of their bodies, and make it unfit for restoration?"** The resurrection of the apparently dead, which is entirely the work of today's physicians, would suffice to prove incontrovertibly the usefulness of medicine. We do not know what life really is; but thousands of resurrected apparently dead, whose saving was once considered the work of some god, bless medicine which was able to bring them back to life.

The great progress which medicine has made, mainly in the last two centuries (since it has indefatigably performed post-mortem examination according to an accurate list of all the phenomena observed in the course of lethal diseases, and endeavors to preserve the organs observed in such examinations in special pathologi-cal cabinets, distinguishing carefully between cause and effect, to place them in the right light, to have them drawn or modeled accurately and to describe them) has shed light to an incredible extent on the nature, the seat, the causes of most diseases that were previously not understood, and thereby also greatly corrected the curing methods based on them. As my excellent friend Antonio Scarpa has already mentioned, almost all the latest discoveries of surgery owe their origin to examinations of pathological anatomy.†

On all sides the epidemics attacking people, and even their cattle, and the endemic diseases occurring in different regions, as well as the successes in their treatment

---

* "Reise um die Welt," Part II, pp. 254, 255.
** "Göttliche Ordnung," Part II, §520, p. 413.
  † Sulle Ernie, Pavia, 1809. Prefazione.

are being carefully recorded, new remedies are tested, and all this is made publicly known, partly by individual physicians, partly by medical associations, to the certain profit of posterity. Although the medical journals and papers, which in our days are so numerous, have replaced a deeper and more thorough study of their science to most younger physicians, instead of which they promote only superficial knowledge and a pitiful conceit of omniscience; although the tone predominating in these sheets is partisan, coarse, thoroughly "sans-culottish," insulting to science and fine education, choking every sprouting writing talent, and sometimes deterring the most experienced and deserving men from further participation in public instruction and really causing much damage that the authorities ought to take note of; although many of our journals only take care to exalt or humiliate some school or other, to promote some teaching system or other, to disparage the north against south or vice versa; although in some of these journals all human passions are let loose to the detriment of humanity; nevertheless, a large part of the mischief is remedied by the fact that in view of the present high price of books, which is beyond the means of most physicians, these journals spread very rapidly the knowledge of every new discovery, of every medicine proved by experience, as well as every useful ordinance concerning public health.

Whereas up to the eighteenth century, the practice of medicine was learned by each young physician after completion of his theoretical studies, whereupon he was left to his own devices, learning with great difficulty and by sacrificing a hundred times more sick persons, this mischief has how been considerably reduced by the practical training given to young medics. This was first begun in Edinburgh, then in Leyden, Vienna, and Pavia, and soon also elsewhere, by experienced men directly at the sickbed, or through the creation of clinical schools, thus providing many students with much important experience which they could not acquire alone in ten years, nor need they now pay in blood for this experience.* However, this institution can yet be greatly improved according to the principles to be submitted in the present work.

If internal medicine has so far gained much and promises, with better care and supervision, to provide innumerable advantages to mankind, the same, if not more, applies even now to surgery. Although this part of medicine, considering that it does not deal with dead mass but with live bodies, cannot boast of mathematical certainty in its acts, to be carried out according to mechanical principles; although the mere extraction of a tooth may cause a lethal bleeding; the amputation of the smallest limb, e.g., a finger, may cause a lethal cramp; although there are sometimes the most serious doubts whether a surgical operation should be performed or not

* In the third century of the common era the clergy also had some sort of clinic. Persons who were baptized in their beds because of a dangerous illness were called Clinici. Fleury, "Histoire ecclésiastique," Vol. II. Liv. 7, p. 280.

and if it is decided to operate, the ensuing death proves the opposite; and although many cripples and disfigured people (even when there was no lack of famous surgeons nor of timely intervention) moving in our midst publicly display the proof of the impotence, and sometimes the mistakes of the surgeon; although it cannot be denied that after great battles and in overcrowded field hospitals now and again people are mutilated without exact indications, or even killed by daring deed, without which they might have recovered; nevertheless, it must be admitted that an art which restores within a few moments to so many citizens their eyesight, lost either through illness or lacking since birth; which controls the most violent inflammations or helps remedy them; which sets dislocated and broken limbs, mostly without permanent disfigurement, and if it cannot save them, replaces them to a certain extent by artificial limbs; which completely closes deep wounds that could easily lead to lethal bleeding; which cleans and heals unclean ulcers and fistulas; which extracts excreted, coagulated juices, or foreign hardened bodies that could easily cause death; which destroys with their roots such disfiguring growths and swellings as may hinder the functions of parts of the body; which in dangerous prolapses and protruded intestines reduces them before they are destroyed by gangrene, etc.; an art which can do all this and more, is not only useful but indispensable to every state.

As regards obstetrics, it cannot be denied that some obstetric schools cause immense damage by teaching that hardly anything can be expected of nature and almost everything has to be expected of the art. Therefore they instruct their students that whenever birth is somewhat difficult, they are immediately to help by turning the child or even by using lever and forceps. In all this there are enough cases where nature can do little, art can do everything; and it is here that obstetrics can render the greatest service to the state, and where it really renders it. When I was appointed to the teaching post of obstetrics in the countries of the Speyer Principality, one out of 85 women giving birth died in childbed. After I had held this post for 10 years and had instructed all the midwives of the Principality, only one out of 125 women died. In the first two years I had spent more time on turning than on explaining the natural processes during birth and the necessity of patiently waiting for them. The result was that when the old midwives were unable to help when the child was in an incorrect position, my younger pupils were able to apply skillful remedy and to help the birth along. Even so, they often turned the child without absolute necessity, and on the whole they lost fewer women giving birth, but certainly more children than the old midwives. However, as soon as I had corrected my mistake in teaching, my efforts were richly rewarded by the most fortunate success. It is not only the actual birth where well-instructed midwives can be of great use; they can achieve much in thorough instruction and guidance of pregnant women, women in childbed, and in proper attention to and treatment of the newborn.

If we examine the tools and means which physicians and surgeons use for treating diseases, or which obstetricians need in difficult cases, we must admit that medical art in our day is much advanced as compared with previous times. Many instruments, which can easily do damage, are cruel, or altogether superfluous either have been completely discarded by today's surgeons and obstetricians, or they have been wisely replaced by simpler, less dangerous, less painful, and much more efficient instruments. It is terrible to think of the many children who were mangled alive in their mothers' bodies by murderous hooks before the art had been learned of turning them skillfully if their position impeded birth, and before midwifery forceps had been invented.

If we consider how many surgical operations were previously omitted even in the largest German towns, operations alone which could have saved the lives of the patients, we see that it was because most physicians were almost completely ignorant of the principles and the great advantages of surgery, and therefore treated their surgeons contemptuously and despotically, as if they were their servants. This was also partly true because almost everywhere even the most indispensable instruments were lacking, especially, however, because there was nobody who could have instructed the surgeons properly. It is easy, therefore, to understand, although even now there is a lack of experienced and trained surgeons in many German and foreign provinces, that in times where this lack was even greater, many patients perished miserably because of lack of courageous and prudent surgical help.

We know very little about the medicines which the ancient physicians used largely because the meaning of the names they used has been lost. It is only now, because of the generally accepted technical language in natural history, that the names of the better described and even illustrated natural products are for ever secured. From what we do know about ancient times, however, we see that many very violently acting drugs were used in antiquity, whereas we now may choose between milder and less ambiguous medicaments and we certainly have at our disposal such that surpass the former greatly. The usefulness of Peruvian bark alone surpasses by far the entire stock of drugs known to the ancients. And camphor, musk, castor, asafoetida, valerian, rhubarb, ipecacuanha, aloe, quassia, Columbo, Senega, foxglove, not to mention other products of animal or vegetable origin, surpass almost everything that has come down to us from ancient medicine. Chemistry, which in our days has been so much perfected, supplies us from all domains of nature with a number of the most efficient drugs, with mercury, antimony and steel preparations, with volatile and penetrating salts and essences, etc. With the aid of this auxiliary science, many mineral sources and baths in all countries were most thoroughly examined, excellently imitated, and applied by physicians with the greatest success. The dispensing art, of which I will speak later, could not, as long as chemistry remained in the childhood stage, acquire more regard and dignity than groceries and confectionery with which it in reality also dealt. When the physicians stopped collecting, preparing, and dispensing drugs of vegetable origin, these were supplied to apothecaries by lowly herbwomen, and for lack of certain botanical principles, which were stipulated as late as the eighteenth century, were often confused by both to the detriment of the sick.

Among the host of human diseases there are such, like smallpox, measles, scarlet fever, typhoid and others, which seize the whole system of the body and do not leave it until they have completed their course. Other ills, if properly treated and in good time, can be considerably shortened if not altogether prevented. Among these are gastric fever, intermittent fever, inflammations, illnesses due to swallowed poisons, etc. Thus by using this advantage, the physician not only saves the patient from prolonged suffering and from the danger of the illness turning into a lengthy and often dangerous one; he also saves him the time which he would have otherwise lost for attending to his profession and the support of his family, and the strength required for this, as well as the expenses he would have incurred for curing a prolonged illness. V. Wedekind says that a thousand sick people cost more than three times as many beggars because not only is the beggar cheaper to maintain, but he also does not need any attention and therefore does not prevent other people from attending to their professions. "If, therefore, the physicians did not achieve more than cutting the duration of each illness by half, even for that they would deserve the eminent attention of the government because the means expended on the unnecessary duration of the illnesses can be used for other purposes."*

Considering the number of incurable diseases, the fate of those afflicted by them would be desperate if medicine were not able, at least in many cases, to mitigate these sufferings, and thus to make their lives not only more bearable but also, to prolong them as far as possible to the solace of their families. It is well known how often the fate of many a household depends on the latter. And where good regents are concerned, those who bring happiness to their people, or experienced and wise ministers and statesmen who are dear to their country, the fate of entire provinces and empires depends on them. How dear to every individual is each additional day of life, even if it is not a happy one, for wise nature imbued everybody with the love of life. Therefore, this service of the art, too, though very limited, must be regarded very highly. The famous despiser of physicians, J. J. Rousseau, says in his "Emile": "They (the physicians) make corpses walk about!" . . . But this is really the greatest triumph of the medical art; if they are able to bind together the threads of life, though not for long, after they have been sundered, this should prove their great power, unless nature itself works against it. A prudent physician must never consider an illness incurable as long as it seems to him that the life organism still exists, and he must never withdraw from treating an illness of the entire system, no matter how advanced it is. Whereas the physicians of late antiquity believed that

* "Über den Werth der Heilkunde," Sect. I. p. 55.

they were entitled to deny their aid to patients whom they believed to be lost,* they must have found their predictions wrong more rarely than latter-day physicians, or they overlooked completely the dignity which the art acquires through the art of mitigating suffering, no matter how infirm the patient. Aesculapius and both his sons Machaon and Podalyrius, who practiced medicine outside Troja, are imputed by Socrates according to a premise, which seems very improbable to me, a mentality which every physician today would abhor.** Nevertheless, some sick people, who had been abandoned by their physicians recovered, sometimes without any help, by old women and quacks, to the ridicule of the rash medics. The fortuitously eliminated apparent death which, as I have found in my own experience, attacks people with very dangerous illnesses, teaches sufficiently how much care must be taken before a sick person is given up. By assuming that there is no longer any hope for his recovery, nature itself, which has supplied us with soothing remedies, hints to us to try everything to defer the end of life as much as possible. It is known that in the last stage of consumption there is no hope of recovery; nevertheless, the physician can alleviate the dry cough, the complete insomnia it causes. He can mitigate for months on end the sweating and diarrhea that quickly weaken the patient's strength, and thus put off for the same length of time the inevitable end. So far, medicine has no remedy against gout, but it mitigates the excess of pain; it knows in most cases how to prevent it from affecting the nobler parts, where it would soon cause death, and if the patient obeys the prescribed regimen, the relapses occur much more rarely. Pellagra, which so far is incurable, can have its fatal outcome put off by several years when lukewarm baths are given, when the nutrition is better, and when the local effect of sunrays, which are dangerous in spring, is avoided. Abdominal paracentesis cures dropsy only very rarely, but through the evacuation of the water that frequently stagnates in the abdominal cavity, the oppressions, anxieties, and even the choking, are relieved for months or even years, etc.

Thus medicine at least alleviates the suffering of the sick whom it cannot save; and if one has once seen these miserable people and has witnessed their gratefulness, one cannot but acknowledge the value of this aid. If one would waive medicine completely, most patients of whose recovery we have a moral certainty, would perish

---

 * "Qui igitur eos reprehendunt, qui victis a morbo manus non admovent, non minus adhortantur ad ea suscipienda, quae attingere fas non est, quam quae fas est. In eoque apud eos, qui nomine tenus medici sunt, admirationem conciliant, ab artis vero peritis ridentur." Hippocrates, "De Arte Lib.," Cap. VII.
** "Cum animadverteret (Aesculapius), in civitatibus bene constitutis suum cuique opus assignatum esse, in quo necessari sit elaborandum: neque ulli otium adeo superesse, ut per omnem vitam valetudinarius, in corpore curando occupetur;—Homines ipso naturae habitu et victus incontinentia, neque sibi, neque aliis existimabant (Aesculapius ejusque filii) utile esse vivere, neque circa illos artis operam adhiberi, eosque esse curandos, ne si quidem Mida ditiores essent." Socrates in "Platonis Republica," Lib. III. Platonis oper. omn. edit, Jo. Serrani, T. II. pp. 407, 408, 410.

miserably of scurvy, venereal disease, or malignant intermittent fever. And those of whose recovery we are less certain would be robbed of all consolation and would be given over to certain despair.

Since, however, people, even in such a state, are forced by nature itself to seek help, they would be unscrupulously left to the mercy of ignorant charlatans and barber-surgeons, and thus in the diligently cultivated field of medicine, instead of the cultivated, well-grafted tree, there would be left only the uncultivated wild tree which, moreover, bears inedible or poisonous fruits.

As there is no doubt about the service which medicine provides for the administration of justice by making available its knowledge of nature in the interest of ascertaining the truth in case of suspicion, or in the actual occurrence of punishable injuries, it can be only mentioned here.* By this assistance, whereby, as it were, it makes the dead speak and reveal the truth, medicine protects innocence and unmasks vice trying to hide from justice. It is difficult to imagine how judges went to work in dubious cases where the highest requirement for a decision were medical principles in the time before this comprehensive branch of medicine had developed.** But, it is certain that often in former times reasons were accepted as proof of crimes as well as of innocence (such as ordeal or the fire and water tests, bleeding of the murdered upon being touched by the accused, wedlock-congress) which were more fit to induce the condemnation of the innocent or free the certain criminal, and unfortunately it did so thousands of times.

But if forensic medicine, as noted by Leyser† and Bodinus,†† which makes the application of scientific and medical principles for the elucidation and decision of dubious legal questions especially for criminal law, an absolutely indispensable science,‡ and provides a not unimportant service even to theology,‡‡ then the science on which it is based, namely medicine itself, must also rest on solid foundations, and should therefore be supported in every way by the highest authorities.

Since I might be considered too partial, being the author of the system of Medical

---

* See Laurent. Heister, "Diss. de medicinae utilitate in Jurisprudentia," Helmst. 1730.

** Johann Heinrich Kopp supplied us with an outline of the history of public medicine which makes one wish he would have treated the entire subject. "Jahrbuch der Staatsarzneykunde." First year of publication, pp. 176–221.

† Polycarp. Leyser. "Diss. de frustranea cadaveris inspectione," Helmst. 1723.

†† Bodinus, "Diss. de non requirenda Lethalitate vulneris," Halae Magd. 1743.

‡ In addition to several writings on this subject, especially the following deserve to be read: "F. Meister's practical ideas on the indispensability of thorough knowledge of forensic medicine, etc.," in Pyl's "Repertorium für die öffentliche und gerichtliche Arzneywiss.," Vol. III, St. 1, pp. 28, 19. Thom. Aug. Ruland, "Von dem Einflusse der Staatsarzneykunde auf die Staatsverwaltung," Rudolstadt. 1806. pp. 6–17.

‡‡ Mich. Alberti, "Diss. de Convenientia medicinae cum Theologia practica," Halae Magdeb. 1732. Ejusd. "Specimen medicinae Theologicae," Halae. 1726.

Police, I deliberately abstain here from proving to my readers the necessity of medicine by the indispensability and the so far undisputed usefulness of this science.

* * *

*In §10, Frank deals with the damage suffered by medicine especially from the numerous
quacks. He provides a picture of their activities typical of the 18th century.*

On the duties of physicians

There are duties which are imposed not only by public laws, but also by morals
and by the interests of physicians themselves. Among these, for instance, is the
inescapable obligation of silence in regard to secrets, either entrusted to them by
patients or come to their knowledge by the mere contact with them or their families,
and often touching upon honor, reputation, and domestic peace. The French
criminal code contains a strict law against those medical persons who abuse the
confidence of their garrulous sick; it enjoins §378. "Physicians, surgeons, and other
health officers, as well as apothecaries, midwives, and all those persons who reveal
secrets entrusted to them because of their rank and their business, except in cases
where the law obliges them to report the secrets, are to be punished by prison terms
of one to six months and a fine of 100 to 500 francs." However, there are also cases
which relate to public security, which the physician, even if not called, is obliged
to report in good time. Thus a physician, who has to treat the first persons suffering
from plague at a place that had hitherto been free of suspicion of this ill, cannot
conceal from the authorities this observation concerning the well-being of an entire
country, without committing a serious offense. Likewise, the surgeon, when called
to persons who were wounded or injured in public attacks or in duels, has first to
provide aid, but is then obliged to report it without loss of time to the police court.

"When undertaking cures, physicians, under threat of heavy penalties, are forbidden to make the diseases seem more dangerous than they are in order to gain
the right to an extraordinary medical fee. They should be satisfied with the hitherto
valid fee, but poor persons, whom they are obliged to advise and help just like the
rich, should be treated with consideration or for the sake of Christian love, according
to circumstances, or their fees waived."*

That true physicians appreciate the magnitude, the dignity and at the same time,
the responsibility of their profession, can be seen from the fact that nobody stipulates
more stringently the duties of their demanding calling than they themselves, and
what is more, also fulfill them most punctiliously. Who can calculate how many
sacrifices the medical profession has made from a burning zeal for the well-being
of mankind in times of plague, during infectious epidemics, in hospitals, military

* Medical Regulations for the Kingdom of Bohemia. Prague, 24 July 1753. Part I, No. 19.

hospitals, prisons, during battles, and in military camps? Did not the murderous war since the last years of the French troubles rob entire German provinces of almost all their most active physicians and surgeons? Yet the advantages granted long since, and rightly, to the medical profession (§8) have been largely abolished, and what has remained is completely out of proportion to the dignity of this science which is so indispensable to mankind.

* * *

On charlatans

No matter how strongly the laws in general, and those in Germany in particular, inveigh against the participation of charlatans in the treatment of the sick*; although now it is no longer permitted, as it was in the past, especially in imperial cities, that any cheap-Jack might appear on public stages, dressed in shining clothes and under the pretense of dispensing pills and essences, sell the misguided people destruction and death; nowadays it is unlikely that a real hangman, like the one in the County of Salem, obtains the right, according to his instructions for service, to heal internal and external diseases in men and cattle, or to be made Royal Physician-in-Ordinary;** and thus only the form changed with us Germans, but not the matter itself.† It suffices to read in the Hamburg, Frankfurt, and some other newspapers about secret medicines which are highly recommended for all cases, and are therefore necessarily in most diseases mutually opposite and extremely deleterious. And who would belive that the laws that are meant to secure the health and well-being of the citizens in all countries are being taken so seriously! The Tyrolese still stroll about carrying their dirty medicine chests, and visit small towns and villages in order to do their mischief among the credulous country folk. There are still apothecaries, grocers, herb and root collectors, barber-surgeons, hairdressers, monks, shepherds, blacksmiths, gamekeepers, and knackers who enjoy a great reputation because of their medical knowledge. Many of our scholars now see demons and spirits again. Chemistry has taken it upon itself to explain all our bodily functions and the origin of all diseases. And the branch, which is very speciously called natural philosophy has taken possession of the medical rudder, in order to cross the great ocean of diseases, completely abandoning the experience of all times in the past, being guided

---

* I would have to fill a large book if I wanted to quote here all the regulations against charlatans; but even one page would be too much to confirm the fulfillment of such just decrees.

** According to Oelrich's report, Frederick I of Prussia made the Berlin hangman Coblenz, court and personal physician. The entire Collegium Medicum was against this, but was unable to achieve anything. It is said that Coblenz's sword, with which he himself had executed 103, his father 19, and his grandfather 68 persons, is kept in the royal armory in Berlin. Reports on the Life and Writings of the Formerly Renowned Physician in Waiting D.G.c.G. von der Mühlen.

† See Raven's "Thoughts on the Utility and the Necessity of a Medical Police System in a State." Christian Rickmann, "On the Influence of Medical Science on the Welfare of the State," Jena, 1771, pp. 148 ff.

only by an a priori magnetic needle. We question hysterical maidens, women, and men who are similar to them, whom we have gently put to sleep by stroking, in order to hear from them the seat and the nature of their ills, and even the remedies which we should prescribe for them against these ills. Another few years, and we will quite seriously gaze at the stars in order to explore their direct and powerful influence on the diseases. I can already visualize the writing in large letters: that certain nations advance in the sciences only so far and no further, and then sink back again into their great-grandfathers' absurdities.

It would be easy for me to complete this picture of the medical system in Europe, and to provide my painting properly with shadow and light. It would be even easier for me to show up in their bareness the reasons marshalled by Dr. Reimarus in the defense of charlatans,* but it is time to set out the causes which still prevent the desirable flourishing of medicine, and the means by which such a great nuisance could be restricted.

§11
On the causes of the inefficiencies of medicine

The lack of knowledge of most superior officers in control of public health about the most common causes of impaired health, or the dignity of medicine, or the ravages wrought by charlatans, or the advantages of a good medical system; the aversion of the cameralists [economists] against expenditures that are not reimbursed immediately in cash, as in the maintenance and multiplication of a healthy population, which is not so striking as ordinary financial speculation; the envy of jurists, who were used for centuries to be exclusively in charge of matters of state, when there is medical interference, though this be based on the most thorough knowledge of the harmful factors affecting the health of nations; the fear in case of improved order of greedy executive officers that they will lose the extra private income derived from their hitherto common protection of quacks, or even from their threats to them; miserable medical factories supplying goods similar to that supplied by ignorant charlatans; quarrels, mutual denigration and defamation of physicians;— all these are the fountainhead which carries off all seeds of proposals that are of public benefit and that concern public health, and turn the soil that could be easily cultivated for their certain benefit and yield the most abundant harvest into a swamp that exhales nothing but poison and decay.

Ignorance and ill-advised, even religious, tolerance on the one hand, greed and fraud on the other, are the most widespread hunting grounds of the quack. Thus

---

* See "Examination of the Presumed Necessity of an Authorized Collegium Medicum and a Compulsory Medical System," Hamburg, 1781. 8. C. L. Hoffmann in his writing from Scharbock, etc., Münster, 1781. S. Scherf's "Archive of Medical Police," III, p. 291, and J. M. Apli in his "Antireimarus, or the Necessity of Improving the Medical System in Switzerland." Winterthur, 1788. 8. He thoroughly disproved Reimarus' paradoxical sentences.

the charlatans can be divided into two classes in regard to the reasons for their criminal activities. Those belonging to the first category, as long as they do not know the consequences of their behavior, may be considered misguided; the others, however, should be regarded as murderous swindlers. There are also graduated physicians and surgeons who, however, out of greed, call attention verbally or in writing, to their fictitious excellence, secret remedies, or their special cures, and thus belong to the class of cheap-Jacks, which has been tolerated so far, but which should receive the disdain it deserves.

As I said before, it is almost an inborn quality of man that if someone asks him for advice concerning indisposition or illness, this advice is given immediately, even if not required, and without further examination of the state, or some medicine is extolled with great eloquence if not altogether forced upon the enquirer. Once, when this propensity of people to give each other medical advice was discussed, a great regent said to one of his minions that he greatly disapproves of such a habit. Soon afterward, the minion held his handkerchief to his cheek. The king asked full of compassion whether he was plagued by toothache. Upon an affirmative answer the good-natured monarch advised him to put on the ailing gum a fig that had been cut in the middle and boiled in milk.—"You too are a physician, Sire!" the healthy minion exclaimed.—Unfortunately, it is not always toothache that is involved, and then rash compliance with the rashly given advice, even if it is only because thus the application of more efficient remedies is missed, sometimes becomes the cause of increased danger or even leads to death. If most persons were not so incomprehensibly ignorant in matters concerning their physical well-being, they would never listen to those who have never learned the extremely difficult art of medicine, nor would they listen to others whom they themselves asked for advice concerning diseases, and who are willing to give advice without knowledge of the matter, which entails the danger that they will kill the questioner.

* * *

No less pressing than the struggle against quacks was the problem of educating the people and enlightening them about such matters of public health as a sensible manner of living.

Lack of enlightenment of the people

One should realize that the common people, as long as they lack the necessary enlightenment, ultimately cooperate in the public health arrangements prescribed by the state only under duress, and as soon as they can evade state supervision (faithful to their old, though obviously deleterious, habits), they thwart them. Only he who is in favor of the people's shortsightedness and prejudices, who does not use any language but the people's coarse language, who has the same habits, and who acts like them, thinks like them, shows the same aversion to all innovations, can count on the people's acclaim and trust. In such a general mood, the coarsest quack, barber-surgeon, urine prophet, blacksmith, and even the knacker, in whose opinion the liver still boils phlegm, the exhalations from the stomach rise to the head, and the uterus, like an animal, rises to the throat, the evil beings, witches and specters still play their games with people, will be able to hold their own against the most experienced physician. However, if the elementary schools did not teach the future peasants and craftsmen utterly superfluous subjects, but in addition to the required religious and moral doctrines also taught the young people important, albeit simple, concepts of the duties to themselves, to their fellowmen and domestic animals, especially that which regards their own and public health, if the deleterious prejudices were uprooted, and finally, if the harm endangering our lives constantly, and the ways of avoiding it were made known, only then could we expect that the public health arrangements would be in greater esteem and would be better obeyed, and that the advantages of true medical men over the spurious physicians would be better recognized. "I believe," says Unzer, "that even if nobody were ill, one would not let the physicians perish. We are really only persons with whom one shows off. It is very rare that we are used for the sake of someone's health: for as regards the rules of life set down by us, everybody knows that they are not being observed, although many diseases may be avoided thereby. Very few patients undergo our cures in order to have their health restored to them. When someone falls ill, he first of all looks on for a while, until it gets worse. When things get bad, one uses all domestic remedies of which one can think, until things get so bad that the town and the family are apprised of the illness.—Thus we do not serve any other purpose than to make death more celebrated."*

When I impute that the lack of popular enlightenment is the source of confidence in charlatans, however, I must also point out that this shortcoming is not confined to the rabble. Even men who are otherwise intelligent, venerable jurists, officials, and even ministers, are often as I have mentioned briefly before, so ignorant of everything concerning the structure and functions of their own body, the natural laws which the body obeys in the healthy and in the sick state, and the causes of its early disorder, that it is not surprising that they are also ignorant of the value of medicine, of the conditions that presuppose its learning, and therefore are ignorant also of the difference between true medical practitioners and charlatans. Even the maintenance and promotion of the public health system suffer infinitely from this gap in the scientific education of future civil servants: for how can someone take up the cause of a subject of which he does not have the slightest notion, if he is not convinced of the utility it can bring and of the disadvantages it entails? This indifference of superiors, based on lack of knowledge of the healthy and the sick human

* "Der Arzt," eine Wochenschrift. 53. Stück.

being, has necessarily the consequence that other decrees concerning public health, and especially laws directed against quacks are very rarely obeyed, and if so, then only in the most indolent manner.

* * *

PART ONE
Section Two

Of medical schools in general

§1

Necessity of improving studies

When I deal here with the arrangement of public instruction of medical students, I must touch upon some points which might just as well be said of other, not medical schools, or of universities, and which has already been partly said. In view of the required brevity, I would have liked to presuppose this silently, but I mention them, trusting in the full confidence and indulgence of my readers, merely for the sake of lucidity and completeness.

As I have mentioned already in Part One (§8), in the renaissance of the sciences, Europe has also contributed much to the promotion of medical science: medical schools, academies, and societies of physicians were founded, and protected, and many a beneficial arrangement was made for public instruction. But, since the art has gained so much by the swift progress of the auxiliary sciences, of physics, and natural science, and has gained so many of its own discoveries, it has, as the saying goes, outgrown its clothes.

* * *

§2

In view of the shortcomings and ills of public institutions of learning which are deeply felt everywhere, many improvements and somewhat contradictory proposals for the improvement of universities have been made, especially in the past and in this century.

* * *

Perhaps the voice of a man like myself, who studied and taught at universities which are unlike as to their religion but equally famous in regard to their subject, will not be thought superfluous in such an important matter. If I sometimes disagree with learned writers in questions of studies, this should be ascribed to my age and

311

to my consequent experience, which is not one-sided, and my frankness should be excused since it ultimately serves a good purpose.

If one can compare parts with the whole, universities are almost like kingdoms and states: some obey a monarchic, others an aristocratic, others, again, a democratic government, and none, despite the different forms, is even wholly good or wholly bad. Yet it seems that a constitutional monarchy at least for large states, is still the best, and I am of the opinion that the same applies to the management of universities. Certainly, there are some excellent ones, where only few regulations govern the course of public studies or limit the freedom of the teachers in determining the instruction to be given and the freedom of the pupils in the choice of subjects. Several men, employed by each faculty, excelling both by their erudition and by their exposition, establish the order, the fame, and the utility of a school, so that acting thus, and by themselves, all that is required is that each is instructed on which subject to lecture and how long the lectures are to last. The curator is not always so lucky, however, in the choice of new subjects; the influx of new students is not at all times so considerable, and then we see that within less than half a century, the splendor of a school is extinguished, except for some flickerings, and regardless of the expenditure made, its renown, order, and benefit vanish.

* * *

Seat of medical schools

It seems that I posed too late the question where medical schools should be established, since they exist wherever there are universities. Yet, after what I have said elsewhere about the necessity of providing a healthy position and all sorts of safety measures in establishing public schools, I want to mention the following in passing: in establishing some great educational institutions, more care was taken of the scientific education than of the healthy physical education of the young men.

Several writers have maintained that the choice of large and populous cities as seats of universities is very injudicious in view of the many dissipations there, and the daily opportunities leading young people astray, as well as the greater mortality. On the one hand, this choice is substantiated by the remark that most civil servants employed in large cities can send their sons to school while keeping them under their own supervision and having their maintenance cheaper; nevertheless, I am of the opinion that medicine cannot be taught better anywhere than in populous cities, where in ancient times the famous teachers congregated for the first time, not, as was said, for lack of small towns, but for much more important reasons. To be sure, the breaking down of universities into small schools as in France, where special schools of jurisprudence, medicine, etc., were established, is open to the reproach that they thus lost the right to call themselves universities. But once a young man is in possession of the preliminary knowledge necessary for learning medicine, he is so busy with medical study to be begun that it is impossible for him to take part in the study of sciences that do not belong to his field and are to be learned at a university. In populous cities there are among the foreign, as well as the indigenous inhabitants many illnesses that are rarely found in small towns; and the many factories, arts and crafts; the extreme misery of the poor; the revelry of the rich and great; the terrible consequences of debauchery, extravagance, of insulated ambition, of envy, and a hundred other passions that are almost unknown to the fortunate peasant or provincial town dweller, all provide for the teachers of medicine, both in large hospitals and during the usual visits of sick and medical councils, many opportunities for lively presentations and daily treatment of all human ills, for frequent dissections of bodies, for discovering the causes and effects of the diseases in them, and for the instructive storage and demonstration of the pathological objects found. They provide equally well for the daily dissection practice of the students, and for surgical operations that have first to be learned on dead bodies. In small towns of barely eight to ten thousand inhabitants, without hospitals or with insignificant hospitals, the teacher of anatomy barely has three or four bodies at his disposal annually, for the necessary demonstrations, and it is a veritable misfortune if at least a few persons every year are not hanged or beheaded there. Of course, in our times endeavor has been made, most commendably, to take clinical measures at the medical schools in such small towns, and to visit sick persons with the students, both in specially designated houses and in the abodes of the poor, and to treat them properly for the sake of instructing the students. This is certainly better than nothing; but especially instructive cases are rare, for one thing: at the most there are some cases of fever or chronic, usually incurable diseases; for another, the narrow, low huts of the poor do not make it possible for more than a few students to enter; and often the students themselves have to bear the costs, at least in part, of such imperfect institutions.

* * *

Even if now and again a student in a large city does not escape the influence of moral debauchery, nevertheless, most of the medical students, who are usually from less rich families and are less sumptuously educated, are less exposed to the dangers of seduction than the youth who has been pampered with worldly riches from birth. Besides, intercourse with various classes of persons living together in a populous city provides many insights into the varied ways of life and habits of the population that are useful to medical students and graduated physicians alike, and teaches them how to behave toward different classes. This cannot be learned in smaller circles and is an accomplishment that many medical men lack. If a medical student studies for several years in a large city, endeavors to refine his behavior, and knows how to commend himself by good behavior and thirst for knowledge, he is also able to make the acquaintance of experienced physicians, who are useful to him because of the instructive contact, or to gain the favor of other learned and noble men who later will be able to help further his career. Here I do not include the opportunities which some poorer candidates of medicine grasp in order to further their careers in large cities, namely, as often happens in Vienna, that they let themselves be used during their studies as teachers or tutors of children of rich or noble families. For in addition to the fact that it would be desirable that fewer poor persons than actually do should devote themselves to the study of medicine (§16), such child instructors spend all their time, which they need to learn medicine thoroughly, on the guidance of their charges, and thus have to neglect either their charges or their own scientific training. Matters are the same in Germany with young surgeons in large cities who usually become apprentices to barbers ostensibly in order to be able to complete their studies within the few prescribed years without further expenditures which they cannot afford, but basically they hire themselves out for menial tasks and have to skip most lectures in view of the need to attend to the eternal shaving of beards, which is both shameful and disadvantageous to the German surgeons.

§3

Qualities necessary for teaching

Experience has long since shown that the best curriculum must fail if there are no good men who are able to conduct it. A very mediocre curriculum is sometimes crowned by the greatest success if several great men undertake to conduct it and to fill in its gaps. But where such men are lacking, even the best regulation comes to nothing, especially if the most important chairs are not filled by suitable appointees.

If I demanded no more of a public teacher of medicine than that he knows his field perfectly, that he has an excellent reputation because of his erudition and his published writings, that there is no well founded doubt concerning his moral character, and especially his conciliatory spirit, that his enunciation is correct and intelligible, that he knows how to give his lectures in good order and concisely,*

---

* Although the judgment of individual students cannot determine the worth of their teacher, nevertheless, experience shows that the voice of the listeners in general proves correctness of the saying "Vox populi vox Dei." A professor may often be more learned than his listeners say, but if he does not know how to communicate his knowledge, it is not unjust to consider him unsuitable to be a teacher. Of course, the first condition for employment as a teacher is knowledge, but presentation in proper order and clarity, so that the subject matter is comprehensible and fruitful to heads of different capability, is only the second requirement, in regard to classification. In view of the short time allotted to academic lectures, the conciseness of lecturing is no less necessary. Without such conciseness the end of the school year approaches and the subject is not yet exhausted. One should take care, however, not to believe that the best orator is also always the best teacher! It is very true what Cabanis said: "Une remarque qui s'applique à tous les temps, c'est que les professeurs les plus habiles n'ont pas toujours été les meilleurs observateurs, ni les esprits les plus étendus. Car il faut l'avouer ingénument, ce n'est pas entièrement à tort, que toutes les fonctions, pour les quelles la facilité de la parole devient bientôt par elle-même, un mérite éminent, ont la réputation de gâter plus de têtes, qu'elles n'en peuvent

that he combines with these qualities robust health which is necessary for his academic activities, these requirements would not be different at all from what is merely required of medical teachers.* But since (disregarding the branches of anatomy, chemistry, and botany, which belong more to natural science proper than to medicine) no other subject is so often the fertile ground for imagination and heated fantasy as medicine; since metaphysics and spurious philosophy produced nowhere but in this field so many dreams, hypotheses, and systems that are so dangerous to mankind in their application; since no art presupposes so much variegated and thorough knowledge, such power of judgment, and such ripe experience as medicine, the following is certainly most important: the teacher to be appointed should not be too young, for youth is more inclined to enthusiasm and less to calm examination, and he should not be too old, for age is often less inclined to accept new concepts that are perhaps completely opposed to the old truths, is more subject to forgetfulness and disgust, and requires more comfort.** It is a great blunder if the curators of universities, only for the purpose of attracting foreign students, appoint as professors the first young writers who are available, and who acquired ephemeral brilliance by new systems, theories and hypotheses taken from the complex realm of imagination. In addition to the irreparable disadvantage accruing from such dreaming,

---

former. On s'enivre des succès de la chaire doctorale, comme de ceux de la tribune aux harangues; et il est assez difficile de ne pas s'entêter pour des opinions qu'on a débité tant de fois avec applaudissement; il l'est peut-être encore plus de ne pas rejeter celles qui y sont contraires, et de ne point chercher à détourner de leur sens naturel les faits capables de troubler la paisible jouissance de certains préjugés pour lesquels on a longtemps combattu." "Révolutions et Réforme de la médecine," p. 179.

* Quelle réunion de qualités distinguées n'est pas nécessaire à celui qui occupe une chaire dans une grande Université! Il faut, comme homme, que son Caractère moral imprime la confiance et le respect, que comme savant, il possède tout l'ensemble et les accessoires de la science dans une grande supériorité de telle sorte qu'il puisse y orienter parfaitement ses auditeurs; comme maître, il lui faut une élocution aisée et agréable, clarté et concision, un tact sur et fin pour reconnaître s'il est compris de ses auditeurs, ou s'il leur faut de nouveaux éclaircissements; enfin, il faut qu'il soit inventeur, ou qu'il ait perfectionné quelque point, soit de la méthode, soit du fond de la science; il faut qu'il soit écrivain, car ce n'est que par ses écrits que sa renommée s'étendra au loin et lui attirera des auditeurs; et c'est en écrivant qu'il s'habituera davantage à approfondir et à ordonner convenablement son savoir." Charles Villers, "Coup d'oeil sur les Universités d'Allemagne," p. 88.

** In every other occupation, a civil servant is employed from his fifteenth year, initially for inferior and easier activities in offices, bureaus, etc., and gradually he may advance to more important work, and thus only after forty normally prescribed years of service, in his fifty-fifth or sixtieth year, he is considered pensionable. But public teachers of medicine before their thirtieth year cannot possess the required qualities for their teaching office involving life-and-death decisions (for general teaching) or before their fortieth year (concerning practical teaching), and consequently, by the time they are pensionable, they would have to reach the rare age of seventy or eighty years. It would be unjust to subject them to the same laws in view of their important service to the state. Therefore, the professors employed at Russian universities are entitled to a pension for life equal to their full salary, not only after twenty-five years of service, but if they published a thorough fundamental work in their science or published in print a discovery, they are entitled to this pension even sooner.

they expose themselves to the danger that the learned meteor, thought to be a sun, will suddenly burst and spread a smell of sulfur that will long adhere to the whole institution of learning. For millenia, philosophers, and for centuries, chemists have aspired to be pilots of medicine, and nobody is versed in the history of medicine who did not notice the shallows and reefs on which this art, not guided by experience but by a rudder influenced by mere hypotheses, foundered. And despite that, not half a lifetime passes in which (as if the distressing fate of humanity wanted it) the same ship is guided to the same destruction by the same helmsman! Indeed, philosophy which ventures outside its boundaries may be counted among the better class of mental disorders! For often it proceeds from principles that refer more to the diseased state of the sensorium than to realities, and testify more to the bad tuning of the strings put into motion for thinking than to their harmonic sound. A saying based on a thousand years of experience comments that there is no absurdity that some philosopher did not teach. For proof of this statement, it suffices to leaf through the history of so-called worldly wisdom. Of course, true philosophy is not prone to this humiliating reproach; it is the science of the causes which explain the phenomena of the physical and moral world and their necessary or possible consequences. But I feel inclined to call today's sophists, who with their high-sounding systems, supersede and disparage each other from one fair to the next, medical moths who deliberately avoid the light of the sun (experience) in order to burn their weak wings on the light of a flickering nocturnal candle.* Where is there a lucrative truth which has not been known for a long time? Where is there a discovery useful to suffering mankind for which in the last twenty or more years we would have to thank such medical flighty creatures? Even the sentence stated with such wordy pomp is not a flower that was first raised in the garden of today's natural philosophers: "That the highest idea of all knowledge and being in the whole universe, a macrocosmos and a microcosmos, manifests itself as the perceptual, as phenomenon and product, and that the various forms with their properties, which the universe represents in its organic and inorganic natural realms, have to be reduced as harmonic parts of a great whole to that highest idea." Plato ascribed the comparison of the Universum with the human body to Hippocrates' writing on human nature, which has been lost to us. "This comparison," says Sprengel, "can be found in several places of Hippocratic writings, especially Aph. III. 18, as it was very common during all of

---

* In my opinion we can apply to most subjects treated so high-soundingly by present natural philosophy what Hebel said of comet stars: "Now, there is much to say about comet stars because not much is known of them." "Treasury of the Rhenish Family Friend," p. 205. "On a dit, et on dit tous les jours des choses aussi peu fondées, et on bâtit des systèmes sur des faits incertains dont l'examen n'a jamais été fait et qui ne servent qu'à montrer le penchant qu'ont les hommes à vouloir trouver de la vraisemblance dans les objets le plus différents et de la régularité, où il ne régne que de la variété et de l'ordre dans les choses qu'ils n'aperçoivent que confusément." M. de Buffon, "Histoire naturelle," Tome I.

antiquity, especially in the Pythagorean school." No great physician has ever thought differently, and what Gilibert said about this as long as 40 years ago* has never been considered as something new. Even the mania of determining everything a priori has not stood in our time only in the way of true medicine based on experience. In keeping with my mentality, which is never inclined to polemics, I made my voice heard on the subject of Brown's system of medicine only late and after a publicly repeated exhortation,** and this, my humble votum, has been considered unbiased by just judges when the final verdict was prepared. I hope therefore that what I, an old physician, but not dead to the sciences, think in matters of natural philosophy, just as dispassionately, though without complex motivation that would lead me too far astray from my main purpose, will not later be put ad acta. My advice is, therefore, that according to my above declaration, young men, usually still greatly inclined to rapture, even if distinguished by brilliant talent, should not be chosen as public teachers of medicine which has so often been abused by idle whims, until they have attained the necessary maturity and, as our German forebears used to say, until they have sown their wild oats. Otherwise the well-being of mankind may again be endangered, notwithstanding all the warning examples.†

* * *

§9

Conditions of teaching

In the curriculum drafted for the medical school in Pavia, I briefly indicated the general conditions on which medical instruction must be based.†† Experience of many years has confirmed the validity of these conditions, and I maintain them, but for greater lucidity I wish to add a few remarks.

1) "The subjects to be taught, which are closely related to each other, must be lectured in connection with each other." Thus in dissecting different parts of a human

---

* "Si vous considéréz la médecine dans toute son étendue vous la définirez par la connaissance des êtres vivants et de leurs rapports. Toutes les substances de l'univers agissent directement sur l'homme et les animaux qui lui ressemblent; réciproquement l'homme ou tout autre animal réagit sur toute la masse de la matière; en deux mots, les êtres sont perpétuellement en action et réaction. En effet tout philosophe accoutumé à saisir l'enchaînement des objets, voit evidemment, que la plus petite parcelle de la matière, quoique considerée isolée, peut étendre ses relations sur toutes les substances créés. Cette importante vérité, developée le plus brièvement qu'il sera possible, va nous servir à coordonner les différentes branches de la médecine philosophique." J. B. Gilibert, "L'anarchie médicinale etc.," Partie III. pp. 189, 196, 197. To this belong "Ludwigii oratio de neglectu contemplationis naturae, causa neglectae medicinae; in adversar. med. pract.," vol. II. Part. I. p. 46.

** Praefatio ad Joseph Frank. Rat. Instituti clinici Ticinensis. Vienna. 1797.

† Concerning this, see G. G. Ploucquet, "Diss. de noxis neoterismi in Medicina et constituendo tribunali medico catholico," Tubingae 1806. 4. Ejusdem, "Diss. de non admittenda reductione Astrologismi in medicinam," Ibid. 1808. 4.

†† Supplementary volumes to Medical Police, Volume I, pp. 178–181.

body, in order to attract the attention of the students to this initially repugnant, or at least not very attractive teaching, and to cause them to remember better, the professor of the dissecting art should make some general remarks concerning the purpose and use of these parts, and thus pave the way for the teacher of physiology. The latter gains so much time in his lectures through the students' preliminary knowledge of the healthy functions of the parts and viscera of the body that in developing them [the functions] he may also deal with diseased or disturbed functions in general, and thus prepare the students for future courses of special pathology. The teacher of pathology, as I shall say below, not only by describing diseases orally from the pulpit, but also by showing them in nature at the sickbed, and developing their symptoms, prepares the students for the therapeutic rules to be taught the following year, etc.

2) "The students must be guided gradually from subjects that are more easily grasped to the more difficult subjects." This rule applies to all teaching of young people, but it is more necessary in medicine which is so difficult to learn. If the young man who is to study medicine has not learned during his philosophical studies the general principles of the teaching of the three natural domains, if he does not have some notion of fibers, skins, vessels, circulation, the position and main functions of the different organs, then the specialized language of the medical teachers, as well as each subject taught, will be so alien to him that it will be impossible for him to follow the public lectures. And as each lecture presupposes the knowledge of the previously explained subjects, the difficulties increase daily, the student becomes sullen, and at the end of the school year only confusion reigns in all these concepts.

3) "No part of medicine should be taught by mere words and feeble drawings if it can be shown in nature and if the understanding of the concepts can be facilitated by the assistance of the external senses." Merely verbal descriptions are like the so-called water colors: even if they are well chosen and well applied, they immediately dissolve upon the slightest wetting and leave only shapeless spots on the canvas. By using dry words we still fall short of finding those stronger colors which can faithfully depict the diseases even in a passable drawing—and when we have found them, that we also know how to mix them properly. Who once saw an object as we say, with his own eyes, may later recall it on the basis of a description that is only half correct; but without any impression at all, we are like a blind person who, after listening to a labored description of the color of a rose that we held to his face and having been asked what notion he had of it, replied that the color of this flower must be rather similar to a quadrilateral. I once led a young physician to a sickbed; he had just obtained his doctorate at a much frequented university which, however, did not have a practical institute attached to it. The patient suffered from a very common, feverish, erysipeles on his left foot. After a long examination of the patient, the physician admitted to me that he could neither determine the nature of the disease nor the required remedy.—I explained both to him. "Oh,"

my student said candidly, "so this is the disease about which I earned the greatest approval of my teachers with my replies at the public examination, and now, that I have it in front of my eyes, I am in difficulties!"—I knew an excellent teacher of practical surgery who was employed by a famous university. Usually there was no opportunity to show to his pupils the surgical operations that he described to them even on corpses, and, therefore, he sometimes used scissors and paper and cut out the required incisions and shapes of the stumps to be left when diseased limbs had to be amputated. At last in our days, the necessity of clinical institutes has been recognized, but they are mostly frequented by students of the practical teacher. The students of pathology, on the other hand, must make do with the verbal description of all diseases, even in places where there is no lack of hospitals, and when they see in the following year the originals of the copies they had studied, they need months until they find some similarity between the two, and the teacher at the clinical hospital is forced to repeat himself at each sickbed which robs the more advanced students of the time needed for more important observations.

In regard to medicine therefore, I cannot agree with what Weber said: "Indeed, the proper boundaries between practice and theory in academic teaching are not so easy to find; it is very important that practice be not mixed too soon or too late, too much or too little. However, it seems that it is less of a disadvantage to start too late rather than too soon, and less dangerous to mix in too little, rather than too much practice." Likewise, Meiners believed erroneously "that practical instruction at universities aims more at drawing the attention of young people through observation and clear instructions connected with them to the methods of their teachers used in operations, births, etc., rather than providing them with a more than ordinary skill in obstetrics, in operating, and in the treatment of diseases." Of course, one must not demand that the teaching of physicians be concluded within three years or even less; but if the students visit a good clinical hospital for at least two years, they can be trained to be, if not perfect, at least very practical physicians. "The young people," says this author, "cannot remain so long at such practical institutes." . . . Why not? He who cannot do that renounces medicine which, being an art of experience, cannot be obtained more cheaply. As is known, I have educated a large number of young physicians who were not satisfied with two years of visits at clinical hospitals, and we have too many students of medicine to confine the study of medicine merely to its theory.

It is hardly necessary to recall that the pictures of diseases should best be made or drawn in nature, and then provided by the experienced teacher with shadows and light and properly painted. The same applies to the parts of natural science and medicine which are a preparation for pathology: wherever it is feasible, the subjects to be explained should be made perceptible to the students by lively representation and with the aid of repeated experiments. Rich and well-ordered museums available in every field and at every hour to the teachers, fortunate injections, which are not always so easy to make on the spot, plaster casts, drawings, engravings, good preparations of both human and comparative anatomy, and especially deformed parts deviating from the healthy state that were found in corpses after the most variegated diseases, collections of every kind both of very good and of bad and adulterated medicines, of herbaria, of various obstetric tools, machines, bandages, both those formerly in use and now abandoned and those now current, all these are the surest means of facilitating all the student's ideas and ensuring that they will forever be imprinted in their memories.

4) "The time that is required for learning medicine in its entire extent by most of the students must be accurately determined."

* * *

It is of course difficult to find a sure scale for thoroughly learning the art of medicine, and the time that different heads will need to do so. This difficulty also seems to touch upon the law that everybody should visit schools for precisely so many years and not less, before being admitted to the independent treatment of the sick. If, however, one takes into account that it is not a question of scientific knowledge only with the young physician, but mainly a matter of experience and a certain skill in the execution of the rules of his art, especially in the most urgent cases which do not give him much time for quiet contemplation, one must admit that even the best talents cannot count on any dispensation in the study of this science of experience. Therefore, it would be only just if a law should stipulate at least five years for the study of medicine. The regulations of the University of Pavia stipulate six years for the study of medicine, but there a year of physical instruction is included because the young man who transfers to medicine must have learned in that year the first principles of anatomy and physiology. At the end of the fifth school year, the candidate who has passed his examinations can obtain his doctorate but not permission to practice alone. Before obtaining such permission, he must have visited either the clinical hospital of the university for an entire year, or a large hospital where his visits are under the supervision of a good practitioner known to the general director, and he must submit several [written] observations made by him, and signed by the supervising physician, and obtain a certificate of his successful activity.

* * *

5) "Each part of medicine must be lectured in its entirety."

* * *

6) "In regard to place, time and arrangement, the order of things must be determined to the advantage and greater comfort of the learning, and only such regulations should be enacted which help bring the pupils most assuredly and most quickly to their goal."

Since the students not only have to listen to the lectures, but must also arrange their contents at home, think them over, and commit them firmly to their memory, one cannot prescribe easily more than four lectures daily, in addition to the anatomical practice which requires more time. Although morning hours are the best for teachers and students, the afternoon hours, and at the sickbed the evening hours especially must also be usefully employed.

* * *

7) "One must not endeavor to heap notions upon notions and thus cause them to be confused, or waste time by fruitless repetitions"; thus, one should not try to exhaust the entire subject matter, but should teach the students only the fundamental concepts, guide them so that they learn to think for themselves, and attempt to acquaint them with the literature of each branch, or with the best sources of the science, as well as with its shortcomings and narrow boundaries.

* * *

The greatest art of the teacher of medicine is to protect his students in time from the dangerous delusion that merely speculative statements are certain, to teach them to doubt everything that is not confirmed by mature experience, and to acquaint them with the gaps, with the known limits of the art, as well as with the best sources from which they can obtain truth in the future also.

8) "The teaching aids provided by the state for public instruction must be made common property, and every teacher and every single student must be permitted to use them as much as possible."

The aids of which I speak here are primarily the public book collections and the various museums: natural history, anatomical, physiological, and pathological.

* * *

9) "The teachers must base their lectures on an appropriate textbook, either someone else's or written by themselves. They must read clearly and without digression, their own explanations, amendments and annual additions, explain more in detail what they have read, and before every lecture, briefly recapitulate the main content of the previous lecture."

* * *

10) "The students must be made to attend the lectures punctiliously and from beginning to end. The teachers, on the other hand, must seek to revive their [students] attention again by the seriousness and the lucidity of their delivery."

11) "The students must be trained in applying what they have learned." The best anatomical representation and description of the parts of the human body is lost from the memory of the students if they are not guided and instructed for years in

the dissection of bodies. Equally, nobody will become a passable botanist through merely being shown various plants, if he does not have to examine them frequently and is not trained to accurately determine their characters. No theoretical physician, unless he himself has observed and treated various diseases under experienced teachers, no young surgeon can succeed in being a true physician, unless he has first learned to apply his tools on corpses, and then on patients, according to the principles he had heard in lectures, etc.

§ 10

Necessary qualities of the students

After having spoken of public teachers, their instruction, and related subjects (§§ 1–5), I now go over to the consideration of the qualities required in a future student of medicine.

That from time immemorial many persons without previous medical training permitted themselves to practice medicine, which can so easily become dangerous, may be explained by the causes which I named in Section One of this part in § 11. But that in our times, except for some great, more northern countries, the number of those who study medicine according to the regulations and make it their exclusive profession has so much increased in most regions that it has led to a veritable flood of authorized physicians, may be ascribed to somewhat related motives, although this is not quite satisfactory. To explain this phenomenon, the saying is often quoted "dat Galenus opes," but it is far from sufficient to resolve this question (as nowadays only a few chosen ones at courts and in large cities prove the truth of this saying, for many physicians, no matter how hard they work, barely make a living, and most of them literally starve). There must be other reasons for the disproportionate increase in the number of physicians. In my opinion, one very important cause of the increased number is firstly, that the nations of southern Europe have been freed of the yoke of bondage under which they had bowed so deeply for centuries, and that in consequence of it, and due to improved agriculture, a greater number of factories, more widespread commerce, higher spiritual values, the number of free individuals of whom the middle-class consists increased everywhere. Thus, I saw in Poland and Russia, where the mass of the common people is still the property of the nobility and of the landowners and none of them can devote himself to science, only foreign physicians or those selected from among the sons of Greek priests and trained at the expense of the Crown. The sons of free persons, however, who do not belong to the nobility, devote themselves mostly, except in Courland and Livonia, to military or civil service where they had good hopes of more rapid promotion. Or they join the commercial profession to which their fathers perhaps belonged. Whereas, formerly the universities admitted to the doctor's degree of medicine only free sons born in wedlock, the number of the young men entitled to study medicine was much smaller than in our days in view of the many serfs. When bondage was abolished, many families from the country let their sons study medicine, and whereas even noblemen could hardly sign their names a few centuries ago, now the number of persons from the middle-class (with their better education) devote themselves to the sciences in general, and to medicine in particular. The number so doing is infinitely larger than in former times. A second and very important reason for the daily increasing influx to medical schools is the lessening of the former inclination to the clerical profession and the abolition of so many monasteries.

* * *

Qualities of physicians

The qualities required in a future physician are partly of a physical, partly of a moral nature. The former can be divided into general and special qualities, depending on whether the physician deals only with internal diseases or also with external defects.

The general physical conditions for every physician are: a firm, healthy body, free of any illness that causes revulsion or fright to the sick, and with no external sense impaired. The life of a physician, especially during epidemics, is one of continuous business, in addition to unceasing mental strain, and it also constantly taxes all physical strength. If the physician wants to fulfill his sacred duties as he should, there is perhaps no hour of the day or night which he can, with confidence, devote to his rest. Ever prepared to rush without delay to the aid of the imploring sick, which may easily be fatal, he must, although almost exhausted, deprive himself of the most necessary sleep and even the minimum of food, in any weather, be it stormy, hot, or bitterly cold, and regardless of the distance, renounce all domestic bliss, and even the education of his children, often for days and weeks. Therefore nobody will deny that in view of such strenuous as well as essential duties the physical capabilities of the physician must be high, especially in the country where usually there is nobody to take the other's place.

* * *

One of the most essential conditions for every medical man, but even more so for surgeons is perfect condition of the external senses, through which we perceive impressions of foreign objects with which we come into contact from far or near and notions of which are produced in us. And just as all external senses can be reduced to mere tactile sense, the perfect state of its tools, the finger tips, is a very important requirement in the treatment of diseases, but especially in surgical and obstetric examinations.

* * *

A fine sense of hearing is a requirement that no physician can lack without being detrimental to the sick. This is true also of vision, the perfect state of which is among the indispensable requirements of the physician both in treating internal and external diseases. In itself, the mere appearance of the patient provides for the experienced physician an idea of the nature of his disease which can hardly be improved no matter how many questions and answers.

* * *

If one has no fervent love of man and a tender feeling for the suffering of one's fellow creatures, the most important quality required for learning and practicing medicine is lacking. Only a feeling heart overcomes the difficulties inseparably bound up with the medical profession, and rewards the physician's self-denial that is so necessary almost every hour of the day. The unfeeling, rough, and hard-hearted physician always lacks the most effective balm which pours from the hands of the philanthropic physician at every visit and heals, or at least brings relief to the despairing patients. A physician who is by nature bereft of all tender feeling will never discover ways for alleviating the sufferings which are visible only to a sympathetic eye. The physician is most often the confidant of the families he treats when they are ill. As such, he enters at all hours the abodes of great and small, friends and foes. Without arousing suspicion, he sees and hears a thousand things the public knowledge of which might have the most unfortunate consequences. Secrets, which one would like to keep even from oneself, must be confided to him whereby often the honor and the future fate of the persons who are forced to this admission by their pressing ills and their foreseen consequences, are placed into his hands, too.

* * *

2

Medical Institutions in Particular

PART TWO
Section One

Of public teaching in the field of medicine in particular

§1

I have already published the curriculum for the medical faculty of the University of Pavia, which I prepared on order of the Imperial Court in the years 1785 and 1786, most of which was retained although the government had changed, and I could easily refer to it here. When a curriculum is devised for a given institution, some things have to be subordinated to local conditions and to customs which cannot be easily suppressed. The reason on which brief decrees are based may not always be made clear; furthermore, after an interval of 28 years, the field of science and medicine had become considerably wider. It is natural that lengthy experience, gathered among various nations, in many respects cools or corrects the views of the forty-year old man when old age approaches. Finally, since in a work such as the present one, various seeds are collected for very different soils, and their selection must be left to each individual, it seems to me all the more justified in the position of giving public instruction which is opening up to me not to apply the curriculum which was drafted so many years ago and under completely different times and conditions, although at that time it did not miss its stipulated purpose. Yet even now I consider it useful to retain parts of it, since my supplementary volumes to Medical Police are fairly generally known, and since I am obliged in addition to give an account to the learned public of important additions and amendments to some of my previous proposals and arrangements.

§2

It is natural that the childhood of medical teaching (excluding the skill to be acquired in it by lengthy experience) required fewer teachers and a smaller number of lectures than after the boundaries of this art had been greatly extended, and after the powerful trunk of this art had grown new and quite substantial branches each of which requires its own cultivation. But apparently the teaching of medicine at many universities, especially in our times, has been split up more because of learned luxury and the pressure the professors feel to earn from their students the living which the state denies them by multiplying the paid lectures, rather than because of true need. I believe that it is right for young men who have already learned the basic foundations of the art in its entire context, and who wish to perfect their acquired knowledge or to become even more qualified for a public teaching post in medicine, to attend famous schools where there is no lack of opportunity for them to achieve their purpose. I even admit that science itself may gain from the fact that its individual parts are lectured on with more learned display and are, so-to-say, exhausted for the benefit of more advanced medical men. But just as a sculptor, wanting to hew an Apollo out of one block, does not begin his work with the finest of his chisels, just so the last refinement by the public teacher cannot be applied to the still rough student, for either the excessively fine chisel cracks on parts which are too hard and require a stronger wedge and a more powerful hammer, or the chisel simply slides off the block and leaves only a lot of lumps, which are only too obvious on most young physicians who are given a superfine finish in our learned fashion factories. If in the course of time the number of branches of medicine increases, it is only fair that these, too, be cultivated by special teachers for the good of the students. But schools for advanced medical studies cannot be attended by beginners without the result that most of their instruction is in vain or, once having taken root, is stifled by its own density. Likewise, never can medical schools be attended by licensed practitioners without the result that these men waste their time which could be put to much better use than listening to long-known fundamentals. In addition, only a few newly graduated physicians are sent by their country's government or by affluent parents on scientific journeys to either important practical institutes that are mostly only in large cities, or to some other universities, in order to hear there in the course of a few months private lectures by the most famous teachers, chiefly remarks and views intended not for beginners but for practicing physicians.

Before universities were established and in the Middle Ages the few young men who wanted to devote themselves to medicine without also entering the Church, had no other way open to them but to become apprenticed to a reputable physician, just as our barbers and artisans do now, and there for a previously agreed price for a certain number of years to learn all that their teacher knew, and then to endeavor to perfect themselves further for a time at their teacher's side or in lazarettos and military hospitals.

* * *

At present the teaching at the newer medical schools is slowly being put into proportion with the growth of the auxiliary sciences and of medical science itself, and at most universities, staffed by full professors, exclusively paid by the state, lectures are held free of charge on anatomy, physiology, pathology, botany, chemistry, Materia medica, pharmacology, general and special therapy, surgery, obstetrics and veterinary medicine, and even clinical institutes are being established. All these parts of the science are publicly taught by a fairly small number of teachers; therefore, as was shown in the previous sections, after the institution of university lecturers and private docents had been introduced, each of the above-named parts of the science were cut up into many pieces, and as I have already proved, the number of academic lectures increased daily, but mostly for the good of the teachers and to the inevitable detriment of most of the listeners because they learned the basic sciences only superficially. It suffices to read the lists of lessons which are published each semester at most of our universities, and it will become clear that the stuff offered is calculated more to increase the income of the learned tradesmen than to satisfy the requirements of the inexperienced buyers who, moreover, do not know much about their own requirements.

* * *

Frank subsequently lists 17 main branches of medicine with which he deals thoroughly in eight sections. Samples from the sections on anatomy, physiology, pathologic anatomy, general pathology, special pathology and therapy, surgery, and midwifery are then given, and these indicate the crucial points of the system of medical instruction at the time of the Enlightenment.

PART TWO
Section Two

Of human anatomy and general physiology

§1

In the second section of Part One, §11, I not only described natural science as the basis of the study of medicine, but I also pointed out the advantages to other sciences, arts and crafts if natural science in its entirety would be the introduction to their study. I had already said, in my expert opinion which I had submitted on 31 October 1798 to the then Imperial and Royal Court Commission for the Revision of Studies which dealt with medical and surgical studies in the Austrian States: "The teacher of natural history is in great contradiction with his profession if, as is mostly the case, he deals less with man than with animals, and acquaints his students with everything except with what concerns them most, i.e., their own nature. Such neglect is again a consequence of our injudicious chopping up of natural history, and of allotting all dissections and physiological considerations to the medical faculty. Of course, the medical faculty must elucidate with great effort and accuracy the structure of the human body. But never will a natural scientist make any progress in his science, never will young people be properly prepared by natural science for other sciences unless they obtain a brief survey of the animal, and especially of the human structure, the main parts of the body, its primary entrails, the circulation through it, its main functions. This knowledge will be of greatest utility to every class, it will best help in combating prejudices and confidence in superstitious remedies, and charlatanry among cultured people. One will no longer hear that jurists and theologians speak of and judge physical matters concerning man, health, predominant diseases, and injuries with an ignorance that could be forgiven only to the rabble. If the teaching method will be thus improved, the student intending to study medicine will already have received the best preparation to this science in natural science, and already in the first year of study he will be able to absorb the higher anatomical and physiological teaching."—The artificial division of animals in general with respect to the investigation of the structure and purpose of their parts is, just like chemistry, part of natural science. The excellent works by Aristotle prove that already in antiquity the utility and necessity of such investigations were probably understood, and already the ceremonious slaughtering of sacrificial animals and the thorough investigation of their entrails regarding their healthy or diseased state must have promoted the knowledge of entrails. Yet the deep reverence which the oldest nations, according to their lopsided religious ideas, felt for the corpses of their relatives and friends, was for a long time an almost insurmountable obstacle to all dissections of human bodies, and although the Egyptian priest had to open bodies, remove the entrails, and apply a coat of balm to prevent them from decaying, this was done so hurriedly and with so much fear of the rage of the superstitious rabble, that this crude dissection did not yield any advantage to science. The natural scientist and the physician bowed to the peremptory delusion of the times and attempted to find a substitute in the diligent dissection of those animals whose structure seemed to them to be closest to that of the human body; but they felt with regret the deficiency of their conclusions based on analogy. They seized on battles and serious injuries to obtain correct ideas, and some great men among them even risked obvious danger to their lives when they secretly dissected human bodies. This seems to be the basis of the popular rumor that they even dissected living persons. Thus ignorance and the superstition based on it oppressed science! For centuries wise men battled against this prejudice, and we do not know how much it cost them to finally win the permission for us to be allowed to be of use to the human race."

* * *

§3

All these teachings of dissection, i.e., physiological, comparative, pathological, and forensic anatomies, must be taught at a well appointed university. Thanks to the indescribable efforts of physicians and surgeons, physiological human anatomy has in our day attained such a high degree of perfection that few discoveries of great importance can be hoped for in this field, but it must also be admitted that this knowledge of practical medicine which has enriched the natural science of man so much, has so far not served in equal proportions. Only pathological anatomy, in which we owe Lancisi, Valsalva, Bonet, Morgagni, Lieutaud, Baillie, Soemmering, Portal, Walter, Sandifort, Camper, Hunter, and others so much, is a never-ending source of new knowledge that is important for practicing medicine. And although it is difficult to distinguish with certainty the effect of a disease from its cause in pathological anatomy, it is nevertheless certain that the immense host of local illnesses, and even part of the diseases of the entire system can never be completely surveyed without a certain perfection of pathological anatomy. Likewise, and this was unfortunately realized too late, is comparative physiological as well as pathological anatomy the only means of assisting human physiology and pathology to forge ahead and to increase our knowledge of animal life, both healthy and sick. It is very risky to entrust to a doctor who has had only theoretical instruction without previous practical instruction and without experience in the forensic dissection of corpses who, sometimes certainly, sometimes only presumably, died by criminal violence, either someone else's or their own.

* * *

'§8

Promotion of pathological anatomy in general

But post-mortem examinations will never attain that perfection which would benefit mankind so much if only universities would perform them, and not all hospitals of the state, and particularly if the bodies of those who died of especially complicated, rare, or unknown diseases are not dissected as often as possible by hospital or family doctors well versed in the human anatomy and its deviations from the normal state. The results of the dissection must then be painstakingly compared with the anamnesis, both carefully collected, and according to the selection of experienced men, the most noteworthy observations made known to the medical public.* It is already a great achievement nowadays that the bodies not only of European regents and their relatives, but also of the great persons at their courts, and other members of the high nobility are most carefully and thoroughly dissected without any objection and even according to accepted custom. It does the Italian public honor that hardly a physician is prevented when he asks permission to dissect a dead patient in order to enlarge the boundaries of his science. Even in France and Germany, although much more rarely than in Italy, the enlightened nobles do not put insurmountable obstacles in the way of this medical thirst for knowledge. I even know of quite a number of sick commoners who, on their own initiative, in the last days of their suffering, instructed their heirs to have their corpses dissected (as they philanthropically put it, for the benefit of their fellow human beings, who suffer from similar ills).** I have never found in Russia, with those who profess the ruling Church, or in Jewish families, the slightest readiness to permit the dissection of their dead. In the public clinical schools in Vilna and St. Petersburg, which had been founded upon my proposal, I could never have counted on post-mortem examination, which is indispensable for practical students, of the patients who succumbed to their illnesses in these institutions, if adherents of other faiths had not

---

* A comprehensive treatise on post-mortem examination is contained in the second volume of the "Dictionnaire des Sciences médicales, Art. Anatomie pathologique," pp. 46, 78, by Laennec and Bayle.

** How much the abhorrence of dissecting human corpses has diminished in Germany, too, can be seen from the precept which Dr. Queitschel gave to physicians as late as 1749: "Familiae permissu, ad indagandam abditam morbi causam, aut potius effectum occultum, Anatomiam pathologicam corporum morbis defunctorum privatim quidem instituere poterit (Medicus); sed caveat, ne id frequentius repetat: secus enim facile poterit accidere, ut a praxi medica, praecipue in pluralitate practicorum, excludatur." L.c. [De cautelis in praxi Anatomiae adhibendis commentatio. S. Selecta medica Francofurtensia," Tom. IV, Vol. III,] pp. 179, 180.

been charitably admitted to them. At the clinical hospital in Vilna, no patient had yet died but what the common people, though mostly consisting of Protestants and Catholics stated publicly that I would even subject living patients to the ana-tomical knife; and I could use only the corpses of members of other faiths for autopsy after I had won over their poor relatives with little presents.

In a country whose ruling, or merely tolerated, religion absolutely forbade the dissection of human bodies for special reasons that are unknown to a layman like me, these reasons, as well as freedom of conscience, which is so sacred to the human race, would also have to be respected in this matter. Yet, there is no cultured nation in Europe which would prevent the courts from viewing and dissecting bodies if there are signs that a man may have been robbed of his life due to mistreatment by himself or someone else, and which would perhaps reveal the only irrefutable proofs of a wicked murder. It seems that we may hope that no religion will lack reasons for approving the dissection of bodies if the overriding interest of human society should require it.

Sometimes the post-mortem examination of persons who died of less known or very complicated diseases is certainly of such interest. The timely knowledge thus obtained may provide swift help to the sick suffering sooner or later from the same states, or at least provide for them treatment that is suitable to alleviate their suffer-ing. Up to the last half of the eighteenth century not an insignificant number of pregnant women died in approximately the third or the fourth month of pregnancy, simply of retention of urine and stool, without any physician finding the cause of such an illness and without being able to find a remedy to restore these natural excretions. Finally post-mortem examination of the bodies showed that this illness was produced by the folding over of the uterus; from then on most pregnant women with this deformity were most fortunately saved by mere mechanical assistance. Often, and even during certain epidemics, people were seen to die miserably and often without the usual symptoms accompanying pneumonia, without breathing difficulties, without coughing, without pain, without fast and irritated pulse, and without impediments to lying; finally dissection of the corpses revealed the nature of the hidden illness and led to its successful cure.

* * *

At present it is difficult to order by law the post-mortem examination of persons who died in the bosom of their families and had not been admitted to a public hospital, except in cases of grave epidemic diseases which have not yet been sufficiently recognized and have been lethal in many cases, and in cases requiring a coroner's inquest. The example of some nobler fellow citizens, however, and improved instruc-tion in public schools in regard to the prejudices that are so deleterious to public health, especially if, as can be expected, post-mortems will not entail any expenditure for physicians, will within a few years gradually defeat the ancient abhorrence of the public as regards the quiet dissection of some of its dead. Only eleven years have passed since I carried out such dissections for the first time in Vilna, by persuasion, but only on the dead belonging to Catholic or Protestant families, and with the utmost preservation of all the decencies. And already my son, who is now head of the clinical institute, can obtain a corpse without hindrance, if only its dissection promises some gain to science, and he can then enrich the pathological museum which had been founded there only a few years ago.

If only a hospital belonging to a university lets the latter have its dead for dissection, physiological and forensic anatomy may gain by that, but pathological anatomy will not gain so easily. For pathological anatomy requires a much larger number of corpses or their diseased parts than the former two; otherwise, the pathological museum will be supplied too slowly with instructive preparations. The curriculum of the University of Pavia says therefore: "The pathological museum is to be enriched increasingly with pathological preparations, even with those that can be found in other hospitals of the state. Therefore all (43) hospitals of Lombardy are to send to the pathological museum in Pavia everything peculiar that their physicians and surgeons found upon dissection of bodies and these physicians and surgeons should be obliged to dissect most carefully the corpse of every patient who died of a strange disease that is worthy of their attention, if it is to be expected that the corpse will yield something of interest to public instruction. The expenditures incurred by the hospitals in purchasing spirit of wine required for the maintenance of the preparations and in sending them are to be refunded from the budget of public instruction.— In that way efforts will be made to collect for the pathological museum everything that may promote the study of the surgical sciences, and to obtain especially an abundant stock of diseased bones, arterial swellings, tumors, renal and biliary calculi, etc. All these specimens, both from human beings and from domestic animals, from all regions of the provinces are to be sent to the aforementioned museum.* A list is to be made and kept up of all the pathological specimens collected in this manner."

In this way I succeeded in equipping the pathological cabinets in Pavia and Vienna and to make substantial institutions of them**; in both I had at first found no more

---

* Joh. Pet. Frank's supplementary volumes to the Medical Police, Vol. I, pp. 206, 226. Hunczovsky says [in his annotated German translation of Hamilton's work, "On the Duties of the Regimental Surgeon"] that in the Austrian army the regimental surgeons are obliged to dissect every corpse from whose examination they may expect something instructive, and if the case is noteworthy, they are to report it immediately to the Medical-Surgical Academy in Vienna, possibly also enclose the pathological preparation. L.c., p. 173.

** In the first volume of my Interpretationes clinicae I have already given several descriptions of them; and should I live long enough, I shall endeavor to add some important items.

than six preparations, but within a few years I thus equipped them to the greatest advantage of my students, as well as for the good of the study of the nature of many previously obscure diseases.*

* * *

* When I was still physician-in-ordinary to the Prince-Bishop of Speyer, he founded out of his own pocket a small hospital according to my design. When an anatomical-surgical college was attached to it, in which I took part, I was already intending to initiate a collection of pathological objects for the benefit of the students and to enhance science, and though the number of beds in this hospital could be fifty at the most, I succeeded. This was so because I also used the bodies of many who died in the penitentiary there, thus within a few years endowing this small collection with very instructive pieces, e.g., a double uterus (uterus bicornis); a flexible skeleton, soft as wax, of an adult maiden; a strange skull, lacking all bones of the palate and nose, belonging to Johann Beck, who is well known to pathologists, etc.; I heard that after I had been appointed as teacher in Göttingen, this small collection flagged again. Upon my appointment in Vienna, my first care was to establish in the general hospital there a pathological museum equal to that in Pavia, and with the support of the highest authority I succeeded within 8 years in collecting a considerable number of the most important preparations of this kind. Professor Vetter, who worked for this museum, had published without my knowledge an incomplete description of the museum ("Aphorisms from Pathological Anatomy," Vienna 1803). In the meantime I had laid the foundations for pathological museums, first in Vilna, later also in St. Petersburg, and it is to be hoped that in these towns the work thus begun will prosper in dignity.

PART TWO
Section Three

Of human physiology and general pathology

§1

If, during their study of natural science, students of medicine have already acquired some knowledge of the animal structure, and if, in addition, at demonstrations of human dissection they have obtained a general view of the healthy functions of the human body and its parts, then (and this I learned from fourteen years' experience at three medical schools organized by me) a detailed explanation of these functions together with a general examination of the most usual derangements, by one and the same teacher, in one and the same school year is fully appropriate. The natural order of things requires that in dissecting a body and describing its organs, the student is at the same time made acquainted with the purpose of these in general, and that a human body is not hacked by its dissector in view of its future use and hung up for display, like cattle by the butcher. Likewise the explanation of the healthy functions of the live human being and his parts cannot be separated from the functions of his deranged, obstructed, destroyed parts, although both have seemingly opposite effects, but depend on the same causes which differ only in degree. Such separation involves contradictions and is detrimental to the learning of students.

* * *

§3

Needed reformation

It is necessary, therefore, on the occasion of describing all the functions of the human body, to mention their disorders also, and thus the general history of the most common diseases and their origin, their remote, and as far as we are able to know, also their immediate causes so that it becomes clear to the beginners how necessary it is to learn physiology as thoroughly as possible in order that they may understand the obscure course of diseases, their symptoms, and their causes. It is only natural that the physiology teacher, speaking of the living animal fiber, its excitability or susceptibility and sensitivity, which distinguishes it from the dead fiber, how it is induced to act by an applied stimulus, and how it expresses life activity, explains at the same time how this excitability can sometimes be blunted, how a

336

certain stimulus can induce a slight motion in the fiber or in the organic part which it composes, or how an excessive stimulus may induce too violent a movement or even exhaust the fiber, and how a separation or some other local fault may prevent or annihilate the activity of this fiber or of the organs. It is natural that this teacher, while explaining the healthy functions of the heart and blood vessels, also demonstrates the deviations of their functions from the healthy state, and at the same time shows the students this or that cause, and under which circumstances this occurs. It is only natural that such coherent teaching cannot be suddenly cut off and postponed for the coming year, to be expounded by a different teacher, usually according to a curriculum that does not match. The excellent Gregory, Professor Emeritus at the University of Edinburgh, already realized profoundly the necessity of combining physiology and pathology in lectures, and I myself have lectured on his Conspectus medicinae to the students' advantage at the University of Göttingen in the years 1784–1785.

* * *

PART TWO
Section Five

Of special pathology and therapy

§1

Once the student is in possession of the foundations of anatomy, physiology, general pathology and therapeutics, pharmaceutics, pharmaceutical chemistry, and the dispensing apothecary art, it is at last time to acquaint him with human illnesses according to all their classes, orders, genera, and species, with their symptoms, characteristics, causes, effects, and forebodings in particular, or with special pathology, but also at the same time, with the principles of medicine or special therapy applied to each kind of disease.

§2

For this purpose, firstly, special pathology must be lectured on by the teacher of special therapy from the clinical hospital itself and by nobody else. In medicine it is necessary that experience based on reasoning, unless it presupposes the conclusion, be correlated with it by one and the same hand, and as closely as circumstances permit. Without close connection between special pathology and special therapy, effected by the same teacher, it is hardly possible to avoid a great confusion of concepts in the students, and eternal repetitions or malevolent insinuations on the part of the lecturers. For in special pathology are the premises from which the teacher of special medicine and clinical physician have to draw their conclusions. If a strange and perhaps practically inexperienced teacher postulates these premises, according to his own lights, and they do not conform to the inner conviction and experience of the practitioner, the latter must either embark upon inappropriate and time-wasting rebuttals, or draw conclusions which are not contained in the premises, and act according to principles which are unknown to the students or which contradict the concepts which they have so laboriously acquired.

Secondly, the students of special pathology must attend the clinical lectures most diligently throughout the entire school year as mere auscultators or as spectators and observers. They must see for themselves the symptoms of the diseases, study the semeiotics of nature, investigate the causes of various infirmities, and judge their result, before they can treat a patient themselves under the supervision of the same practical professor, and as probationers, which they should be permitted to do only in the second school year.

Thus, there is no doubt that the school year of special pathology is spent really usefully and that the students learn with great ease at the sickbed the science of diseases (nosology) as well as that of the causes (etiology), and the science of symptoms (symptomatology). As regards the science which teaches the determination and application of all phenomena of life and death in the healthy and the sick state (semiotics), it is to be explained especially diligently by the teacher of physiology and general pathology. However, the sickbed is really the place where this science can be learned most thoroughly; everything that is said merely from the pulpit concerning semiotics is much more easily forgotten by the students than if they see at the sickbed itself the import of every phenomenon and the prognosis from it confirmed by the result. Therefore, the new constitution plan for medicine in France says: "Semiology cannot be treated separately without exposing oneself to innumerable repetitions and a great confusion of ideas, for the explanation of symptoms in general belongs to pathology, and the explanation of the same effects, viewed as symptoms, supplies the characteristics for nosology, whereas, the professor of practical medicine, after having put it in order, applies observation in order to sum up his description."

* * *

§4

Both must be taught at the sickbed

However, as I have said before, it is senseless to teach the students of such important subjects as special pathology and special therapy according to a feeble copy if one is able to demonstrate to them the original. It therefore happens that students, after having heard the description of the diseases merely from the pulpit, and perhaps from a man who himself saw few, if any patients at all at the sickbed itself, hardly recognize the object of the description. Previously, medical practice was even taught in lecture halls without any patients, and the result was that when young physicians came home from university, they were hardly able to recognize erysipelas, and consequently they treated it quite haphazardly for years.

* * *

§8

In hospitals

"Public hospitals are the best schools for future physicians;—some military campaign or other is for a young surgeon the Non plus ultra of practical instruction!" —Of course, if only the number of sick seen or the number of arms and thighs cut off could be instrumental in training good practicing physicians, this would be correct. Even assuming that all the physicians in charge of civilian and military hospitals and their curative methods could be a model for young people, however, the number of patients to be attended by them daily, as I have mentioned before, is so considerable and the time for visiting them is so short, that it is nevertheless impossible for beginners to keep up with them in observation and to put their notions in order. Those among them who were not guided for several years by specially appointed teachers, who are sufficiently paid for their work and are under the supervision of an alert school administration, treating fewer sick but a sufficient number of them at a slower pace, are made by mere hospital practice into raw empiricists.*

Things are quite different when young doctors, after having enjoyed instruction at a well-appointed clinic for two years, endeavor to perfect themselves and gain more skill in the treatment of diseases in hospitals which, as I shall show later in this work, have also been established for this purpose, or with excellent town physicians who have at least twenty years' experience and have been approved by the medical authority for practical instruction. This endeavor cannot be prescribed by law, but it deserves to be especially recommended to young doctors by the government, and should be considered a reason for future preferential promotion.**

* I therefore agree with Pinel who says: "Les hôpitaux, à leur origine, servirent plus à satisfaire la bienfaisance pieuse des Chrétiens, qu'à perfectionner la médecine, et les études eurent lieu, comme aux époques précédentes." "Dictionnaire des sciences médicales," Tome V, p. 365.

** "Il est très inutile sans doute d'insister sur les avantages des écoles cliniques en général: on sentira très facilement aussi combien la multiplication de ces établissements dans les hôpitaux de malades, peut devenir avantageuse. D'abord les malades de ces hôpitaux seront mieux soignés: quand ils sont le sujet d'observations utiles, ils sont aussi l'objet d'attentions particulières. Le médecin, plus directement intéressé au succès des traitements, les combine avec plus d'attention, et les dirige avec plus de soin; il prend plus de précautions pour que les effets du régime concourent avec ceux des médicaments. Sous ses yeux, et presque sans sa participation, se forment de jeunes élèves dont l'instruction est d'autant plus solide, que la nature elle-même en fait, pour ainsi dire, les frais, et que cette même instruction est, jusqu'à un certain point, indépendente des talents du professeur. (?) Dans cet exercice continuel de leur sagacité et de leur jugement; à l'aspect de tableaux, tous composés des faits, les élèves contractent l'habitude de les mieux voir, et le dégout de tout raisonnement qui ne s'y conforme pas; ils acquièrent, en quelque sorte malgré eux, le véritable esprit philosophique: qui se fonde en médecine, sur cette habitude et sur ce goût. Des récueils complets d'observations sur toutes les infirmités humaines, se trouvent bientôt tout formés, dans les journaux tenus par les professeurs: et de leur comparaison résultent les règles les plus sûres touchant les modifications qu'exige le traitement des mêmes maladies, à raison des lieux, des saisons, de l'état, de l'air, de l'âge des malades, de leur tempérament, etc. Les épidémies générales, ou communes à différents pays, et les épidémies particulières, ou propres à certains lieux, sont observées avec plus de soin, dans leurs variations et dans leurs retours; elles sont décrites plus scrupuleusement dans leurs phénomènes les plus fugitifs. Enfin par de nombreux essais, on vérifie la puissance et l'utilité de tous les moyens connus, on hasarde des tentatives indiqués par l'Analogie; il s'établit des correspondances, ou des communications rapides entre cette foule d'observateurs, tous également intéressés à ne pas enfouir le fruit de leurs recherches, et de ces riches matériaux doivent sortir nécessairement des corps de doctrine plus complets, plus réguliers, plus exacts, qui chaque jour se rapprocheront de plus en plus de la nature, et qui plus susceptibles de se plier et de s'adapter à toutes les circonstances, réuniront aux avantages d'un sage dogmatisme, tous ceux du véritable empirisme rationel." Cabanis, ["Révolutions et réforme de la médecine"], pp. 360, 362.

I resume my subject again in order that I may continue here about the two kinds of public and special pathological and clinical instruction at the sickbed.

Although the advantages of outpatients' departments, as admitted above, may be ever so great, I believe that they alone are far from sufficient for the desirable training of general practitioners. And no matter what has been written in praise of some universities, without a practical school equipped like a hospital, no university will succeed in supplying the state with perfectly trained physicians who will be able to practice satisfactorily upon leaving the university. Therefore, even those universities which seemed to set the greatest store by their dispensaries always endeavored, and this must be said in their honor, to possess also a practical institute similar to the clinics in Leyden, in Edinburgh, in Vienna, in Pavia. Otherwise, their contentedness, which contrasts so much with the true interests of a university, can be explained only by the certainty that in view of the complete lack of hospitals at their not very populous and often poorly endowed seats of the Muses, such a useful institute can hardly ever be attained. What I have said here about the shortcomings of policlinical institutes for physicians, applies also to similar institutions recommended for obstetricians.

§9

If an educational institute for clinical practice is to fulfill as much as possible its purpose concerning the well-being of all the citizens, it is necessary (in addition to the conditions concerning the teaching and serving personnel, partly dealt with and partly to be dealt with later) that there be first a suitable place where all students can simultaneously and comfortably congregate at the sickbed. Secondly, a sufficient number of sick of every age and sex is needed, the number, however, being in proportion to the gradual acquisition of thorough and lasting knowledge; thirdly, an unlimited choice of diseases, both acute and chronic; fourthly, the moral certainty that the prescribed curing method will be strictly obeyed; fifthly, the opportunity for observing also during their requisite convalescence, the patients who have been saved; and sixthly, the opportunity for dissecting those dead who died of their diseases, in order to confirm or correct the ideas harbored or expressed by the teacher and concerning the seat, the causes, and the effects of the disease, and in order to preserve objects found in the bodies which are instructive and highly conducive to public instruction.

* * *

The decision stands therefore that the basis of all clinical establishments must be a hospital that is sufficiently provided with patients of all ages and both sexes, or several houses destined to admit them, and the unlimited choice of patients who are to be treated under the view of students.

Experience teaches, however, that this free choice of the sick [to be transferred] always meets great obstacles, if at the same time the teacher of the clinic is not recognized as the medical superior of the hospital which was assigned to him for his practical school. Human mentality being what it is, a hospital director will not easily acquiesce to seeing the professor of the clinic daily scan the journals of admittance, walk through his sickrooms at any time, examine the patients and, according to his judgment, remove them from his supervision. Even some of the physicians employed by the hospital will resist arbitrary investigations of their previous curative methods by a strange physician, especially if their director secretly supports them, and they will be inclined to denigrate any cure he effects, which may be directly opposed to the treatment hitherto applied.

It has been argued that a teacher at a clinic is so busy with this work that it is not safe to let him direct a large hospital as well, without detriment to both institutions. Of course, if the same superior who, as an expert, is in charge of the hospital policy, and is also charged with the hospital economy, with which a physician is rarely conversant, and which consists of a thousand time-consuming details, and was therefore consistently rejected by me, then such an office composed of such heterogeneous parts can hardly be mastered by one man, without neglecting one service or the other. Therefore, when Joseph II was pleased to put me in charge of the hospital in Pavia, in addition to my professorship, the economic administration of this considerable hospital was given to the distinguished Marchese Malaspina. As is generally known, soon afterward, and as protomedicus, I was charged with the general management not only of all (43) hospitals, but also of the entire public health in Austrian Lombardy. After having fulfilled these functions for ten years in Italy, I also combined the office of practical teaching with hospital administration in Vienna for the same length of time; and the honorable testimonials of the Italian and German public, which I have to this day, seem to prove what has been contested for a long time, namely that combining in one man the supervision of a hospital with the professorship of the clinic is as practicable as can reasonably be expected.

* * *

§12

On the clinical school

Although twenty-five years' experience in clinical teaching, and even the creditable opinion of the public, have confirmed the applicability of my hints "how to teach publicly practising medicine with good success,"* I nevertheless gladly submit

* Joh. Petri Frank, "Oratio inauguralis de instituendo ad praxin medico," Göttingen 1784, written in the 3rd volume of my "Delectus opusculorum medicorum." "Plan d'École clinique, ou méthode d'enseigner la pratique de la médecine dans un Hôpital académique," par Jean Pierre Frank, Vienna 1790. This publication was translated soon afterward into Italian by one of my former students, Dr. Careno in Vienna: "Piano di scuola clinica ossia metodo d'insegnare la pratica della medicina in un ospedale academico, del. sign. Giovanni Pietro Frank etc.," Cremona 1790. 8. As is well known,

that my plan for a clinical school is far from being as perfect as would be not only desirable, but possible, if the state were in earnest in its desire to aid medicine (just as can be said that no matter how skilled a master-builder, if he does not have to build a completely new residence but only to improve an old, irregular building, he will be very limited). What I have to improve in this work of mine or what I have to add to it, will be seen from the following considerations.

Necessary doubling of the clinic and its teachers

As it is impossible to establish at every university a true graduate school which would be worthy of its name in every respect, it is necessary to appoint two public teachers for the clinical subjects, each with his medical and surgical assistants, and to establish a double clinic at least at those universities which are attended by many candidates of medicine. At Edinburgh in Scotland generally three teachers are appointed for the clinical school; they usually relieve each other after three months. In my opinion this arrangement is not very good: for if the students observe the same teacher at the sickbed for three months only, they rarely completely absorb his way of curing, and thus they usually learn from each teacher something, but not so much as they would learn from a good practitioner whom they could see in action for a whole year. It seems impossible that in one school year a teacher could lecture on the entire system of special pathology and therapy and ensure the required extensiveness and accuracy. Even if he devoted several hours a day to this, in addition to the hour he must spend at the sickbed, it could not be expected that the students would follow him, remember what he said, and consult the books recommended for reading. The matter is not solved by means of a superficial presentation of the clinical subjects, for here all the teaching presented hitherto concentrates, here all must be applied and reduced to the stipulated final aim, the curing or alleviation of the diseases, and such work is not a matter of one school year. But if one teacher alone spreads his subjects over two years, e.g., to lecture in the first year on the acute diseases, and in the second on chronic diseases, or according to some other curriculum, there are nevertheless many new students every year, and they arrive and start just when the first course is over so that when they reach their second year, they have difficulties in understanding the teacher, because they lack the knowledge of what had been taught in the first year course and is not repeated. But in a great medical school, founded in a capital, there is also another reason that makes it desirable that neither of the two teachers of the clinic be ever idle. The large number

---

another of my former pupils, Dr. Titius, professor at Wittemberg, who has since died, published this and two other of my works in German under the following title: Dr. Johann Peter Frank's etc., three treatises on matters belonging to medicine: 1. Draft concerning the establishment of a clinical school; 2. Draft concerning the establishment of a medical-surgical college in Pavia; 3. Regulations for Apothecaries in Austrian Lombardy. Leipzig 1790. 8.

of students makes it impossible for many students to approach the sickbed, or at the least they are excluded from themselves treating the patients under the supervision of the professor, which is extremely important. When I inaugurated the clinical school at Pavia in 1785, there were no more than 24 students who were bound to frequent it according to the prescribed regulation. The clinical building was in proportion with such a number, or even with twice that number of students. But within a few years, the number of clinical students, partly native, partly foreign, increased fourfold, and now several of the small and too low rooms, intended for male patients, had to be turned into one handsome and higher sickroom, just as had been done with the women's rooms under Tissot. Upon my appointment in Vienna (1795) I found approximately the same number of clinical students as I had at the beginning in Pavia, but this number, too, increased within a few years so considerably that more than 300 students accompanied me daily to the sickbeds, in my last year, and as to accommodating them, some years previously the four sickrooms that had proved too small were turned into larger and higher halls.

Too, if the instruction at the sickbed is not perceptual, and the student cannot observe each phenomenon with his own eyes, the clinical school loses infinitely in value. The patients themselves suffer when there is such a large number of students: partly because of so many persons about them, especially in raw winter when doors and windows are closed, and on humid and hot summer days when the air around the sickbed loses much of its cleanliness; partly because the required silence cannot be expected when there are so many young persons about; and partly, also, because the patient eventually tires when so many individuals want to feel his pulse, inspect his tongue, etc., and his state of health deteriorates. However, if there are two facilities for clinical instruction, and if each of the two clinical teachers instructs the students alternately, and for a whole school year in his own clinical hospital, the students become well acquainted with teachers' curing methods, the number of students of each teacher diminishes, and students and patients are relieved.

Of course, it may be expected that the most diligent students, in order to observe more patients and make use of both teachers, will visit the prescribed institute and the other one as well; and such a commendable intention should be promoted by having the two schools of the clinic at different hours.

* * *

How one teacher would suffice

It cannot be expected that two teachers will always be of the same opinion regarding the same subject matter, but now, when the more mature students are so far advanced in science that they have their own views on differences of opinion, this is not so important. It is even useful in that a constant competition between the clinical teachers may lead to viewing the subjects with different eyes and further development. The treatment of the sick in two clinical institutions under the care of these two teachers, if they contradict each other, will also soon show, by the success achieved, whose principles are supported by experience.

However, the employment of two teachers for special pathology and special therapeutics, as well as the creation and maintenance of a double clinic in universities would be too expensive in a small state where maintenance is without contributions by the students. And, unfortunately, since medicine is taught today in very few places with such large hospitals that two clinical institutes could be kept with all the exigencies required by public teaching, it will be necessary to make do with one clinic. So far, even in large capitals, the authorities confine themselves to one such institute, obviously relinquishing some advantages. I myself, in the course of 24 years, had to teach alone special pathology and special therapy at Pavia, Vienna, Vilna, and St. Petersburg, and in addition to provide clinical demonstrations. I was fortunate to have been able to provide education commensurate with their great calling to a large number of young physicians, of whom by now many have excelled as personal physicians and public teachers. In any case, this teaching assignment is so important that not less than two years are sufficient for it. Where only one teacher is available for such a professorship, he would have to hold two lectures daily (so that students who had arrived a year before would not be deprived of a more advanced lecture because of his giving a lecture to new students) in addition to his clinical demonstrations. I myself (loaded down with other, no less important, official tasks) never held these double lectures, but as far as I could I made up for them each year in the clinical demonstrations as follows: e.g., when in the previous year I had lectured on fevers, inflammations, acute and chronic rashes, discharges, and in the subsequent year I dealt with the other classes of diseases, in this last year of school I explained directly at the sickbed the previously cumbrously described pathological, as well as therapeutic principles as far as necessary, to enable the students to comprehend the occurring fevers, inflammations, rashes and discharges. This effort, lasting so many years, made me realize how unseemly it is that seven or eight professors are kept for the mere theory of therapeutics, whereas at universities, where the fees for the lectures are such that no competent teachers albeit only theoreticians, are lured to lecture on a clinical subject, only one teacher is usually employed for that part of therapeutics which really represents the main purpose of all the previous academic studies, i.e., for special pathology and special therapeutics.

However, if special pathology and special therapeutics are to be profitably lectured by one and the same, or by two professors, both these parts of medicine have to be merged into one, and the latter, special therapeutics, has to be dealt with in the introduction and appended at the end, as I did in my "Epitome de curandis hominum morbis." Thus, as soon as each of the two clinical teachers has held his theoretical lectures on special pathology and therapeutics which concerns sickness and recovery, and is dealt with most thoroughly, and where part of therapeutics is also dietetics, he leads his students, accompanied by his assistant, into the rooms that are earmarked for instruction at the sickbed. If the teachers conform to these rules, their students who have been charged with the treatment of some patients under the teacher's supervision, have to visit them before the lecture and without the company of their colleagues, so as to be able to report to the professor in the presence of all on everything that had passed since the last visit to the patients. If this prior visit of the sick is prevented, possibly due to the length of other lectures the student has to attend, it is advisable that the professor, before he himself opens the clinical demonstrations, grants to his clinical students the necessary time to examine their patients. The watching students and those probationers who do not have to treat any sick at the time all remain in a specially appointed, spacious forechamber of the clinic until the teacher arrives so that his lengthy sojourn of so many young people without proper supervision, which is usually noisy, does not permit the atmosphere to be polluted even more, the patients' rest to be disturbed, and sometimes, especially in the women's room, the decencies to be mischievously violated. Such a proposal should not be considered petty! It is based on many very unpleasant experiences to which, however, there is less occasion where only a few students are admitted to clinical demonstrations.

Altogether, the clinical institutes at universities are so new that it can be seen in all of them that their initial appointment is due either to a lack of accurate knowledge of their true requirements or to a parsimony, which is obviously contradictory to the former, unless, despite all the learned splendor, the real reason is the poor state of the university exchequer. As I have already mentioned above, most of the sick rooms allotted to the clinic are too narrow and too low, and they bear no relation to the number of patients required by such an institute, nor to the number of students, which in our days is higher than it used to be. Handsome hospitals are indispensable magazines of well-appointed clinical schools. If poor helpless patients of every kind are entitled to be received into them, they must be chosen according to the requirements of public instruction and at the teacher's discretion at the hospitals, and in some cases must be permitted to be transferred back to them. But most clinical institutes of universities in small towns are in reality only hospitals which, at certain times, do not lack patients, but lack the variety of diseases and of opportunities necessary for a good clinical school, and are unable to remove a patient, who may be incurably ill and occupying without any profit and for months on end a bed that is public and therefore scarce, to some other place where he could receive treatment. The number of beds in a medical clinic should be no fewer and no more than twenty. No fewer, so that the students do not lack opportunities for gaining experience and to give the teacher sufficient time, and no more so that the notions of the beginners are fortified and do not get confused. The beds should also be divided evenly between the sexes. Whereas in ordinary hospitals, because of savings of space, the distance between bedsteads need not be more than three feet, the distance between bedsteads and between bedsteads and walls in the clinic must be no less than six feet so that many students can approach the sickbeds and observe everything thoroughly. It is always good if three or four unoccupied beds, in addition to the mentioned, are kept in readiness at the clinic for the reception of available [patients with] important or rare diseases. But if 20 to 24 patients suitable for public instruction are to be selected and constantly maintained, a hospital containing at least 200 sick persons constantly is required. The more patients of every kind such an institution has, the easier it is for the clinical teacher to make an interesting choice among them, both for the benefit of his school and for the sake of science, a task which also belongs to his duties.

It is very important that the clinical institute be near the hospital: so that the clinical professor and his assisting physician have all the more often time to visit in order to select patients; so that the patients that are to be transferred to the clinic or back from it can be brought there without great hardship; and so that the institute, which is to be erected next to every hospital and should serve for the post-mortem examination, could also be used by the professor of the clinic, without having to transport the bodies far. If there are several hospitals in town, even if somewhat distant from each other, their patients must also be delivered comfortably, if required by the professor of the clinic because of the importance or the rarity of their cases, provided their transport does not involve any danger. The professor of the clinic must also be entitled to enable poor patients who wish to enter, not the hospital, but the clinic, if the teacher considers their state of health important for his instruction.

Most clinical medical schools also lack, in addition to adjacent lecture halls and some premises for the installation of the pathological exhibits which are often used during the lectures, the requisite number and the proper separation of the sick rooms. Almost everywhere there are only two halls, one for males and one for females. Yet I am convinced that if we want to improve these clinical institutes seriously and make them correspond to their ultimate purpose, much more will have to be done for them than has been done so far anywhere.

* * *

Examination of the sick

Since the sick who are to be received at the clinic for public instruction, so that their state and the best treatment for them can be correctly determined, have first of all to be examined thoroughly, it is most necessary that the teacher of this school (or in special institutes where there are two teachers, the one who is appointed to instruct the beginners or students of the first year) should begin with the rules of the art of how to examine patients properly, before visits to the patients are arranged. These rules of a difficult art, an art which often determines alone the happy or sad result of the disease to be treated, can well be summarized in a few lectures. We have a large number of rules which young physicians may blindly follow, and in their zeal to find out about the illness they may, by a hundred or more questions, which are meaningless and sometimes even ridiculous, tire out the weak patients, drain their strength, and themselves become confused in the end. An inexperienced jurist, who wants to determine the truth, may question a man who is charged with, or suspected of, one or several crimes or a real criminal who endeavors to evade a confession of his unlawful action by cunning or stubbornness; that jurist has to prove guilt, and often fills a whole stack of paper with indecisive questions and answers, whereas an experienced criminal judge, through expedient investigation, either establishes clearly the innocence or the crime of the accused in a brief protocol of a few sheets. Equally so is the difference between the investigative method of an inexperienced physician and the method of a trained medical practitioner who is already acquainted with the speech and the physiognomy of diseases. Common sense, lengthy intercourse both with healthy and sick people, acquaintance with the origin, age, status, work, way of life, passions, influences to which a person is exposed, existing ills, previous illnesses—all these, rather than a whole litany of questions, guide the prudent practitioner toward a clear insight into the true nature of the sick.

Just as the students of the first year at the clinic ("Auscultanten") do not treat the patients, so are they also excluded from examining diseases, up to the following year in which they, as practitioners, are admitted to the sickbed. In the first year they are only exhorted to pay continuous attention and are instructed how to examine sick persons and what conclusions can be drawn from the replies and from the symptoms of the disease. If the patient is able to describe the history of his previous and his present state, no matter how roughly and incompletely, he saves the physician a host of those tiring questions and provides him with a hint with which he, without taking roundabout paths, can approach the truth. If the sick person is already too weak or bereft of speech, his friends or relatives, who accompanied or delivered him to the clinical institute, will be partly able to substitute for him. Now the teacher turns the patient over to one of his practitioners for public examination, and guides him, with the utmost consideration and speaking Latin, a language incomprehensible to the patient, both in the propriety and the modesty of the questions. When they are finished, and he has obtained what is necessary for judging the illness, its symptoms, the difference between it and others that seem slightly similar to it, the student has to give his opinion on the nature of the disease and on the prognosis, indications, and plan of treatment, based on them. If the teacher finds the student's opinion substantiated, he then prescribes the indicated medicines under supervision and slight modifications. On the other hand, if the student erred completely in his opinion, the teacher guides him gently back to the path indicated by experience and reason. Here the teacher tells his charges the reasons why he rather applies this cure in the present case and not another one. He will quote both his own and other people's experience to clarify the matter better, and he will also have recourse to the latest discoveries in order to experiment, using the greatest possible caution, with new remedies which after honest and repeatedly confirmed private experience promise to have a healing effect.

Immediately after the first visit to the patient, the young physician to whom the patient was entrusted should enter the patient's name, country of origin, profession, duration of his illness, and its nature on a special numbered chart suspended at the head of the sickbed. The name of the practitioner treating the patient must also be entered there. The formulas of medicines to be sent to the pharmacy are written on special slips of paper on which are also written the number of the hospital room, and of the bed [patient] for which the medicine is destined. The diet prescribed for the patient is written on special printed cards which are affixed to the chart.

With such a procedure, the first examination of a patient proceeds but slowly, and thus, when a clinic is being opened, only three or four patients can be admitted daily; all the beds in the clinic can be fully occupied only after several weeks have passed.

The history of each patient, who has been examined as described above, is to be written down the same day by the practitioner assigned to him. This should be done in Latin with the utmost accuracy, and on the following morning it is read at the sickbed. During each new visit the practitioner has to make his report publicly to his teacher, mentioning everything that happened with his patient since the last visit, and then continuing with the case history. If the nature of the illness and its probable consequences were ascertained during the first examination of the patient, and stated with sufficient accuracy, the case history must be complemented by the remarks of the teacher. Day by day, this will now be continued by the same hand, and this will also record most accurately all the accidents and changes observed in the course of the disease, as well as the medicines and foodstuffs prescribed against them from time to time. This continues up to the hour of discharge of the patient from the clinic, or his death. Since the bodies of those patients who died in the clinic have to be opened, almost without exception, to discover the seat, the causes, or the consequences of the fatal illness, the students have to record the findings of these post-mortem examinations lucidly and faithfully at the end of the case history. In any case, within eight days after the end of the illness the student has to deliver to the teacher a legible, signed, faithful copy of the case history recorded by him. The professor of the clinic, after perusing each of these case histories, has to keep them as faithful protocols of all the cases treated under his supervision and guidance. To put them in order, and to prevent any of them getting lost, he should have them bound in several volumes every year.

In addition to these detailed case histories to be written by the practitioners, an accurate register of all the patients admitted to the clinical institute, separate for both sexes, has to be kept by the physician assisting the professor of the clinic. In this register, to be kept in tabulated form, the name, age, home, trade, the state of the patients, the day and hour of their admission, their discharge, transfer, their death, the name of the student treating the patient, and the delivery or default of the case history, have to be entered. The medical assistant takes care altogether, in the professor's absence, that his dispositions made at each bed are carried out; he takes care that the clinical institute is in good order, that the patients are well treated by their attendants, and that the prescribed medicines are scrupulously administered. After school he reads, corrects where necessary, and signs the medicinal formulas prescribed by the students upon instructions of the teacher, sees to it that they are sent in good time to the pharmacy, supervises the correct and rapid preparation of the medicines, and checks the correctness of the signatures determining their application and the bed numbers. He visits frequently and unexpectedly, especially at meal times, but even at night, the sick rooms, and he is ready at any time to come to the patients' aid without loss of time in case of unforeseen occurrences. During pathological postmortem examinations he aids the teacher, the professor. If the professor is too preoccupied with the pathological changes found in the body, he sees to it that the parts of the body that deviate from the normal state are accurately marked by a student to whom this task was assigned, and he, in addition to the prosecutor, sends whatever is worth keeping to the pathological museum. Upon demand by the teacher, he also orders from the museum those pathologically changed objects which are sometimes needed during lectures for purposes of demonstration, and after their use he sends them back undamaged.

A very important observation about practical instruction, both in medicine and in surgery, is that a great deal depends on the assistant who is assigned to the professor. It takes years for a professor to train his assistant, and, as I have already advised, not only should the choice of assistant be left to the professor himself, but his appointment should also be made so lucrative that he should not be forced to leave this post as quickly as possible. The point is that as soon as such assistants find a better post, which usually does not take them long, they hurry away from the clinical school. And until a new assistant is trained, public instruction suffers badly, for he has to look for almost all the suitable patients, with great effort and danger, in all the rooms of the hospital, and in the professor's absence or in case of illness, he has to supervise by himself all patients, attendants, and all the incoming students who yearn for scientific instruction. If each clinical teacher in his entire lifetime trains only three men to be perfect assistants, and these are encouraged to ever more useful activity, then the state has gained in them a constant source from which it can obtain in its own country at any time suitable individuals, when appointments are to be made for clinical teaching posts.

* * *

Mode of instruction at the sickbed

Should the clinical teacher at the sickbed speak not only about the present case and its proper treatment (as I often did with rare or very complicated illnesses), but also point out on this occasion related illnesses, and give from the wealth of his experience everything that is useful and could contribute to the enrichment of the art and the broadening of the students' outlook? Or should he (as is mostly done at Edinburgh) confine himself at the clinic itself to only what concerns the present patient, and voice his secondary considerations only at his clinical lectures?

There are objections worthy of thorough consideration to each of these procedures.

The first method seems to result in a lack of time to be spent by the teacher of the clinic on other patients at the institute, and because of this shortage of time it is to be feared that undue hurry would arise which would be detrimental both to patients and students. Besides, it seems that not only the pronounced and lengthy teachings of the professor must be very taxing for the patient, but that due to the presence of so many students surrounding the sickbed, the close confined air must be also somewhat deleterious to the patient.

With the other method, it is certain that a few words said at the sickbed by the teacher will make a much greater impression on the students, and what is most important, a lasting impression, than what he could achieve if he lectured from his chair for hours, and no matter how learned that lecture were. The somewhat pro-longed view of a still rather unknown disease, which is rich in important phenomena and sheds light on other related ills, offers the experienced teacher, who is inspired by a really practical genius, a unique opportunity to develop concepts and inductions which perhaps can take root only at the instant when all the students' senses are concentrated on the subject and are receptive to a powerful and lasting impression.

* * *

The best teaching method, also at the sickbed, is the Socratic method, and what Marsilius Ficinus said about it in regard to his teaching post, I was also able to say as teacher of clinical medicine.* A learned dissertation of some medical subject may be held from the chair but certainly not at the sickbed, and nothing attracts the students to practical medicine more than when, on this occasion, the teacher by shrewd questioning, so-to-speak, puts the replies in their mouths, the correctness of which they may flatter themselves to be able to ascribe to their own cogitation. If the clinical teacher finds from the student's answers that he missed a decisive circumstance in his review of the illness under consideration, this will also be sub-mitted to thorough consideration, and among some of those standing nearby a kind of medical council will be held, in order not only to stipulate as accurately as possible the nature of the illness and its surest cure, but also to prepare the young

* The following was written by this man, who was so deserving of the belles lettres in Florence, to his friend Uranius: "Non tantum mihi adrogo, ut docuerim aliqua, aut doceam; sed Socratico potius more sciscitor omnes, atque hortor, foecundaque familiarium meorum ingenia ad partum assidue provoco." Vid. "The Life of Lorenzo, Called the Magnificent," by Roscoe, Vol. III, pp. 69, 70.

medics for the Consilia medica, which await them in the future and for which only few show a certain adroitness.

When the students read their case history publicly, the teacher has to see to it in particular that all the pertinent circumstances are correctly presented, in an orderly manner, and succinctly. Many physicians show in their written reports, counsels, or even in anamneses intended for print, that they did not have the benefit of instruction in preparing such treatises in their youth, and did not learn to handle the brush while painting their pictures.*

In training young physicians at the sickbed, it is most important to see to the following in addition to matters concerning the progress of the studies: good manners, gentleness, compassion with the sick, modesty, especially when treating females, secrecy, and compatibility with one's colleagues. Far from mocking all theory, as is beginning to be done again, the teacher of the clinic must derive it more and more from experience, but everything which does not pass this fine-meshed sieve has to be discarded as mere chaff.

I have already spoken of the importance of performing autopsies (§6). Therefore, every time a patient at the clinic succumbs to his disease, and the time stipulated by the funeral laws draws near, unless there is reason to fear contagion, the body must be delivered to the anatomic theater, and there the practitioner who treated the patient reads his case history aloud in the presence of the teacher and all his students. After that the prosector, under the professor's instruction, and after thorough inspection of the exterior of the body, begins dissecting it in order to trace as far as possible the real seat of the fatal illness, its causes and effects. The above-mentioned practitioner, as the witness standing nearest the body, and under the supervision and instruction of his teacher, makes a true and detailed list of all the pathological changes found in the corpse. When he has finished, he reads it aloud to those present, signs it, and attaches it to the anamnesis of the late patient. When the dissection is completed, the teacher in a brief and concise discourse makes a careful comparison of the former symptoms of the fatal illness and the findings in the body; he will correct previous, perhaps erroneous, concepts of the illness without a trace of unkind blame, but with the openness of a man and true scientist who loves his science more than his own fame. Or conversely, this new pathological proof will confirm his findings concerning the seat of the disease, its nature and its ending. As I mentioned elsewhere, now the parts deemed worthy of keeping are prepared by the prosector, as necessary, for better preservation and for exhibition for instructional purposes, delivered to the pathological museum, and there its custodian or custos records them in detail in the register of the cabinet, according to the instructions given by the teacher.

* * *

* See what I said on this subject in the academic speech "De conscribendis morborum historiis Ticini," 1791. This treatise is contained in Volume X of my "Delectus opusculorum medicorum."

PART TWO
Section Six

Of surgery

The superficial division of human diseases into internal and external ones has become the source of the greatest disorder. By limiting the physicians and surgeons in the application of their knowledge, which stems from the same principles, and confining their skill within narrower limits, by causing between these two closely related sciences continuous quarrels and misunderstandings, the worst consequences have ensued to the citizens' well-being. There are few external diseases of some import which do not also affect the inner organs of the human body, and the internal diseases cause external illnesses too often to permit a dividing line to be drawn between physician and surgeon in the future. The former, largely by ignoring the course of external diseases, lost thereby the opportunity, if which the ancient physicians made use to such great advantage, of judging internal diseases more correctly. Such are, e.g., constipations, the excretion of juices, inflammations, suppurations, internal swellings, which cannot possibly be understood if there is no endeavor to draw the correct conclusions from what occurs on the surface of the body. There is only one medical science, which may be called medicine or surgery, since the seat of the disease is different and requires this or that help. But intrinsically, there is no difference, and the same knowledge is required in the case of both external and internal cases. Or else one means by surgeon, a man who only applies plasters, bleeds, and carries out similar insignificant remedies. It is not true that a man deserves the honorable title of surgeon in the full sense of the word if he is not at the same time a physician, and the latter will always have to be regarded as a very imperfect being if the mere skin if the human body determines the boundaries of his knowledge. It cannot be denied that there is a great difference between mere theory of these sciences and their practice, but this applies to all arts and sciences. To be applied and executed with success, they always require on the part of the artist or scientist a certain talent and a certain skill which are not attained without constant practice. Nevertheless, it is beyond any doubt that every good physician must be in possession of the theoretical knowledge of surgery, and it is absolutely necessary that a surgeon must be acquainted with all the principles of medicine if he wants to heal successfully the frequent complications of external diseases by internal illnesses.

However, if both surgical and medical knowledge and experience are essential to every medical man who is to be worthy of this title, it cannot, on the other hand, be denied that for the country folk and for the class of soldiers, the unification of both sciences in one and the same man is entirely indispensable. Neither in the country nor in warring armies can two individuals be found and kept suitably, of whom one would be able and entitled to practice only medicine and the other only surgery. Who could provide for each department of the armies their physician and surgeon? Imagine village people and peasants living in widely scattered farm-steads, especially in mountainous regions, when falling ill, having first to visit a distant physician, and if he prescribed bleeding, an enema, the application of a catheter, a remedy against blisters, suppression of a prolapse, opening of an abscess, would have to call an equally distant surgeon. And only then, when each of these medical men had prescribed medicines, what those two prescribed would have to be brought from an equally distant pharmacy, whereby the cost would be triple, in addition to the carrier's fee and the loss of time. What annual salary could a perfect physician and an even more perfect surgeon command in order to subject themselves patiently to the innumerable discomforts of war with armies on the move, or the sad life, bereft of all opportunities for bringing up children, of all comforts, being condemned to wandering about day and night in pathless regions and to live in dirty huts, without any of the economic advantages which can be attained in towns with less effort? It is clear from these few remarks, and from what I have said publicly on this subject long before* what is to be thought of the prize question put by the Academy of Useful Sciences at Erfurt in 1797, namely: "Whether it is necessary and useful to unite again both parts of medical science, medicine and surgery, both in learning and in practice, which were the causes of their separation, and what are the means of their reunification?"** Röschlaub therefore says rightly: "What is being taught and practiced as part of medicine, is not at all real medicine. Medicine exists only as an inseparable whole. A separation into parts, of which each would still be real and true medicine, thus, does not exist at all. From this point of view

---

* Curriculum for the Medical Faculty of the University of Pavia, Section XI, §1, "Oratio academica, de chirurgo medicis auxiliis indigente, habita Ticini," 1787. This speech appears in Volume IV of my "Delectus opuscul. med. argum.," p. 146.

** Among 14 candidates for the prize, Dr. J. Stoll (reply to the given question: "Is it Necessary and Useful to Reunite Both Parts of Medicine, etc.?," Giessen 1800. 8) and Math. Mederer v. Wuthwehr ("Necessity of Reuniting Both Medicines," Freyburg im Breisgau, 1782. 8) were the only ones who declared that the unification of medicine and surgery was desirable and necessary. The prize was won by J. H. Jugler. His paper appears in "Novis actis academiae Electoralis Moguntinae quae Erfurti est," Tom. I, and it was simultaneously published in German translation (Erfurt, 1799, gr. 18).

therefore the (above) question is senseless. For if there is to be unification, there must be a real separation. But as has been proved, true medicine exists only as an inseparable whole, and ceases to be medicine upon every separation. Therefore, assuming that there is a real separation, what exists is not real medicine but different branches of medical bungling, and unification cannot give rise to a harmonic whole that would deserve to be called medicine."*

* * *

§4

How both sciences are to be united again

To eliminate at last such sad consequences for science and even for mankind, it is necessary: 1) that between physicians and higher surgeons there be no other difference than the practice of this or that branch of medicine; 2) that as long as lower surgery (niedere Chirurgie) has to be tolerated, especially in the country, its members should be rendered as harmless as possible by better training and stricter supervision.

§5

As regards the first point, the curriculum for the Medical Faculty of the University in Pavia has already ordered that the students of both medicine and surgery alike attend the surgical institutions, i.e., attend lectures on external diseases: the indications given by their nature, causes, effects, symptoms, and the rules based on the successful experience of a large number of surgeons, although these may not seem to have any connection with any hitherto known theoretical system.

* * *

§6

Surgical clinical demonstrations

Only after the students have frequented the above-described surgical institutions for a whole year, and have both seen all operations on bodies performed by their teacher and have performed them under his supervision with their own hands (during which time they may attend the surgical clinic only as watching students), are they considered clinical students, and as I said of the medical practitioners (§10), they are admitted to subordinately treating patients at the clinical institutes.

At many universities, clinical institutes were opened for young surgeons much later than for prospective physicians.

* * *

Whereas in a medical clinical demonstration, twenty patients with the course of their illnesses suffice to provide daily material for useful observations by the medical

---

* "On Medicine and its Relationship to Surgery," p. 108.

students and for important conclusions by their teachers, a surgical institution of this kind requires almost double that number of patients because many surgical diseases are so important as to attract the students' attention before and during rather than after the indicated actions. Even if the period of convalescence deserves the full attention of the pathologist, the practical student has more need for a variety of the operations during the short time of his instruction. Thus, setting of broken or dislocated bones, the piercing of large abscesses, amputations of limbs, breasts, etc., which merit the student's complete attention in most patients, are rather similar and have easily recognized symptoms and do not keep the surgical students busy enough for weeks, and it would be desirable for the sake of better instruction to have more frequent changes in the operations, to give students greater opportunity to become acquainted with each type of them.

* * *

PART TWO
Section Eight

Of midwifery
"The great importance of the Science of Midwifery, whether considered in a moral or political view, is sufficiently evident; and was its utility only confined to the preservation of women and their offspring, that alone would effectually recommend it to all who are tenderly solicitous for their safety; but, by a review of its several advantages, it appears a necessary branch of Philosophy as well as Physics, the public administration of Justice, under certain circumstances, calls for its assistance; and even the cause of Religion itself has been promoted by its extensive influence. It may, therefore, be truly said, that it contributes to the good of society and the general interest of mankind in a manner superior to all other Science."

> A lecture introductory to the "Theory and Practice of Midwifery," by John Leake, London 1776. 4. pp. 59, 60.

§1

After having spoken of the lower physicians, I now pass to the instruction which should be received by those who are charged with assisting during delivery.

I have already proven elsewhere that skilled midwives and accoucheurs are essential.* At least I have not heard from the public in the different countries in which I have lived the same loud, violent, yet justified, complaints about the lack of skilled midwives and accoucheurs as I have heard about the scarcity of good physicians.**

---

* "Medical Police," Vol. I, Part III, Section 3. Of the necessary care for women giving birth and in childbed. Vol. IV, Part I, Section 1, §6. The following also deserve to be read: A. Platz, "Diss. de sanitatis publicae obstaculis." —Ch. Aug. Langguth, "De cura qua respublica prosequi debeat rem obstetriciam," Viteb. 1782—1789, and Joh. Aug. Schmidtmüller, "Conspectus politiae obstetriciae," Erlangen 1801.

** Concerning this, see mainly Gebel's documents on the possibility of eradicating smallpox and improving medical institutes in the Prussian states. Breslau, 1802, pp. 129 ff. "In Silesia 286 women died during childbirth in 1798, 514 died in confinement, and 135 of hemorrhage; 2562 children were stillborn, and 1904 died in their first year. In 1799 there were 292 women who died during childbirth, 492 in confinement, and 260 of hemorrhage; 3138 children were stillborn and 1908 died in their first year;

But what could be more mortifying, more outrageous than the sight of a fertile woman still agile some short time ago, who under excruciating birth pains, fell victim to or was literally butchered out of ignorance.* In Sparta pregnant women who gave their lives while bearing the country a citizen received the same honor of the epitaphium as warriors who, with sword in hand, had died facing the enemy. What a contradiction in countries which make the most edifying but costly arrangements for the blessed demise of their fellow citizens while on every side they bar the entry of posterity! . . .** Of course, the birth of the most thick-headed of all animal creatures, the human being, who is provided with such abundant brain mass and is able to effect such wonderful spiritual feats, is also more difficult, and sometimes more dangerous. If, however, there were not the worst prejudices, the most senseless superstition, the injudicious speeding up of labor and of the extraction of the afterbirth, if there were not the restless behavior, the foolhardiness of our crude and only half-educated barber-surgeons and barbers, the daily malpractice of turning, the head drill, lever and forceps applied by ambitious and super-clever accoucheurs, in short, if, with otherwise good position of the fetus in a well-formed pelvis, Lucina or Nature were the sole assistants of the woman giving birth, we would not have to complain so much about the difficult process of the human birth compared with other animals.

Not so much; but not too little either (which is due to a large extent to the faulty physical and moral education of our daughters, their excessively early or excessively late marriage, their untamed passions, the excessive exertions of the poorer mothers); there is unfortunately too much not to call loudly for assistance to the governments in view of the thousands of women who every year are on the brink of death while giving birth and their posterity threatened.

* * *

§9

To whom in the country midwifery should be entrusted

Except for the illnesses of women giving birth, midwifery, as the work of hands or of instruments, belongs to the surgical field. But just as a good obstetrician cannot

---

189 women died during childbirth in 1800, while 591 died in confinement, 126 of hemorrhage; 2966 children were stillborn and 2322 died in their first year." L.c. p. 133. How many children died in France for lack of good midwives can be seen from the Learned Reports of Göttingen for 1771, 47 St. Supplement, p. 393.

* Hence the pious exclamation: "Phoebe fave! Laus magna tibi tribuetur in uno Corpore servato, restituisse duos. Tibull."

** Stoll's reproach, though hard, is justified for the country that deserves it: that whereas in several large cities the ladies of pleasure freely find opportunities of getting rid of the fruits of their debauchery in comfort, the wives of country dwellers often give birth with pain without skilled midwives, and not even on an appropriate bed. "On the Medical System," Part I, p. 166.

be ignorant of the illnesses threatening pregnant women, women in labor, women in childbed, and their tender embryos or children, as well as the remedies for them, physicians cannot dispense with the knowledge required of an obstetrician (although many physicians lack the natural talent and the skill that can be acquired only by much practice).

Although midwifery now belongs to surgery, it would be desirable that a surgeon destined for the fine and dangerous practice of his art be forced only rarely or never to fulfill the difficult task of an obstetrician where his hands must soon lose their suppleness and steadiness (not to mention the time they must devote to the woman in labor). We therefore find that in populous cities the employed accoucheurs desist from all other functions carried out by surgeons. I know of a famous accoucheur, who also taught practical surgery in a large capital, who when he had begun to operate on a patient at his clinical institute, had to ask the surgeon assisting him to finish this doubtful business because his hands shook so greatly. Of course, in some small towns and in some regions of flat country, there are not so many difficult births requiring great efforts of the hands, nor such frequent very fine surgical operations with which a skillful regional surgeon could not deal as long as his age is not too advanced. And it probably can be required only on paper that in every, usually overloaded country district, in addition to the physician and the surgeon, also there be a special salaried accoucheur who would desist from all surgical action, and thus also waive the profit derived from it. If it is proposed that "those who as authorized physicians are in addition subjected to a strict examination in midwifery, and have acquired not only theoretical, but also practical knowledge, and have attended or were in charge of a sufficient number of births, be awarded by universities the title of Doctor of Midwifery, and that only these doctors of midwifery should be called to difficult births," I do not see what could be gained for the good cause by such an easily obtained title. Sacombe expressed the same opinion in this matter.*

If only in this respect, it is necessary that young physicians who are destined to become regional physicians later should learn midwifery and acquire the necessary skill for it at the universities. Therefore, I also proposed not to employ any district physician unless he is also an accoucheur.** For if midwifery is to be learned per-

---

* "Le grade ne sera jamais qu'une vaine formalité digne tout au plus d'égayer la scène sous le pinceau de Molière, tant que le titre de Docteur ne sera point aux yeux du public un garant assuré du mérite de l'individu qui en sera décoré." "Le Médecin accoucheur," Paris 1791.

** "Of the improvement of midwives in the country," p. 26. Jac. Staalkopf, "Commentatio parergica, qua medicum in casu necessitatis munere obstetricis fungentem a decori regulis non deflectere ostenditur." This treatise is contained in the 9. Vers. der Bressl. Samml., September 1719, pp. 386–392. John Leake says correctly: "Some of the medical profession there are, who, with more vanity than solid sense, think it below their dignity to exercise a manual art, or endeavour to save the life of their fellow creature by any other means than that of directing medicines or feeling the pulse; means too often vague and ineffectual without the interposition and assistance of Nature herself. But let it be remembered, that learned man in all ages have not only studied this art themselves, but also recommended

fectly, it requires a scientifically trained man.* This part of medicine, too, presupposes knowledge that can be drawn only from the entire store of medical knowledge, no matter how mechanical the functions may seem, for the object of the [accoucheur's] actions, decisive for life and death, is a living body, nay two living creatures, closely joined together by a mutual relationship. This, in the meantime, has been realized by physicians of the first rank,** and midwifery made such rapid progress in England only because there the most famous physicians endeavored sooner than in our country to practice it solely and even to teach midwifery in several maternity hospitals.

* * *

§11

The post of midwife is so burdensome, it hinders all domestic work of a mother of a family so much, carries with it so much responsibility, and is held in such low esteem, especially in the country, that only the lowest women in every community and consequently those whose education has been most neglected, can be induced to take on this service. Although in antiquity, as I pointed out above, the position of midwife was held in honor, less than a hundred years ago, the sons of midwives were still excluded from the guilds, and even today a midwife in the country is hardly considered above the wife of a herdsman in most regions. After the woman in labor has given birth, the midwife is considered by her and her children as a mere attendant, and in many places she is obliged to clean the first laundry.

It is not rare that either because of the late onset of labor or because of some obstacles hindering the relief of the woman in labor, the midwife must be awake for several nights, and for such a service she obtains less than a female day laborer.

* * *

But if the midwives in the country will be relieved of the humiliation that has hitherto been tolerated almost everywhere, if as sworn servants of the state, appointed for the safe introduction of our descendants, they will occupy the well-deserved rank

it to the attention of others as a curious branch of natural Philosophy, which will afford the highest entertainment to a contemplative mind, and as a thing of the utmost importance to the community. It is not, indeed, necessary that a physician should practice midwifery; but if he is utterly unacquainted with that science, he is less entitled to the name, which implies a general and extensive knowledge of the healing art." A lecture introductory to the "Theory and Practice of Midwifery," p. 3.

* Joh. G. Roederer, "Oratio de artis obstetriciae praesentia, quae omnino eruditum decet, quin immo requirit," publice dicta d. 18. Dec. 1751, vid. ejusd. opuscul. med. Goettingae, 1763, 4. pp. 1–16.

** "Ruysch, that laborious investigator and promoter of anatomical knowledge, not only practised midwifery, but was appointed professor of that art, by the states of Holland. The learned Astruc, Royal Professor of Physics at Paris, and physician to the French king, gave public lectures on midwifery; and also Albinus, an illustrious Professor of Anatomy and Surgery in the University of Leiden." J. Leake; l. c. p. 4.

immediately after the wives of the persons in authority in the village, to which villagers are not indifferent, if they and their husbands will be freed of tributes and services, if a moderate rent for their house will be refunded, there is no doubt that not only the class of miserable, incomprehending, awkward, female day laborers who have already been robbed of all feeling by excessive work, but also the class of better educated women, at least those able to read and write, will not easily disdain the post of midwife. And if they will receive a moderate remuneration from affluent women in childbed, they will consider themselves sufficiently rewarded for the free service they give to poor women giving birth.

* * *

3

Medical Institutions of Learning; the Examination and Confirmation of Medical Practitioners

PART TWO
Section Ten

Of the examination and confirmation of physicians

§1

With regard to subjects of such importance for every state as medicine and the schools required for teaching it, it is necessary and time for men of mature experience and unambiguous intentions to reveal their thoughts; the more so this after more than six hundred years' existence of the present university system, and in view of the present volume of sciences in general and in particular. This I did for myself in the sixth volume of this work which due to the amount of subjects to be treated, and with the subsequent sections, consists of three parts. It seems probable to me that our descendants will be able to judge impartially my reasons for seeing the need to improve the teaching system; from this aspect alone, I believe my copiousness will be deemed an advantage.

A very considerable part of the constitution of our universities has remained the same. This constitution was granted mainly by various popes, bishops, and members of monasteries, and confirmed by princes who at that time were not very knowledgeable in sciences, and it has remained the same despite the profound changes in states, habits, and even religions that have occurred in the last half millennium, and despite all the changes in the old school usages that have gradually occurred.* Already in the second part of Volume Six of the present work, I have proved the necessity of some not immaterial improvements in medical study no longer suitable to the conditions of our time.

§2

Importance of examining institutes

However, no less than this, the hitherto applied procedure in examining future physicians requires a complete review based on the circumstances, which have changed

---

* E. Meiners. "On the Constitution and Administration of German Universities," Vol. I, section 6, pp. 325–364.

very much, and on lengthy experience. Once a medical student has fulfilled the conditions prescribed by the lawful curriculum according to the testimony of his teachers, he is, as is well-known, entitled to present himself for the necessary examinations, and if he also passes these by a majority of votes, he has acquired the right to receive his solemn certification as physician. However, the acquisition of this right is conditioned upon the student's first—before being entered into the register of academic graduates—submitting proof as to his qualities* and previous knowledge, prescribed by law for medical students. The second condition is that the state may rely both on the student's morality as testified by the teachers, proven in the entire course of his studies, and on his diligence as confirmed by his attendance at all the lectures, as well as on the rigorous examinations he has passed according to the judgment of at least two-thirds of the examiners.

* * *

§6

Causes of the failure of examinations

Even from a brief historical description of medical examinations (§3) the general conviction of all legislators and philanthropists becomes clear: that it is necessary to safeguard as much as possible the well-being of the sick members of society by effective regulations for examinations. After what I have said elsewhere of the disadvantage of spurious and unworthy physicians,** it would be superfluous here to give further proof of such a well known matter, and to reveal my own conviction of the indispensability of medical examinations, no matter how loudly I protest against their misuse and bad applications. But by grievous experience of at least half a millennium it is clear that the problem of how medical examinations may be more suited to their final purpose is far from being solved. Thus, it is still worth the endeavors of mature men who have experience both in medical subjects and in the administration of the medical system, to investigate the failure of so many regulations and to discover the causes of the failures and of the means of saving a limb, be it only by its bloody severance, previously attacked by inflammation.

I devote my first considerations here partly to the decisive examination to which students must submit, and partly to the examination which graduate physicians have to pass in order that they may practice freely, and I point to the cause of their low value, which at some places has fallen so greatly, or even, possibly, has rarely existed.

1) Through the traditional transfer of the business of examination to those who are strangers to the students, and the dependence of the students on the professors from whom the students have hitherto received their lectures, and to whom they have given recompense;

---

* L. c. §1, pp. 549–588.
** "Medical Police," Vol. VI, 1, §§10, 11, pp. 212–252.

2) In the examination, doctorate, and license taxes which the students have to pay to either their foreign or domestic teachers, or to those who have to examine them again after they have graduated as physicians;

3) In the abundance of universities, some of which have been founded out of financial considerations only;

4) In the excessive number of examiners which has nothing to do with the time of examination;

5) In too favorable an assessment of a brilliant word memory, which is considerable in most young persons against the power of judgment of examined individuals, who express themselves shyly after more reflection;

6) In the division into classes;

7) In the Latin language of examination;

8) In the written papers.

To prove these statements, I refer mostly to what I have already said elsewhere.

Thus, firstly I have proved sufficiently that it is improbable for teachers from other schools, who are paid by their students and are forced to live almost exclusively on the proceeds of their lecture fees, to examine students impartially, and, also, less scrupulous examiners from other schools, might quietly pocket the examination money, instead, and perhaps with a sneer.

* * *

I have already spoken elsewhere* of the third source of the low esteem of academic examinations, i.e., the proliferation of universities that aim only at financial contributions, lack the most important means, especially those required to train practical physicians, and therefore are not adequate for satisfactory examinations.

Fourthly, as regards the disproportion between the number of examiners and the duration of the examination. This is not unimportant, as the examiners in the past in Vienna were four rather than eight who examined later,** while the examination lasted for three hours at the most, although this is very long for the student.†

* * *

Therefore, the aforementioned royal Prussian decree of 1 February 1783, pp. 23, 24, says, not without cause: "Since judging the ability of the candidate, and especially the lucid posing of questions require of the examiners a certain skill which can

---

* "Medical Police," Vol. VI, 1, pp. 292, 293, 330–335.

** "Primo examini intersunt facultatis Praeses, Decanus et quatuor medicinae Professores. In secundo examine, presentes sunt: praeter Praesidem, Decanum et quatuor Professores, bina facultatis membra." John's Lexicon, Part 6, p. 600.

† Also in the regulation published as late as 8 December 1818 at Munich, the duration of the examination is stipulated as 3 hours, and that of graduation as only 2 hours. Schmelzing. [Repertorium der älteren und neuesten Gesetze über die Medicinalverfassung im Königreich Baiern], pp. 204, 205.

be acquired only by practice, we hereby wish to introduce and establish a special permanent examination committee. This committee is to consist of a director and four members; the latter, for preventing all errors in rank in seating and signing, are to alternate at every examination in such a way that the member who was first at the previous session, is to take the last place at the subsequent session, etc."

Although I recognize the great value of this reduction in the excessive number of examiners, I may be permitted to express my doubts whether the gift of lucidly posing questions and the skill in examining students can really be acquired by exercise. There is no lack of experience at the universities which deal all the year round, if not daily, with at least weekly and semester examinations in great numbers, in addition to very strict examinations of very many students. Just as clear and easily grasped delivery of teaching is a special natural gift that sometimes is not attained even after years of academic lectures, so likewise is daily experience with lucidity in examinations. Therefore, just as a professor whose lectures are clear and easily understood despite his great learning—and such professors are rare and should be all the more carefully sought—likewise, he who is appointed as examiner must have, in addition to proven honesty, the gift of examining which is not bestowed on everybody who actually examines. To disdain this gift (because of unjustifiably confusing the comprehensibility of the questions with their unimportance, or even with the unpardonable intention of incorporating the reply in the question itself) so that the students, who do not have a clear idea of the dangers and consequently of the effort required, do not attain their purpose, is in my opinion as despotic as it is cruel. For the ignorant, no matter how brightly he is questioned, will never guess right, and because it would be unjust to put such insurmountable rocks deliberately in the only feasible path of immature youth.

* * *

Fifthly, as regards overestimating students' memorizing words against their ability to make judgments, there is no denying that in many examinations, both in school, and the final examinations, the former gift of nature is taken more than the latter as the measure of the candidate's scientific value and as an assessment of his qualification. It is very difficult, unless one has much experience, to beware of this fallacy. I, myself, must admit that in the first years of my teaching career I overestimated some of my students solely because of their better word memory, whereas this judgment later proved wrong, while I did not do full justice to those who were more deliberate than garrulous, but whose talents were brilliantly confirmed later. Once the student knows that his ability will be judged merely by the literal repetition of what is written in his textbook or in his copybooks, he relies, like the eight-year old boy with his catechism, on mere memory. And, as the constant memorizing of different subjects does not favor the superficially absorbed concept taking root, all the student's so-called knowledge lasts only until after the examination, and like an actor, he forgets his part as soon as the curtain has dropped, and immediately commits to his memory another part and rattles it off on the stage. What may be preserved in the mind and held in honor while being not amenable to proof of mere reason but, rather, supported by entirely different, albeit unobjectionable, reasons and surrounded by insuperable boundaries (like a sacred treasure), such is necessary for social man to know, and may be committed to his still tender memory without participation of his power of reasoning! It is known that in the Middle Ages almost all education, scientific education included, could be obtained only at monastery schools, and that instruction consisted more in the constant exercise of youthful memory than in the earnest efforts of reasoning powers, which awaken in adolescence. It is known also that medicine at that time was practiced almost exclusively by the clergy, and that it was first taught in monasteries. It is not surprising therefore that the first universities, established under the undeniable protection and superior guidance of the Roman court, continued to teach in the old spirit of instruction, and taught the young man science in the same way as the boy was taught the catechism, and to endeavor later by endless examinations to imprint the matter more on the memory than on the reason.

The intention of these schoolteachers was commendable as long as memorization only was trained thereby but because it was so limited, no peremptory conclusions were drawn about memory for substantive matter, or about a healthy, even excellent, power of judgment and true talent. I myself had a very weak verbal memory from my youth onward into old age, but my circumstantial memory was as good as anyone could wish. As a boy I attended Jesuit schools which were certainly excellent for their time. I was diligent and attentive. Every day in these schools the pupils had to write papers and learn by heart several pages of useful textbooks so as to be able to recite them. Almost every week, those who had written the best papers were allotted the first seats in the room. I was almost always one of the fortunate; however, the humiliated boys who had been relegated to the last seats were permitted to challenge to recitation of oral exercises their colleagues who had been given preference because of better composition. If they won, they could gloriously exchange their despised seat with that of the vanquished, and I was, unfortunately, soon relegated again to the donkey's bench, red in the face (friend Gall should explain this to us!) but never improved. Bowed low, I entreated the strict judges in vain that although certain words may have slipped my mind, their sense was always faithfully retained in my memory, as was always proved by my written papers. But the principle was established once and for all that victory went to word memory, and there was nothing I could do except to reconquer my place of honor a short time after with the aid of my faithful pen.

I realize how unimportant this tale of my boyish victories and defeats is, and I would not have imposed it on the respected reader, were it not that it provides a small contribution to the history of examinations, and thus proves from experience how easily a talent, that will later be so beneficial to the state, can be misjudged by coarse examiners. How easily can it be stifled, when the ordinary examination eventually decides according to these principles, and how unjustly mere word memory is preferred over the more mature power of judgment which, however, expresses itself shyly in careful steps. However, even when these worthy fathers endeavored to promote memorization in boys by giving it preference, it did not have equal weight at the examination at the end of the school year, when it was determined whether the pupil had the necessary knowledge to advance, or whether he should be obliged to repeat the class because he had not grasped the teaching sufficiently. Yet, throughout the lower schools the outstanding memorizer was entitled to administer humiliating cuffs to the better talent. And things were the same in the earlier schools, which had been established according to the oldest monastery schools in which there was no end of determinations and disputations, and where the smooth tongue won the palm branch rather than the brain.

* * *

§9

All the teaching arrangements made in the nineteenth century at most universities, which had been established by the state itself for the gratuitous instruction of students, certainly reflect the noblest intention of helping medicine. Firstly, that in regard to the preparatory sciences both the subjects and the time devoted to them will be increased; secondly, that only the better heads among the students of philosophy will be permitted access to the infinitely difficult study of medicine; thirdly, that the students will be continuously trained by their teachers, either through daily, or through weekly and half-yearly examinations, and that thus at the end of each school year, like sifting wheat in a screen the chaff will be separated and only the healthiest seeds will be used for the new harvest. And, in a strict examination, an even more fine-meshed screen will be applied, and under the conscientious supervision of seven or eight experts in the art, only the most nourishing fruit will pass for the benefit of the public. Finally, among these there was also the endeavor to determine the inner content, to sort the grains and to sort them into certain classes.

The question now is (and no government can reasonably resent this question in view of the daily experience that not a few innovations, no matter how brilliant they may have seemed at first, caused more harm than good in the long run), what advantage really has been made by so much care and strictness in order to attain only the best? Of course, the reply to a question that is so important to every state requires more space than I am free to grant here. However, what I have said so far about the subject permits me to be brief, and I add only the following:

1) All prejudice put aside, one must admit that at universities where the students have to pay a certain fee for the lectures they attend, most teachers have been appointed without public aid, but they are widely recognized and fully deserve their

fame. They need not envy any professor of other state supported medical schools because of his skill. If complaints are heard from some schools that examinations and promotions of the students are too easy, I believe I have proved that this is not the fault of the professors, but that the fault lies in too great a freedom of the students who are permitted to arrange their studies according to their own judgment, and to finish them as quickly as possible. The fault lies even more in the system which forces the teachers, because of the paucity of their annual salary, to live on the fees for their lectures, and thus do not wish to spoil their relations with their students. That, despite all the bad "wares" supplied to us by such doctor factories, we also receive, without so many preparatory and obligatory studies, with such frequent examinations, excellent physicians from them; where the opposite occurs, this is not so much due to the skillful handling, the abolition of weekly or half-yearly examinations, but to the rawness of the material itself, or the premature shipping of the wares under the same stamp.

It is high time to compare the chaos of subjects with which boys and adolescents have been burdened in Germany for more than a quarter of a century, with the success of the teaching, which by now has ripened, with the influence on the progress of the higher sciences, especially medicine, and finally with the daily increasing deterioration of the once great esteem of the learned abroad. One will thus easily be convinced of the truth of my statement which offends our national pride, namely, that in the matter of education we have gone astray. We stuff the tender brain of our youth, like the Jews stuff the stomach of their closely confined geese, with superfluous nourishment, and like the greatly swollen livers of these fattened birds, which on a somewhat hotter stove immediately run out and collapse, the overstuffed brain of the young man also collapses upon the approach of the torch of thorough knowledge, and only the darkness of broad knowledge remains. Would it not be better to feed the heads of the boys only so many spiritual meals as they can digest now, and to teach them only so much as may be required for grasping the correct notions of higher things at a more mature age? Would we Germans, after such great progress made in all fields of science in the eighteenth century, have sunk so low in the esteem of enlightened nations that our rising generation (provided mostly with only superficial knowledge patched together from mere journals and encyclopedias) throws itself again so hurriedly into the arms of the silliest superstition and the most contemptible mysticism?

2) That only the better heads among the students of philosophy be admitted to the study of medicine, I find so just, in view of the very excellent talents required for this difficult and distinguished field, that I myself also proposed such a law. In the meantime, I beg my readers who may be charged with the execution or administration of such an extremely important investigation, not to disregard my not irrelevant remarks, and at the same time to see to it "that, as I remarked elsewhere, every free member of civic society has the right according to legal order to choose a profession

and in it to act for the general and their own good, and not be limited by purely despotic means." But considering that, firstly, not all teachers (not even the field of philosophy excepted) possess sufficiently the gift of being able to ask as lucidly as is necessary; secondly, that a shadow falls on some student, who is either too timid or is not endowed with an excellent memory, because of his replies given to the teacher at the private examination, which shadow he deserves much less than some more courageous young men who may be endowed with a better memory than power of judgment; thirdly, that in view of the excessive number of prescribed subjects at some universities, even in philosophy, it has not been proved that more than one is of use in the study of medicine; fourthly, that between each individual teacher, and each of his students, there is not the same degree of empathy, even assuming that the teacher himself does not know the cause of this mood, and consequently the teacher's way of examining, even if it does not show a possible passion, nevertheless may not be accompanied by such an attractive confidence as in the case of others. If I consider all this, I am of the opinion that (with due respect to the testimonials of the professors who have to teach the preliminary subjects to very different sciences) the student who applies to be admitted to medical studies should be examined by several teachers of medicine before his admittance.

* * *

... and so it seems very expedient to me that, in order to avoid pupils being rejected because of inability after one year of medical studies, and to spare their parents unnecessary expense, the young men who present themselves to study medicine should be subjected to a strict examination as to whether they have the physical, and the moral, and scientific abilities required to learn this art.

* * *

Examination for the free practice of medicine

The centuries preceding the foundation of clinical institutes may have produced some great physicians, nevertheless, there are reasons to say that if these talented men, even after they had successfully passed however strict theoretical examinations, without previous instruction by an older and experienced physician, and instruction lasting several years, if these men were permitted to treat on their own serious diseases, before they could justify their later fame, they would have filled, through no fault of their own, more than one cemetery. Nowadays most universities have introduced instruction at the sickbed for all medical students, and therefore the danger to the gravely ill is much reduced when these patients permit young medics to treat them, the medics having been previously trained at the clinical school. The boundaries of clinical medicine, nevertheless, would be underestimated, and the skill of the teachers, no matter how experienced, would be overestimated if it would be expected that whereas three years are required for learning merely the theory of medicine, perfectly trained and fully equipped physicians could be turned out after two such years of instruction at the sickbed. It must be borne in mind that the medical student has to attend in these two years a total of twenty months of various lectures, has to write in detail the case histories of the diseases treated by him in the clinic, and that he has to make use of almost every hour to recapitulate all the theoretical subject matter because of the impending examinations which are decisive for his future fate. Everybody will understand that in view of these tasks, he cannot concentrate all his mental powers on that which is most important, namely the practical. To this we may add the consideration: most clinical institutes, both medical and surgical, especially in sparsely populated towns that lack large hospitals, are very poorly appointed because various diseases and injuries do not occur there; even in larger clinical institutes, only a very modest number of important, especially chronic diseases, are received in the course of 20 months. There are lucky years in which even in large hospitals there are either no epidemic diseases or only the same familiar ones. There are hardly any opportunities in clinical schools to treat children's diseases; there are very few cases of pregnant women and maternity cases, and even less of demented people. Among the very large number of practical students, of whom I had to guide to the sickbed up to 200 or more every day, only a moderate number can be charged with treating the sick or carrying out surgical functions, while the rest can watch the patients only from afar, amidst diversions that cannot be completely avoided. If all these difficulties are taken into account, it must be admitted that even the best clinic, medical, surgical, and obstetric, although rightly highly esteemed, can lay only the first though undoubtedly the most durable foundations, in the training of young medics, and that we greatly overestimate the value of new institutes for the training of practical physicians, praiseworthy though they certainly are.

I ask now: What can be concluded from the skillful treatment of one or two to three patients at the clinic by a student who is close to his examination? At best that he saw a few, mostly very distinct forms of disease, just as he saw very similar ills, probably a short time ago, to be diagnosed and treated by his teacher, and that under his encouraging supervision, he recognized them correctly, properly followed the instructions of how to heal them and wrote passably the case history. But there is a whole host of acute and chronic ills, of which only a small part has so far been received in clinics and treated in his presence, and as mentioned earlier, there are innumerable illnesses of children, pregnant women, women in labor, women in childbed, demented, etc., that he knows not from personal experience, but at best remembers from having heard merely their verbal descriptions in the therapeutic lectures. No matter how accurate these were, when the medic is separated from his teacher and sees them for the first time, some symptoms being similar in quite different cases, he nevertheless does not know what to call these diseases or how to treat them. And then, where is the skill, so important to the clinical physician, which can be acquired only by frequent practice lasting several years and through seeing the same illness repeatedly in its various forms due to age, sex, temperament? I agree that a student who visited a well-equipped clinic diligently and attentively for two years, and there observed several examples of the diseases that are to be received each school year, and if he then and now still studies the theory of medicine, and answers satisfactorily the questions of his teachers at the oral examination, such a pupil may deserve the doctor's hat, for what it is still worth today. Yet, before he has acquainted himself with a large number of various diseases and their proper treatment for at least another year in a respectable hospital or under an older, experienced and respected physician, I would not like to take responsibility for entrusting him alone with the fate of patients, even if the academic body was unanimous in passing him.

Apart from the teacher at the clinic, the hospital doctors are largely those who, when properly selected and instructed, are most suitable for reaching the stipulated ultimate aim. After them come the town and country physicians who, through many years' experience and fortunate treatment of patients, are given preference, and therefore receive authorization from the medical college to instruct future physicians. Especially in large towns it sometimes happens that young men, either by dint of their other mental abilities or, if these are not outstanding, by their outward appearance, if not by underhand means, win the trust of the people, especially of the fair sex, already in the first years after having gained their doctorate, and thus obtain a larger practice, at least for a few years, than they can deal with by themselves. Then it is not a rare occurrence that such young Aesculaps, who, moreover, hardly ever open a clinical medical book because of their eternal running about, and who at best leaf through a medical journal, and as superficially as possible at that, and who like to gain the respect due to teachers or to lighten their work by entrusting it to inexperienced medical assistants, let themselves be used by equally young or slightly older physicians as instructors at the sickbed, or because of lack of time and because these patients are not very profitable, they let treat them afterwards themselves, or only after a few hurried visits with them. It is easy to guess what kind of physicians graduate from such schools, and nobody can deny that such mischief cannot be tolerated in future without harming society; and that my draft bill, according to which an instructor of medical practice must have an honorable career of at least fifteen years, is not exaggerated.

§10

Is the academic title of Doctor sufficient for a free practice?

The hitherto mentioned decrees concerning examinations and authorization (§§3–9) differ both from the curriculum prescribed for the Medical Faculty in Pavia in 1787, and from the gubernatorial decree in Milan, issued on 28 April 1788, on the occasion of the establishment there of the Direttorio medico. This decree stipulated that students spend two years attending the clinical institute, the first year as mere observers, the second year as participating practitioners who have to produce accurate descriptions of the diseases. For the candidates to be admitted to the (single) stiff examination, they had to submit the testimonials of the professors concerning diligent and attentive attendance at all the theoretical and practical lectures contained in the above-mentioned curriculum; yet before the stiff examination, it was out of the question that there should be a public examination at the sickbed, because the mere academic title of Doctor in Italy in general, and also in Pavia in particular, does not suffice that the graduate can immediately begin treating patients by himself. Instead, according to the medical constitution introduced in Austrian Lombardy, every graduate physician is required to obtain practical experience for at least one year, either at the clinical institute in Pavia or in a large hospital, under the supervision of a renowned and skilled hospital physician, after which he is permitted to apply to the Direttorio medico for the last examination pro libera praxi, concerned only with practising medicine, submitting as proofs of his career thus begun, the diaries of diseases written in the course of it. The part which I had in drafting the two medical decrees (replacing only recently the decrees on medical studies introduced in the Austrian hereditary countries since 1804–1808) entitles me to quote here the sentences concerning the practical examination of young medics who have already graduated,* as does the possibility that not all my readers have its translation at their disposal.** Finally, I am convinced that these decrees are of great value and that their correctness has been confirmed by the greatest success over a period of almost 30 years.

1) "To be able to practice in every branch of medicine, it is indispensable that the candidate be publicly approved. This approbation cannot be granted to all physicians and surgeons, even though they have previously graduated, all apothecaries, laboratory assistants and druggists, insofar as they trade with medical wares, and midwives—without a previous examination which all have to pass if they want to settle in the province to practice their art. Nobody, no matter under what pretense, can evade this law, for by the highest command all titles and privileges are abolished which were once granted to a society of individual persons who thus obtained permission to practice publicly part of medical science. Whosoever shall dare defy this law, is to be punished the first time by a fine of 15 scudi (six ducats), the second time by double that sum. However, should a greater offense take place, the Imperial and Royal Government (Gubernium) is to be informed because the special circumstances require a greater punishment."

* * *

* Chapter 3 of this draft contains the sentences inserted here.
** Johann Peter Frank's (Privy Councillor in Milan and Professor of Clinical Medicine in Pavia, etc.) three treatises concerning medical matters: 1) Draft for the setting up of a clinical school; 2) A medical-surgical college in Pavia; 3) Decree for Austrian Lombardy concerning apothecaries. From the Italian translation by Professor Titius in Wittenberg. Leipzig, 1790. Also in John's "Lexicon of the Imperial and Royal Medical Laws," Vol. 6, pp. 3–55, there is a German translation of the "Piano del Regio Direttorio medico di Pavia," 1788.

SUPPLEMENTARY VOLUMES TO MEDICAL POLICE, OR A COLLECTION OF VARIOUS SPECIAL TREATISES CONCERNING THIS SCIENCE

Volume One

INTRODUCTION

Supplementary volumes to complete works are published additionally either by their authors or by scholars who endeavor to make writings of this kind more complete. However, in view of the many obstacles to the completion of my system of Medical Police (Medicinische Polizey), in view of my premonition, based on my great age, that this intention of mine may be thwarted by death or feebleness and illness, in view of the uncertainty in our turbulent times as to what fate is in store for my articles dealing with state medicine, and written on various occasions, mostly upon prompting from above, and finally because of the justifiable fear that after my demise some of my less important writings, fallen into strange hands, may be turned over to the press by eager persons who are not used to making a selection that would do honor to the deceased, I decided myself to collect the most important articles from among those dealing with state medicine and to make them available to the public in several volumes. If my end should be near, and thus prevent the publication of the remaining parts of Medical Police, these individual articles dealing with subjects of Medical Police proper, which still remain to be elaborated, will nevertheless reflect the spirit in which my system was written, and our descendants will find the key to various arrangements which have been made in different countries upon my proposals. That such an intention of mine will not be considered presumptuous is vouched for by the favorable reception and the many editions and translations of my Medical Police, although if I had been more mature and at an age that ensured more experience, I should have drafted my work in a form more worthy of the public attention it received.

What remains for me to say about Medical Police proper is so extensive and so weighty that it would be impossible for me to compress it all into two volumes to attain the desired brevity if I could not refer to the writings published in the present supplementary volumes.

I think too highly of the spirit of our enlightened age and of the well known wisdom of the governments under which I had the honor to serve to come under the slightest suspicion for publishing articles which I drafted, sometimes upon their instructions, and which I am always entitled to view as my properly acquired property. Of course, treatises dealing with the health and well-being of a great nation belong to the whole of mankind; and if others contradict and hold the opposite opinion, nevertheless, stating the reasons of both sides is a gain for a science which can only be perfected by the detailed consideration of all the difficulties encountered in the implementation of the principles. The state of hospitals and homes for foundlings, of medical schools, etc., have nothing to do with the political conditions of a country which for every servant of the state must be a sacred secret; and even if, upon consideration of these subjects, now and again a weak spot is discovered in the traditional conditions, or if a prejudice dating from previous times is attacked, or a criticized method is manfully rejected, or arrangements made are courageously defended against malicious attacks, the state remains untouched by such considerations and is at most a medical servant of them, yet remains aloof with regard to its opinions or methods, of the delusion of its infallibility which, after all, is not given to any mortal. Altogether, good proposals in the community are like money and treasures: part of them is in constant circulation while the rest, sometimes even the richest, is kept in iron chests, jealously or anxiously guarded, completely unused, or even buried several feet deep in the ground, and is brought to the surface only by accident when digging.

There are in various archives under thick layers of dust reports and recommendations concerning public health the earlier use or public knowledge of which could have saved the state thousands of useful citizens. Therefore no philanthropist can oppose the search for, or the publication of, such articles if this occurs with modest consideration of the conditions which are specific for each state and are not always suitable for public discussion. And every government even must be concerned that nothing be lost or suppressed which may have a considerable effect on the success of public instruction in medicine and on the health and well-being of the citizens. Also, the history of Medical Police stands to gain if the more important proposals concerning health matters are prevented from falling into oblivion, even if they have not always been executed. It could then be seen with how much insight, even in earlier times, some individual and frequently unknown men endeavored to serve the good purpose; and how often the prejudices of certain ages, the ignorance or even the impassioned action of others foiled the execution of the beneficial proposals. It should only be remembered what happened in various countries during the introduction of inoculations against smallpox and of vaccination: how much effort and how many human victims it first cost before these two great discoveries were used as they deserved. The system of predestination of the Muslims still prevents all sensible measures against the plague. And since this system is so closely bound up with their religion, there is scant hope that Europe will soon be relieved of the necessity of guarding its boundary with Asia by such an expensive military cordon, even when there is peace.

During my eleven years of employment in the Principality of Speyer, after I had been entrusted with the supervision of the medical system there, I initiated several measures concerning this important subject and proposed several more. In such a small country, however, with its limited income which, moreover, is ecclesiastical, I could not let my ideas roam freely, which would soon have brought them beyond the borders. All my measures had to be conceived on too small a scale for me to be able to make an important contribution by publishing them for the sake of improving the medical system in large states. However, even the painting of miniatures has its merit, and for me the small but very successful attempts were a preliminary exercise for larger enterprises that would be better secured by more extensive financial means. In both countries, Baden and Speyer, there was only one midwife who had been trained at Strasbourg for several months. In my own country my proposal for establishing a midwifery school had been forgotten, to put the mildest interpretation on it, until after the merger of Old Baden with the Baden Durlach countries when this school was founded and I was appointed its teacher. However, my former circumstances had been so little considered that I was unable to refuse the appointment in Bruchsal, which I received just at that time (1772), although I was loath to leave my country. The Prince of Speyer now demanded that in addition to my office of town and country physician, I also undertake the teaching of midwives according to my own draft curriculum. I fulfilled the wish of this energetic man as far as I could, without having the use of a maternity institute available, and notwithstanding the scanty means, this institute was so successful that the Prince's confidence in my proposals greatly increased. Now he decided to found a hospital in Bruchsal with his own means and another on the left bank of the Rhine at Deidesheim. My opinion on these was also required. I explained that in such philanthropic foundations, the government must invest its capital so as to get the highest possible returns.

These, I said, in establishing a hospital consist in addition to the gratuitous treatment of the sick, also in training of skilled physicians and surgeons so that medicine is advanced through experience beneficial to the community. According to the express wish of the ecclesiastical Prince, the two hospitals, which were not exactly large, were staffed by monk-hospitallers. These were sent from Vienna, and among them was a very skillful practical physician, Joachim Wrabez. After I had been appointed physician-in-ordinary to the Prince, I proposed Doctor Bierenstiel, and he was appointed hospital physician. As is well known, this very skillful and prematurely deceased physician had submitted to the public a reckoning of his arrangements which was very favorable to the author. The bodies of those who had died were used for anatomical, and simultaneously for pathological, explanations; I shared with Wrabez the public teaching and laid the foundations of a pathological museum. Also the pretty considerable penitentiary, as well as the prisons, had to deliver their corpses to the anatomical stage; thus, the young surgeons, who congregated here, had the desired opportunity to train in dissecting; Wrabez lectured on surgical principles, carried out the most important operations, both on bodies and, when cases occurred, on patients, and taught instructively on surgical dressings. The students lacked only physiological knowledge, and I undertook this important task and combined with it general pathology. But there was no instruction in botany, which is so necessary. When this lack was mentioned in the Prince's presence, he became indignant, and I had to listen to charges that I intended to establish a medical school that would be beyond his means. This was not my intention; but I bore the reproach. You have your luxuriant court garden, I told the Prince, and in it the most magnificent hothouses. What harm will it do them if some exotic plants will be put there and taken care of by their skillful gardener? If you like, give me one of your vegetable gardens. For a mediocre botanist like me it will suffice for planting the most ordinary medicinal plants and for teaching the elements of botany, etc. Here I also prevailed, and thus the most necessary was provided for the teaching of country surgeons, without their having to contribute anything more than their diligence.

However, I believe that little can be gained by divulging proposals for institutes in small countries, no matter how fruitful they are, especially when these countries, after having merged, have become larger and their institutions then are too small and insufficient for them. Nevertheless, they [the proposals] should not fall into oblivion since they are the first attempts at improving the medical system by modest means, especially by one who was encouraged by their success to make greater projects and was supported and strengthened more in their implementation. I also used these, my early, experiences in greater projects, always trying to avoid dressing the adult man in a boy's coat, however, and I shall also use them in the future editing of the remaining parts belonging to Medical Police. When I came to Italy, I was acquainted with the constitution concerning medical study introduced in French, English, and German universities and which of course was very different, my having been, albeit for a short time, a teacher at one of the most famous universities of my country. In Italy I had hoped to be for a time, or forever, only a witness observing the quality and course of public instruction and of the medical system altogether, but a few months after my arrival there, I was ordered by His Majesty, the late Emperor Joseph II, not only to devise a plan for the improvement of the hospital at Pavia and to take over its implementation completely, but also to submit a proposal to the Government and to the Imperial and Royal Court as to how medical studies at this famous university could be adapted more to our times and brought nearer to perfection. As soon as I had finished these important matters, the Emperor, who was incredibly energetic in ensuring the well-being of his nations, ordered that from now on the management of the public health system was to be conducted from Pavia, the center of medical studies, and according to a draft submitted by me; consequently, the office of Protophysicus, with which I was charged, was also to be transferred from Milan to Pavia. As the foundation of the plan to be newly devised, the hitherto valid medical constitution of the country was given to me with an intimation as to what should be retained. Although such caution may have been necessary, since each country has its own peculiarities, with which I, a stranger, might have been less familiar, nevertheless, I felt in this work like a builder who is ordered to retain several pillars and wings of an old building and to construct a new one; in consequence, he must often subordinate his plan of the building to the plan of his predecessors.

Soon afterwards, I was also put in charge of the department for medical subjects at the Milan Royal Government (Gubernium), and thus had the supreme supervision of all hospitals in Austrian Lombardy.

With matters thus arranged, and since I was needed in all important cases concerning public health, I had plenty of opportunity to test with the touchstone of experience, both what I had so far thought and written about Medical Police, and, more especially, what I still had to lecture concerning Medical Police proper. After ten years of work of this kind, I was unexpectedly called to Vienna to take part in the proceedings of the Military Sanitary Commission which had been established by the Court in 1795. After this work, which dealt predominantly with health matters of the poor, I was appointed director of the general hospital in Vienna, and public teacher of practicing medicine. In addition to many tasks concerning these institutions, I was charged with numerous other tasks as well. Among these, the most important were those concerning the new system of studies to be arranged, shortly, plague institutions for the Austrian states, as well as some concerning the most important epidemics. Thus, after I had spent my best medical years from the age of forty to sixty in Austrian service amid the greatest activity, fate propelled me to the cold north, after having previously thrown me from west to south. There, too, both in Lithuania and soon afterward in St. Petersburg, I was needed for important work, especially in connection with institutes of learning. But here my previously strong physical constitution was badly shaken, and I saw that at last the time had arrived to do also something for myself, and to use whatever strength I would be able to regain under a gentler sky for ordering and completing my writings which hitherto have been received with so much indulgence by the public.

However, I did not want to write my biography here, though for young physicians it may not be without importance; I only give a very brief excerpt so that my readers may have a foretaste of the treatises contained in the present work, so that, however imperfect they find it, they may kindly attribute it to the excessive amount of my previous professional duties.

Only rarely has one and the same physician, like myself, had an opportunity to work on a large scale for public health and well-being among so many different nations. Whatever I did not achieve, my conscience tells me, was due not to lack of goodwill, but time and narrow limits of the strength of a private person.

Freyburg im Breissgau, 19 March 1811.

SUPPLEMENTARY VOLUMES TO MEDICAL POLICE, OR A COLLECTION OF VARIOUS SPECIAL TREATISES CONCERNING THIS SCIENCE

Volume Two

PREFACE

The present writings were already announced by the late author in the preface of his fifth volume of Medical Police and in the preface of the first supplementary volume; therefore, there is little I can add, and thus I let it now be published.

The material was sent at the beginning of 1823 from Vilna to Leipzig by the worthy son of the author, State Councillor, etc., Joseph Frank, to one of his old friends because he himself was prevented by other work from devoting as much time and attention to it as it absolutely required; the work was accompanied by the wish that the friend should look after the orphaned child.

There is no doubt that in Frank's crucible his grains of gold would have assumed a more compact form, and though it is my pleasure that the papers in question were turned over to me at the end of 1824 with the full consent of the owner, I regret that this famous scholar of our academy could not undertake the work.

I consider it an extraordinary honor to pay homage to the shade of a great man to whose classical works my scientific training owes so much, and to finish that valuable work which he carefully tended as if it were a loved child. While I perceive and recognize this with the strongest feelings of my soul, I expended every effort to develop my best forces for this work.—Convinced that only by premature spiritual conceptions, just as by bodily ones, are abortions and premature births produced, without value, or only weaklings which are prey to decomposition soon after birth, I spent much of my time devoted to the sciences to prepare the way bestowing much care and concentration on my favorite subject, namely state medicine, when a scientific journey took me abroad; I lectured until 1819 on this subject at the university here, and now that the fruits of my endeavor will soon enter reality, I flatter myself that I was unprepared for approaching the present task.

I had complete freedom in deciding what materials to use and how to use them. State Councillor Frank stipulated only two conditions, which are certainly most reasonable:

1) not to bring in anything that could be disagreeable to some government; and
2) not to compromise anybody in any way.

I believe that I most conscientiously met both conditions, but I could not avoid mentioning several honorable names in various connections. If, entirely against my expectation, this should cause the slightest embarrassment, I apologize and declare in advance that it was neither my intention nor my will to hurt a person's feelings or to aggrieve anybody.

In editing the material belonging here, I took as example the first supplementary volume, which contains similar works and of which the present volume is the direct continuation, and I remained faithful to the chronological order. The experts' opinions were fairly completely available in the Brouillon; they only required thorough revision, and now and again some slight polishing. The documents, which I listed accurately in the index, were appended in copy, or in more comprehensive excerpts than was required for our purpose. In using them, I had in mind the double purpose of reporting as much of them as was necessary for a better insight and for a better appreciation of the experts' opinions based on them, and not overlooking what should be equally important and interesting for history.

The learned public will not object to my having included several short treatises since the system of Medical Police was not devised for one country but for the whole world; the public will receive them with approval all the more so since, according to the pronouncement of several critical public journals, nothing that is not important can come from Frank, who gained much fame teaching at five famous medical schools three of which he organized and laid the foundations of their subsequent lustre.

Fortunately this great man lived at a time and in a state where an enlightened government, striving for the good, combined its goodwill with energy and, giving Frank an opportunity to implement his great ideas, the government itself became a bright star on the horizon of medical science by improving the medical schools.— It was equally fortunate for this wise government to have among its great men someone like Frank, who, as regards such a highly important subject so closely concerned with the well-being of mankind, could and did prove most useful with his mature experience and his precise intentions. He was called from Italy to Vienna to take part in the deliberations of the Court Commission for Military Medicine and Revision of Studies, appointed in 1795 by the Royal Court to improve schooling. This gave rise to the origin of part of these masterworks, from which it is clear not only how much the classical judgment of the author was valued, but also how some states derived great profit; thus, even now these works appear at a suitable time.

There is no doubt that state medicine in Germany is a part of the culture; I know from my own experience that even foreign nations recognize this. But Medical Police (Medicinische Polizey) is handled so badly in some German states that one finds everywhere diseases and shortcomings which seem to belong to the cruel Middle Ages. The frequent complaints which we hear from various places concerning the locust-like armies of bad physicians and the bad position of the better physicians in the state, make us presume that in certain countries things are once more almost as bad as in the first period of human society, when anybody who wished to treat sick persons was permitted to do so. The only difference is that at that time the consequences of such nonsense were soon noticed and prevented, whereas now one is deaf to it with healthy ears and blind with seeing eyes. When will it be admitted (and what else can one do?) that there is no class in the world of which the state requires as much as it does of the physicians? And that, therefore, there is no class in the world which would be more justified in claiming the state's gratitude than the medical class. It cannot be denied that sometimes the point of view from which the true medical practitioner should be regarded has become quite disturbed.

This is not the place to reveal more of these truths, and there have been men (Michaelis, Gilibert, Meiners, Stoll, etc.) who have recognized the causes of the cancerous growths in some state administrations and have recommended true remedies against them. These consist in the vigorous application of a purposeful Medical Police, and in the reform of old universities that are corroded by centuries of rust. It was Frank, with his typical love of humanity, who touched upon a subject that concerns so closely all mankind, and here (I, II, III) he alludes to it again.

Whatever remains for me to mention in regard to the other treatises has already been done in the few added notes; I wish only to point out VI, the treatise concerning a widespread disease, venereal disease, which contains much of value also for practical medicine.

I could have greatly augmented the references to the system of Medical Police (Medicinische Polizey), and perhaps I should have done so, but since I shall append to the last volume a subject index for the entire work, such references here become dispensable.

Now I have only to add what must not be missing in such a comprehensive and complete work and for which the material is in my hands. These are: hospital system, arrangements against plague, against yellow fever, against smallpox and other diseases, which I intend to publish at the end of this year.

Leipzig, Easter Mass 1825.

Voigt.

INTRODUCTION

It is of the utmost importance that in elaborating on subjects which have such a direct effect on the fate of many millions of persons to first state the right point of view from which the whole can be easily surveyed, even by those who, not being physicians themselves, have to conduct the medical and health system according to fixed principles that are in harmony with the accepted system of government. This work could well have prefaced the remarks by the undersigned concerning the new curriculum, but even though the highest state authority is still engaged in considering the proposed draft for the future institutions of learning, such considerations are not now belated, and they are perhaps in their right place when the teaching of obstetrics and army medicine is under discussion.

What is medicine, what is the physician to human society?... This is a question which must seem of the greatest importance to a state administration acting according to certain principles before it deals with costly institutions for medical study, physicians, and a health system. It would imply a certain partiality for a physician to undertake answering this question, if that very physician had not made public his creed more than sixteen years ago and thus prevented the suspicion that he is more concerned with his guild than with mankind.

Medicine is that part of science which deals with investigating the natural laws governing living beings, chiefly man and his domestic animals. It examines the origins of both healthy and sick functions and of death, and according to these causes, it teaches how health can be preserved longest, sickness prevented, or where this is no longer possible, how it can be recognized in time, distinguished from other sicknesses, correctly diagnosed, cured, or at least mitigated, and thus delay death as long as possible.

The scientist who knows only the fundamentals of this science is a theoretician, but if he is also able to apply them skillfully, he is a practical physician.

The exploration of the origin, development, nature, varied functions and relationships of living beings, chiefly of man, is infinitely vast, comprehensive, and difficult.

Innumerable are the causes which put into motion the animal mechanism which obey laws that are quite different from merely mechanical laws, and which, depending on the moderate, too weak, or violent effect, make it traverse the path of either well-being, sickness or death.

The goal, all the wishes of individual persons, and of nations is the determination of the rules, based on reason and experience, according to which the creation and multiplication of a strong posterity is ensured, the present state of health maintained, lost health replaced by a procedure almost approaching creation, and death and decay relegated to the outermost boundaries of an attainable age.

This is what medicine means to the state, regardless of how much it has lagged behind in its growth, even over thousands of years. This is so because the beneficial plant often lacked the tending hand of state administration, because dark and barbarous centuries throttled its blossoming, as they did with that of all sciences, and because for so long spurious philosophy and idle passion for disputation and hypotheses inhibited all useful attempts and a calm course based on experience.

Of course, the law of mortality, which has been imposed on every living thing and which directly follows from the structure and nature of living matter, will never enable medicine to satisfy man's unbounded wishes. We are often subject to causes of death which cannot be eliminated by mortal hands. Although medicine has always a broad field of usefulness, as a daughter of natural science, it lacks the heritage of mathematical certainty. It nevertheless has, in common with most of the most useful arts and sciences, a very justified claim to the esteem and energetic support of the state.

Medical science does not recognize narrower borders than those imposed by nature. The application of its principles proceeds with slower and less assured steps, however, because of the darkness which often hides the causes of diseases. For all that, it is not rare for medicine to make the finest discoveries predicted by theory long ago, but without much hope of their use; thereby, and also in consequence of pure chance, it broadens from year to year its sphere of activity. Thus each truth found in the realm of this science is an important contribution to lessening human misery, and no matter how insignificant the discovery sometimes seems to be, it may develop into a means of saving suffering mankind, just as the magnetic needle, which was initially considered a toy, became the surest guiding star of ships on all, and even unknown, dangerous seas.

From this point of view the state must regard the broadening of teaching of theoretical medicine, although it is costly! Of course, it was said long ago that the most learned theoretician often achieves least at the sickbed. For more than one reason this statement was based on truth. For as soon as medicine left the path of experience, the path proposed by Hippocrates as the only one, idle hypotheses were heaped one upon the other, and mere fads and abuses of human reason were thought to be the best theory of this science. Not until two thousand years later did Baco Verulamius point out (what the saddest results had long since taught mankind) how senseless this procedure was; finally the long-abandoned road of truth was resumed again by

Sydenham. The hypothesis mania fought on to retain its long reign in the field of medicine, but just as physics and natural science had in the meantime emerged from the mire of the dark centuries, medicine also saw the beneficial light. Now ashamed, it cast off in indignation the dirty garment, and recognizing its own bareness and want, it finally became simply adorned by pure truth.

From then on (of course, still by only a small number of men who had been born for science) only confident consequences from facts were considered genuine theory of medicine; and no matter how slowly work of this kind progresses, we already see the fruits of a more prudent use. Experience at the sickbed no longer is contradicted by theories twisted out of their original meaning. But even assuming that somebody knows only the theory of medicine and is therefore not suited for curing the sick, this means no more and no less than that in this art, as in everything else, only practice imparts the required skill.

As regards the practical part of medicine, however, that is of the greatest importance, on which the watching eye of the state should chiefly be fixed. At universities the principles of practical medicine must be taught at the sickbed, but it cannot be expected that many students remain there long enough nor within so short a time acquire such skill in curing that they learn this most difficult, and easily the most dangerous, of all arts so perfectly as public security requires. Although the principles of all this science are the same for all classes of human society, nevertheless, the class of warriors, as well as the peasantry, has its peculiarities with which the physician must be acquainted in practice if he is to treat them appropriately. Without the greatest simplicity and the strictest economy, the remedies which the state has to expend on the sick defenders of the country—and which the peasant has to himself expend for his own support—do not suffice to fulfill this just expectation. Both these classes require the physician and the surgeon in one person, and in such numbers which correspond to the varied distribution and mobility of soldiers, and the settlement of the rural population in so many, often remote, villages and farms. The army physician and the country physician must acquaint himself in advance with the way of life of his future patients, as well as with the causes which give rise to most diseases in the field and in the country. The field [army] physician must also be acquainted with military discipline and the necessary subordination; all this, he can learn only among those for whom he is destined, only through instruction of experienced men in garrison and field hospitals, only in hospitals founded for the poorer class, and only by his own work and fulfillment of all the duties expected of him.

Therefore (although five or six universities are probably sufficient for teaching medicine and surgical science in the entire Empire), in addition to these universities, in all somewhat important garrison, field and civilian hospitals of the various provinces, clinical provisions must be made, or practical medical and surgical schools must be established. In any event, only the most experienced men such as staff and regimental physicians and civilian physicians in large hospitals must be appointed teachers.

Only by such appointments and by better organization of the medical system, can the state train such men as it needs for the correct treatment of the sick. In view of the present state in some countries, it would perhaps be better on the whole to follow the example of the Romans and forgo all medical attention rather than permit anybody who is intent on enriching himself by practicing medicine, or at least to earn his living by it, to rush in to treat the health of the gullible populace, and, without getting into conflict with the law, play with the citizens' lives after a few lazy years spent at a university, and then passing there an equally lethargic examination, without acquiring any experience or any skill in curing. Of course, thousands have to thank the hand of their experienced and diligent physician for their lives; and such a savior in adversity is for suffering mankind a jewel of inestimable value! But how small everywhere is the ratio of true physicians to those who only mock the name of this rank! And how enormous in every community is the number of those killed to the number of those saved!

If, then, the state wants to obtain from medical science all the advantages that it can yield, it must use the physician not only for curing but also for preventing the diseases which threaten the great mass. Among the causes of these diseases are many which neither the physician alone nor the individual citizen can prevent or cure; only a Medical Police, provided with the proper power and authority can implement the rescue plan which medicine has drawn up. As late as in the last century the so-called Stuttgart fever was known to all physicians because of its deadliness. Few of those who contracted it were saved, and almost every year many persons were killed off by this native foe. Finally it was done what the physicians could only propose but were unable to implement: through the authorities' direction, the swamps near the town were drained by ditches and were turned into meadows rich in flowers. For a long time physicians more or less cured persons suffering from natural smallpox; nevertheless, this disease robbed society annually of innumerable of its most promising members. Finally inoculation for smallpox became known to Europe also, and was recommended by the physicians, but what use would have been this remedy to the prejudiced nation without the example and active support of the powerful state? From time immemorial the plague has been the most terrible calamity of mankind, and it was rare that medicine saved a victim marked for its rage. However, this science did not confine itself, as its name suggests, to curing alone; it investigated the sources of the impotence of the so-called medicines; it discovered that the plague poison, which suddenly chokes off the vital energy, was of foreign and not European origin, that it was not produced by native seed, not dissolved by air over large stretches, but that it was necessarily conveyed from elsewhere, mostly from the Orient by direct contact of someone infected there, both living and lifeless tinder, more suitable for catching this poison, and was so-to-speak transmitted from hand to hand. It is now up to the care and action of state administration to put a stop to the plague epidemic that comes from afar and is immediately recognized by physicians. All infectious human diseases and cattle pests could be suppressed with equal certainty, immediately upon their first outbreak and before they have spread. Thus the beneficent mother of medicine, physics, conducts the lightning, which smashes everything and the quick killing effect of which its weaker daughter cannot prevent, by means of a thin wire away from our heads. This daughter alone would be able to save mankind from innumerable accidents, if one would demand not only medicines from the curing physician but also more preventive advice from the science, and follow it without jealousy, without misplaced economy, and with the required dispatch.

However, the state administration should be able to arrive without loss of time at a knowledgeable judgment in all matters concerning public health; this, as has already been mentioned elsewhere, requires a medical board in all provinces as well as in towns where the country authorities have their seats, and as a supreme board in the capital of the Empire. The supreme group should be composed partly of theoretical and partly of practical physicians with the addition of some businessmen; this would direct the entire health system in the name of the supreme authority of the country. These boards would investigate most thoroughly all subjects concerning the health and well-being of the countries, and they would submit their findings therewith to the supreme state administration for review and appropriate direction. They would ensure the punctilious fulfillment of the duties of individual physicians, such duties stipulated in accurately drafted regulations, so that doubts, contradictions and shortcomings in certificates and attestations by individual physicians concerning physical occurrences would be eliminated or corrected, as would also injuries due to violence, and other subjects concerning Forensic Medicine and Medical Police and thus administer the entire public health system according to unified principles and to the certain benefit of mankind.

As for medical study in the Emperor's hereditary countries, this is too closely connected with the other subjects taught for it to be transferred without regard to this relation to the Supreme Medical Board (Medicinisches Oberkollegium) which is already charged with so many important tasks of a quite different nature. If, therefore, a separate permanent court commission were appointed to be in charge of all teaching subjects, a still active and confident physician could be appointed as member of the above commission or as principal of medical studies. Such physician would need be well versed in all parts of medicine and no less so in the teaching subject by his own practice and experience. He would be charged with the supervision of the most punctilious fulfillment of their duties by teachers and students, with proposing suitable subjects for newly endowed or vacant professorial chairs, and everything that concerns the perfection of medical science.

After this brief outline of the true viewpoint from which can best be viewed and judged all expected drafts by this court commission for the revision of studies concerning the improvement of medical studies and the health system altogether, the undersigned turns to the questions which were submitted for consideration by the aforementioned court commission.

* * *

In the following assessments, Frank deals with the very special questions concerning the organization of the Vienna Medical Faculty and of the Joseph Academy, as well as with problems of more general interest such as establishing registries for marriages, births, and deaths, and the control of syphilis. As examples of such assessments, we chose those dealing with the organization and work of a supreme health authority of 1799, and the prevention of suicide in 1802.

Supreme Medical Board
(Medicinisches Oberkollegium)

Now, as regards the medical boards about the necessity of which much has already been said, their establishment should consist of the following:

A Supreme Medical Board, to be established in Vienna, would check all existing regulations concerning the medical profession, draft instructions for physicians, surgeons, apothecaries, and midwives, and supervise all medical colleges in the provinces, and consequently the entire medical and health system in all the emperor's patrimonial dominions, except teaching institutions. This Supreme Medical Board would consist of:

1) a director who would be a voting member of the supreme authority of the country;

2) the following members of a medical teaching staff: two professors of medical and surgical practice; a professor of pharmaceutical chemistry; a professor of forensic medicine and Medical Police;

3) two of the most distinguished physicians, one of the best surgeons, and one apothecary well versed in his profession from the capital;

4) several professional men who would be invited when their presence would seem necessary, and they would be questioned about subjects having a bearing on their sphere of activity; these would be, e.g., a member of the criminal court, the police, the welfare commission, etc.

This Supreme Medical Board (Collegium Medicum) would sit on certain days once or several times weekly, depending on the requirements and amount of the business in hand, and would issue all its decrees and decisions under the jurisdiction of the highest authority of the country.

At the place where the country's authority has its seat, each province would have to have a medical board which (with the exception of the teaching institutions subordinated to the administrator of studies) would have to deal with all subjects concerning the medical profession and health system in the entire province. This board would consist of:

1) a director, namely the chief medical officer of the province, who would be a voting member in medical matters and reporting physician to the supreme authority of the country;

2) the district medical officer;

3) in towns with a university, two of the public teachers of medical and surgical practice, the professors of pharmaceutical chemistry, of forensic medicine and the Medical Police;

4) one of the most distinguished physicians, one of the most skillful surgeons, and a skillful apothecary from the town;

5) several professional men connected with some profession as other as in the supreme college.

In Vienna, where the professors of medical and surgical practice, pharmaceutical chemistry, and forensic medicine are already employed in the Supreme Medical Board (Collegium Medicum), the town physician and the Magister Sanitatis would be at the director's disposal in their place, but in towns where there is neither a university nor these medical authorities, some of the most learned and at the same time most experienced physicians and surgeons would serve in this capacity.

The duty of these medical boards would be to make an accurate list of all persons in the province belonging to the medical profession and authorized to practice medicine or parts thereof. The lists would contain: name and surname, country of origin, age, professional career, residence, employment, salary, transfer, death. At the end of every military year, a list would be sent to the Supreme Medical Board. Young physicians and surgeons who had received their doctor or magister diploma from their universities and after that had diligently observed patients for another year in large civil or military hospitals under the supervision of a publicly employed physician or surgeon and who had, in addition to that, a certificate from the teacher of the clinic appraising their assessment and treatment of three patients who had been publicly entrusted to them at the practical medical school, and who wished to obtain permission to practice their art alone, would need: to appear before the supreme authority or the Collegium Medicum in the capital, where the Supreme Medical Board is, and in the provinces, where there is a university for the last or practical examination and to submit the stipulated number of case histories. If found suitable by the proper authority they would receive the Diploma pro libera praxi and would be entered into the list of physicians and surgeons authorized to practice their art. In the provinces which do not have any universities, and in the capital, where the Supreme Medical Board has its seat, the medical boards should not conduct practical examinations of physicians and surgeons because public professors of the profession do not sit on them. With the exception of lower surgeons, they [the medical boards] should confine themselves to have submitted to them the stipulated diplomas obtained from the Supreme Board or from the medical boards on which public professors sit.

Furthermore, to touch upon some of the subjects concerning the official duties of the medical boards, they would have to see to it that the required number of district physicians, surgeons, accoucheurs, apothecaries, and midwives would be gradually employed in their provinces; that they fulfill their duties most punctiliously; and that the poorer class, as far as circumstances permit, does not lack either gratuitous and kind assistance by skilled physicians and surgeons or the necessary remedies; that no physician, surgeon, apothecary, or midwife who has not passed the stipulated examinations and cannot produce the prescribed diploma settle anywhere; that the apothecaries both in towns and in the country are examined most strictly at random times at least once every two years by the director, the pharmaceutical, and another member of the board; that the regulation for apothecaries, to be drafted by the Supreme Board, is painstakingly obeyed, that the present pharmacopoeia or one yet to be stipulated is strictly obeyed, that the public is most conscientiously served day and night as regards preparation and variation of medicines; that nobody, no matter who he be, sell secret remedies; that an accurate topographical description be supplied of all districts to which a district physician has been appointed, as well as of individual towns and places where there are physicians, the description containing the state of health of the inhabitants, the existing hospitals, baths and mineral waters, swamps and stagnant waters; that a watchful eye be kept on infectious diseases of human beings and cattle, appearing abroad or at the frontiers, and the necessary measures taken; that the endemics and epidemics occuring from time to time among human beings and domestic animals, as well as extraordinary and little known or unknown diseases, are described in detail, the remedy applied and its success or lack of success recorded, and an accurate copy of these important remarks sent to the Supreme Medical Board; that in such epidemics the required measures for their suppression or alleviation are immediately taken, as well as for the recovery of the victims and the future prevention of similar ills; that in each town or village and in each district and in the entire province as a whole, yearly lists of births and deaths are made and the causes of excessive mortality be carefully examined, especially that of pregnant women, women giving birth, women in childbed, and children; that descriptions are given of important and extraordinary natural phenomena, such as monstrous births of human beings and animals, of strange discoveries in corpses, that all these, which are important for medicine are not only immediately reported but as far as possible, monsters and rare pathological objects found in bodies, together with a description of the lethal disease, are sent and transferred to the museum of the state medical school, the unavoidable expenses being reimbursed; that habits, prejudices, and superstitions that are detrimental to the health of people and domestic animals are sought out and controlled with the greatest possible prudence; that medicines and cures, widespread among the people and sometimes extremely effective and confirmed by long experience, are accurately determined, and the application of domestic and often effective medicines are given as much preference as possible before foreign ones; that the vaccines, which saved so many people for the state, are actively promoted, and that the good cause not be harmed by careless and inexpert vaccinations;

that foodstuffs brought for sale are examined according to the principles of Medical Police, that deleterious and suspicious ones are immediately removed; that beer, wine and other spirits be examined whether they are spoilt or mixed with harmful ingredients; that public houses and cellars, and even fountains be examined often and unexpectedly for the content and healthy condition of the water, these examinations being carried out from time to time, but especially after important natural phenomena, e.g., after earthquakes, after continuous and widespread rain, upon extraordinary drought and drying up of the rivers; that newly built, still wet, and unhealthy apartments are not prematurely rented and occupied; that ramshackle buildings the collapse of which is imminent be restored or demolished without loss of time, with proper care of the passersby, and that bridges and paths be kept in good condition; that people do not ride or drive fast in the streets, that drivers do not leave their horses and oxen in the streets unattended, and that they are strictly punished in case they do; that pits and precipices, if they endanger the passersby, are properly protected; that dangerous and virulent animals, as well as ownerless and freely roaming dogs are killed; that the regulations pertaining to the sale of poisons are strictly adhered to, and that poisonous plants noxious for human beings or their domestic animals are destroyed as far as possible, or that the people are at least acquainted by accurate descriptions with their deleterious effects; that nobody is buried or dissected before the time stipulated by law, and especially before his death is absolutely certain; and that, on the other hand, corpses that are beginning to rot or spread infection are no longer left unburied or are publicly exhibited; that people and domestic animals who were bitten by rabid dogs, cats, etc., or by such animals suspected of rabies, as well as accident victims and the apparently dead, receive everywhere the quickest and most adequate help; that public cleanliness in general, but especially that of places of assembly, theaters, churches, schools, jails, penitentiaries, workhouses, and hospitals be promoted with the greatest care, etc.

Expert's Opinion On Suicide

In the broadest sense, the number of suicides in every state is far too great for such a law to apply to all of them. The great masses shorten their lives more or less by debauchery, excesses, intemperate passions, by daredevilry, etc., and perhaps this kind of suicide is the most unpardonable of all, although it is not given this name because it is based less on a physical or moral impulse than on lust or rashness. Only the intentional suicide, or at least the intention of committing it, is subject to legal measures, and if it were possible to always judge correctly the mainspring of this intentional endeavor or procedure, our measures against such an undertaking, or the punishments stipulated for it, would not have to fear well-founded objections.

Yet, in which case is the endeavor to commit suicide, or the actual self-destruction, the inevitable result of derangement in the organs of the inner senses? On the other hand, in which case is this action the consequence of a free, i.e., punishable, way of thinking? These are questions which are neither answered well enough by physicians on the basis of autopsies performed by them, nor are they confidently resolved on the basis of the previous mode of life of the dead (except those cases who became their own executioners in order to avoid infamous corporal punishment, obviously due to their crimes), because madness sometimes sets in suddenly or because sometimes only one string of the mental instrument is too highly strung and the dissonance is not heard until this string is touched.

These important questions can rarely be decided by reasons satisfying a fair judge, yet the undersigned is of the opinion that the penal law against suicide would affect the innocent more often than one would think, on the man who acts merely according to the hidden precepts of a slowly or suddenly deranged phantasy, i.e., the demented person. But how can it affect him, who has already inflicted on himself the greatest punishment which can ever be meted out for a crime! Yet according to our ingrained notions, the punishment for suicide affects the relatives of the suicide more than him, for the law cannot catch up with him anymore. And because of a [suicide's] relations to distinguished families, the legislator may be induced to make exceptions, so that the entire weight of the law will be borne only by the lower classes.

If it could be said that the penalties for suicide would deter the living from imitating this act, there would perhaps be some cause for the full success of the law of the

Milesians: that the large numbers of probably hysterical girls who hanged themselves should be buried nude and with the rope around their necks.* Yet of what importance is to most people for whom life is worthless, the judgment of those who are left behind? And is it to be approved that the insensitive remains of a person who ended in suicide, probably out of insanity, and his tearful family should be the object of public derision, so as to deter the living by punishing a corpse, even more than suicide itself can do?

As regards those who were on the way to suicide but (out of remorse or because of an unforeseen feeling of pain in such a mode of death) desisted on their own from their terrible intention without outside aid, experience has shown that they rarely confine themselves to one such unsuccessful attempt. Such a person usually repeats his attempt at the next occasion when he is somewhat agitated, and it is rare that he then fails to reach his ultimate aim. The reason here, too, may be some kind of periodic, spontaneous weariness of life the first incidence of which was interrupted by the terror of the unsuccessful act, but a future, somewhat more violent attack, may lead to a repeated, more fierce, and successful suicide. If, after the self-inflicted injury has healed, a weak-minded person may expect a summons to court, it may only be cause for him to repeat his first attempt quickly.

In consequence of all these considerations it is therefore the considered opinion of the undersigned:

a) that all measures taken by the police against suicidal mania should be confined exclusively to the careful elimination of the cases** which often underly these acts;

b) that all other penal laws, except those ordering a close confinement of a suspect or convicted suicide, to last until the person is fully reconciled with life, either in a hospital or in some other suitable place, could easily miss their purpose;

c) that if somebody has committed suicide (for whom there is at least the suspicion of previous insanity, and because with death all dependence on the laws ends), nothing is to be enacted that could attach a blemish, albeit based on prejudice, to the deceased's family.

---

* Aulus Gellius, "Noctes Atticae," L.XV, c. 10.—Plutarch, "De vita mulierum."
** "System of Medical Police," loc. cit.

SUPPLEMENTARY VOLUMES TO MEDICAL POLICE, OR A COLLECTION OF VARIOUS SPECIAL TREATISES CONCERNING THIS SCIENCE

Third and Last Volume

PREFACE

While I herewith hand over to the friends of Medical Police the last part of the literary legacy of the great Frank, I must at the same time apologize for having fulfilled this pleasant duty somewhat later than promised. Whosoever has prepared a similar indexing work will have no doubt that I suffered more delay than I could have foreseen, even after the material had been excerpted from the original. Yet I admit to myself that I worked very diligently and I flatter myself that I thereby fulfilled the requirement.

Frank's system of Medical Police is a veritable mine which is far from being fully utilized, as it should be. Perhaps the reason is also partly due to the fact that this great treasure of work, which will remain the first for many decades, has a poor and excessively modest index, and therefore that those whose conditions do not permit them to spend much time with a multi-volume work and to study it constantly, come up against many difficulties when searching for individual subjects. Therefore, I undertook to make a complete index, and I should not like to abandon the hope that I was thereby useful and made the work easier to use.

The first treatise of this volume was intended for the article "On Hospitals and Infirmaries in Communities" which is often mentioned in the great work. In addition to some details, the material found consisted of two drafts written in French: "Mémoire sur les établissements destinés pour le traitement des pauvres malades" and "Mémoire sur les hôpitaux," and complete service instructions for the personnel of a public hospital. The author drafted the latter for the General Hospital in Vienna, which also explains why these instructions are so similar to the instructions published in the 5th and 6th volumes of the Yearbook of the Imperial and Royal Austrian State.

The other treatise was destined for the article "Measures against Epidemics and Contagious Diseases among People," which is also touched upon several times in the great work; but it pertains to only four kinds of epidemics: plague, smallpox, yellow fever, and cholera.

Both works are unfinished. Our unforgettable friend titles them with one work, written shortly before the end of his sojourn on earth, as can be seen from the freshness of his pen's strokes: "Beginning" etc., and, as mentioned before, he wanted to execute them according to a grand design. I am far from being sufficiently vain so as not to regret with pain that the Lord was not pleased to leave us the great and magnificent friend long enough for him to place the highest seal also on this unfinished work. Nevertheless, I cannot but regard it as more than a beginning, a preliminary work, and if most of the experts and scholars should be of a different opinion and not receive this gift in as friendly a spirit as the one in which it is offered, I should truly be mistaken!

Voigt.

I

PROJECT OF EQUIPPING HOSPITALS*

> If a soldier may design fortresses which cost millions
> in order to protect countries; why should not a physi-
> cian be permitted to propose a hospital in order to
> save people from devastating diseases?
>
> J. P. X. Fauken**

INTRODUCTION

§1

No state in the world, no state administration, however prudent, can prevent the
existence of a large class of persons whose circumstances are less fortunate than
their requirements. However, as long as age, straight limbs, health, and not too
numerous a family of this poor class permit, and as long as there is sufficient opportunity for them to earn their living by manual work, they do not feel the harshness
of fate as much as persons who live in plenty and have been educated softly and are
then deprived of some comfort or other, and must suddenly do without their habitual
luxury.

§2

Then poverty begins to make its terror felt, either when the number of children
of a married couple becomes so considerable that their earnings no longer suffice
to support the family, or if there is a lack of opportunities for parents and children
to obtain remunerative work, or when the prices of food and other necessities of
life rise so high that they are out of all proportion to the ordinary earnings, or when
the diligent father, the industrious mother of the house, or even both at the same

---

* A well equipped hospital has a threefold purpose: curing poor, sick people; perfecting medical science;
and educating good practitioners; therefore, the present treatise does not deal with clinical institutes
since the author in his "Project of Equipping a Clinical School" (written in Italian and translated by
Titius in 1794) and in Volume VI of Medical Police spoke of it in detail in several places, mainly in
Section II, pp. 217–307, and 341 ff.

** "Scheme of a general hospital," p. 34. Vienna, 1784.

time are taken away by death from their still uneducated children, or when, either because of great youth or because of old age, the strength required for work is lacking, or when illness, infirmity, or organic defects paralyze the father's strong arms, and the now sparse source of livelihood dries up while at the same time all possibility of essential care and of restoring the lacking health by suitable food and medicines suddenly disappears.*

§3

Under such circumstances, it is the duty of the country's authorities to care for the maintenance of the useful members of society, and that of the state's revenue, and the classes of the rich and of the workers contribute from their savings and surplus to the support of their helpless subjects, fellow-citizens and relatives.

§4

As the number of people who are unable to provide for themselves in each community may so greatly increase under certain circumstances that the working class is hardly able to provide for them properly, the laws must make sure that mere idlers do not don the mask of real distress, and that the lazy wasp does not shamelessly rob the diligent bee of the laboriously collected honey that is required for its own livelihood.

§5

Meanwhile, if the state busies itself with such an important and noble task as the support of really needy persons, this must be done according to certain steps and a certain order, so that each needy person is assigned his own place, and after he has stated his most pressing needs, aid is provided. There are poor persons who are unable to do any kind of work; others can and must earn at least part of their own support through an occupation which is suitable to their strength and other abilities.

Both categories contain those who either, because of great youth or old age, or feebleness or deformity, are not able to provide for themselves sufficiently, or not without exciting general loathing among the healthy; and for these there are the foundlings', orphans', work- and poor-relief homes, or merely relief funds from which certain sums are granted.

But the first category includes mostly the really sick persons who, depending on the kind of illness and other conditions, have to be provided for either in their own homes and in the bosom of their families, which tenderly care for them, or in public hospitals, either completely or partially at the expense of the working multitude.

§6

Sick persons who live with their relatives, and have the needed care, such as children with their parents, or parents living with their adult children, unless they suffer

* "System of Medical Police," Vol. I, p. 17. Footnote.

from an infectious or terrifying disease involving raving and madness, and unless not too many suffer simultaneously from the disease, are best cared for at home. For this purpose, they are visited by salaried district or town physicians and surgeons, and through charitable contributions, they are supplied with the required medicines and suitable foodstuffs free of charge. It is impossible for hired attendants in hospitals to make up for the natural tenderness of the closest relatives, and the hospital air and constantly lurking danger of infection in large hospitals make it riskier for the patients to be received there than does the lack of a certain, often only ostensible, cleanliness and mechanical punctuality in the indifferent attendance upon suffering humanity that have been introduced in hospitals. The mortality in private homes in general cannot be compared with the mortality in hospitals, especially large ones. There were, therefore, distinguished physicians and philanthropists who doubted the usefulness to human society of all hospitals without exception, and who maintained that it is better to let the poor live without exception outside hospitals and be looked after in their own miserable dwellings.

It is certain that a tender mother will not easily leave her infant, nor a poor widow her as yet uneducated children, without great harm to them and to her household; on the other hand, in spite of their grief they can still care for their dependent families to a certain extent, and provide at least the most elementary necessities. One pound of meat, which is given daily to such a poor sick woman at the poorhouse's expense so that the weak woman may have broth made from it even if she cannot otherwise make use of the meat than by drinking the broth, may also serve as the indispensable sustenance for several of her hungry children. The mere separation of the children (who cannot be treated in a hospital, while at a tender age, anyway) from their parents, or of the parents from the children, is the cause of some aggravations in persons who have been taken to a hospital and have to be treated there among many unknown sick persons who may be noisy or repellent. As soon as sick persons in the bosom of their families have somewhat recovered, they never lack useful activity, which is commensurate with their strength and at the same time of advantage to the household; whereas in hospitals, convalescents lie idle in oppressive boredom, and they have to be maintained completely at public expense for longer than necessary, and sometimes even at that stage they are attacked by a contagious disease and succumb to it, etc.

However, there are certainly many cases also which, especially in populous towns, must not be treated except at a well equipped hospital. Contagious diseases quickly spread to entire families who live in excessively crowded conditions. Cases which cause an intense stench become insufferable to all those present in a confined dwelling, and are also deleterious to health. Melancholic, raging, mad patients cannot be entrusted to the uncertain care of inexperienced or careless persons without danger to themselves, their relatives and the general public. Evils which appear in society by fearful change or ills which by their hideous aspect make a most adverse impression on very sensitive persons or on pregnant mothers, cannot be permitted to stay in the center of human society.—When several persons fall ill simultaneously in a hut, the necessary treatment is usually lacking, and the healthy must lie with the sick. Then there is a large number of persons who have no dwelling of their own and no close relatives, and who consequently do not receive any attention; for such persons hospitals are quite indispensable.

It should also be borne in mind that well equipped hospitals in large cities are the best school for training skilled physicians and surgeons,* because the most wide-spread diseases and other cases are seen there in large numbers and in the most varied modifications, and therefore, the young physician and surgeon has the excellent and valuable opportunity of observing, under the supervision of experienced men, what he would hardly see in the course of many years of private practice, and what he often would have treated at the expense of mankind because of lack of his own experience. Another reason is that well appointed hospitals offer the best opportunity of perfecting the art and expanding the science, for pure observations are not distorted by disobedient patients or by secretly taken food and medicines; here each new drug is tested and its worth is reliably assessed, and the causes of obscure and mysterious fatal illnesses can be sought in the bodies without hindrance, etc.

§7

It is important, therefore, to decide accurately which poor sick are to be accepted free of charge in hospitals, and which have to be kept in their own dwellings either completely or partly at the expense of the community. If this accurate distinction is not made, or if the prescribed order is not adhered to in this respect, the hospitals, especially if they are known to be well equipped, are soon filled with all kinds of complaining persons, the beds are often occupied for years by the same persons who at home could earn a little or could have obtained the necessary support from their relatives; and finally, there space is either lacking for receiving poor sick who suffer from more pressing ills, or the costs of the support rise to such a level that they cannot be met any more, even if the contributions of the working class are ever so generous.

§8

But not only must those persons be excluded from hospitals who can be supported equally well or even better in the bosom of their family, with the addition of charitable contributions; the same applies to some persons who cannot support themselves. Of course, such a hospital as the General Hospital in Vienna, which is also open to paying patients, need not make any or only few exceptions because of these, but regarding persons who are to be treated free of charge, the hospital can receive them or not depending on the category of illness.

* Cf. l. c. Volume VI, Section I, p. 339 ff.

Predominantly curable diseases of poor persons are those that are to be accepted at hospitals; but they must really require personal assistance: partly because the assistance which they receive in hospital would otherwise predominate over their requirement, and society would be robbed of even that part of their independence to which such persons are still inclined; partly because hospitals, no matter how good their situation and equipment, never have the cleanest of air, and they must, therefore, be filled with persons who cannot otherwise be provided for without great harm. Thus the submission of certificates of real poverty and illness is not sufficient to entitle a person to be received at a hospital. At a place where good institutions, apart from the hospitals, are available for poor sick persons, it must be decided, especially in cases of chronic diseases, whether the ill person is really bereft of all possibility of contributing to his maintenance by his own remaining activity and can be provided for in his own dwelling.

No matter how large a hospital is, it will never suffice to accept all the patients who ask for it. Certainly the intention of such charitable foundations is to assist the largest possible number of wretched persons; therefore those who consume the assistance without any advantage whatsoever, which could be beneficial to others and also could be of advantage to the community, must not be admitted.

Thus completely incurable patients never belong in an ordinary hospital, unless they are near the end and cannot be cared for in any way by their relatives. But care should be taken so that completely incurable diseases are not confused with those illnesses for which the outlook for curing is only grave or doubtful, for in addition to the advantages which persons suffering from such illnesses may still expect from correct treatment, such cases may also be viewed as subjects for the possible broadening and improvement of medicine.

There are diseases which must be treated in isolation from other ills, both because of the nature of the cure and in order not to endanger other patients. But for such ills most hospitals lack the necessary space and suitable opportunity. Of course, the Vienna General Hospital has a considerable advantage in this respect because it is so spacious, but even this institute does not contain all the required departments, because in addition to the lunatic tower, the lazaret, and three small rooms in which are kept patients paying daily 1 guilder for their care, and pregnant women, there are only large sick rooms with 20 or more beds in each; these cannot well be occupied by one or two sick persons and provided with special attendants without the costs required per patient rising beyond all the possibilities of this pious foundation.

If poor patients suffering from contagious diseases cannot well be left in their own houses because of the easy spreading of the disease, an even more justified fear of deleterious consequences applies to hospitals. There the danger of contagion is even much greater in relation to the number of persons lying close together, and the difficulty of maintaining the required cleanliness and healthy air when so many sick of all categories are assembled. A weak woman in childbed in a common room of the hospital has hardly escaped mortal danger when a woman suffering from terrible scarlet fever comes to lie next to her, and the [lying-in] woman, who believed that this pious foundation would be her salvation, contracts the scarlet fever which she never had before, and in the most critical time of her life at that, and must succumb to this terrible epidemic.—There are two hopeful young men suffering from inconsiderable intermittent fever, and there comes to lie between them a third one who had been brought to the hospital on the verge of death of an infectious nervous fever, and those two inherit from him an ill that for them also is soon fatal. A wounded man, not at all in a critical state, is placed next to someone who is suffering from hospital fever; on the third day the former is attacked by the same fever and his wound infected by a fatal infection.—Are these not the daily consequences of the improvident mixing of contagious diseases with less critical ills in one and the same sickroom of a hospital?

For those suffering from scabies and venereal disease, the General Hospital here [in Vienna] has a separate department for each sex; but how difficult is it for one case of scabies to be cured within as short a time as would be possible under different circumstances than his being among twenty or more persons suffering from the same ill, and having to live and deal with them daily. How improper is the community of patients in the case of venereal diseases, partly because not all the infected persons have completely lost their feeling of shame and morality, partly because of the almost inevitable quicker mercurial salivation in a spacious common room in which so many and variegated persons have to help themselves to mercury.

However, not only contagious diseases cause such devastation in common sickrooms; it is the same with some patients with terrifying cases which have the most powerful effect on the state of the other wretched patients present. There are several hysterical persons there now who are just at a time of the period peculiar to their sex, six or seven others who are just now in the most dangerous epoch of a feverish illness, and at that moment an epileptic is brought to the same room; several times a day she is seized by her terrible attacks involving loud shouting and the most terrifying gestures and contortions of all her limbs. Who can foresee the consequences of such terrible occurrences in a sickroom without shuddering?

And what must be feared from patients who rave violently either because of high fever or some other cause, who rage for entire days, and nights on end, and with loud howls interrupt and altogether banish the so necessary rest of some dangerously ill and weak patients? There are even the very sad examples of such raving persons who, before the attendants could intervene, violently attacked patients lying nearby and choked or beat them miserably to death in their slumber.

Running sores, burns, and other ills which spread a violent and penetrating stench and cause persons to excrete unconsciously and constantly, sometimes for months, how much do they pollute the air, even with the most scrupulous supervision, in one or several adjacent sickrooms. At the same time, how questionable to have such wretches in the same room with other patients, and how burdensome to the latter.

Therefore, all these and similar ills cannot be accepted in hospitals without obvious contradiction to the principles of a good Medical Police, unless there are facilities for separating patients who do not belong together. Moreover, even if a hospital adheres to the principle of excluding completely incurable diseases, contagious diseases, diseases inducing terror, and loathing, and diseases accompanied by violent stench, and even if it is well equipped, the facilities for separating patients are all the more indispensable because it cannot possibly be prevented that such diseases originate in the hospital itself and require early separation. It has been said that, except at times of epidemics of a contagious nature, there are not always so many patients, but that a whole room could be occupied without greatly increased expenditures by patients suffering from each disease (and the danger of infection would be greatly increased to physicians, surgeons, father confessors and attendants). From this, it follows that a number of small, well ventilated rooms is needed where patients suffering from contagious, bad-smelling and terrifying diseases or those involving raving can be treated, as is done in the guilder [paid] rooms; these patients can be entrusted to the care of one or two attendants living in the joint anterooms. As long as such arrangements are not made in this hospital, however, it is necessary to transfer to some particularly spacious rooms at least those cases spreading a violent stench that cannot be prevented by any measures of cleanliness, e.g., those rooms intended for incurables. Of course, these cases will spread the same stench here, too, but it is better that it be spread in only a few, and not all, sickrooms, and it is less of a contradiction for persons who are as good as lost to human society anyway to suffer this hardship rather than to endanger patients who may still be saved.

§9

So much on the intention or the final purpose of public hospitals, and on the class of persons suitable for admittance. But every philanthropist must put to himself the question: what was the fate of poor sick persons before there were the so-called hospitals. Let us then look briefly at the times before our own, and when we thus become acquainted with the quality of the institutions catering for the sick, we shall see all the more easily what the present hospitals should be like.

As soon as such a weighty matter as the gratuitous support of poor sick in hospitals comes under the direct supervision of the government authorities, the requirements of the sick must be well considered and satisfied most conscientiously and punctually according to well proven principles. However, as every state has so many pressing needs and unavoidable expenditures that defraying them could become exorbitant without the most painstaking economy, it is necessary to prevent waste caused by: building sumptuous buildings that are only conspicuous; purchasing equipment that is dainty rather than useful; employing superfluous clerks, physicians, surgeons, and servants; supplying foods that are not necessary, and expensive medicines that are nevertheless ineffective; keeping already cured patients too long, and then to limit all expenditures to the barest necessity so that the required assistance can be extended to a larger number of unfortunates. The requirements of poor patients admitted to a public hospital and to be maintained there concern mostly their healthy, secure, and quiet residence, purposeful and good equipment, and the best possible care and treatment of the sick, so that they regain their lost health, the highest of worldly goods, as quickly as possible and in a way that is least difficult and costly to the state. These subjects are to be treated further in the following chapters.

* * *

In the following Chapter One, Frank gives a historical survey on the principal hospitals of the world.

Chapter Two

Location, type of construction, and equipment of a public hospital*

§1

If we gladly admit that the philanthropy and compassion of rich individuals toward the poor and miserable among their brethren laid the foundation stone of the first hospitals, we cannot suppress the remark that the design of such buildings was sometimes due to vanity and ambition, as well as to ignorance of the equipment that buildings with such a noble purpose should contain. People looked at the foremost hospitals in Italy: a lofty and brilliant exterior proclaims the royal palace; the admiration of passersby was bought by squandering of immense sums, and even while too much attention was devoted to the exterior, too little was given to the interior. But should misery dwell in palaces and should luxury devour millions when thousands are lacking the means to alleviate the most pressing needs of many miserable and sick people?—If the poor wretches are to find a friendly reception at a public hospital, more comfort and cleanliness than they have in their miserable huts, satisfaction of their most elementary needs, the necessary attendance to and help against their ills, neither the unnecessary splendor of the exterior nor costly ornaments and splendid equipment contribute anything, whereas a healthy site and efficient design of the hospital, and good arrangement inside and painstaking administration are the best and the only ornaments of such a charitable institute.

§2

If a hospital is to receive the sick from an entire province, it should be situated as near its center as possible. It would be too great an inconvenience for the most distant inhabitants if they had to drag their sick from one end of the province to the

---

* On the best siting and design of human habitations see: "Medical Police," Vol. III, Part 4, Sections One and Two.—See also Vol. II, p. 436.—Best equipment of hospitals see: Murray, "Practical Library," Vol. III, St. 2, p. 166 ff.—A. W. Plazii, "Dissert. de Sanitatis publicae obstaculis," pp. 17–19.—Leroy in Scherf's Archives, Vol. II, No. 13.—M. Malaspina di Sannazaro, "Osservazioni sugli Spedali," Pavia, 1793. Translated (with supplements) by S. C. Titius, Leipzig, 1798.—Tuke, "Practical Hints on the Construction and Economie of Pauper Lunatic Asylums." York, 1815.

other. Some would be afraid of the long transport and rather perish at home, and for others, a journey especially in very cold or very hot weather would again be very deleterious, although under certain circumstances a not too lengthy journey does some sick no harm but is rather good for them. Dangerous illnesses the course of which is very rapid require this consideration even more once they have to be treated in hospital. If the hospital is destined for the inhabitants of a town, it need not be in the center of that town, but outside it or at a distant part of it. Large and populous cities need more than one hospital anyway, and small- and medium-sized towns need not complain of excessive distances. The selection of such a site outside the town, however, must be such that the inhabitants of that town are not endangered by the hospital. It is best if the hospital is situated in the northern or eastern part of the town. It should never be situated between the town and the pre-dominant wind, so that its mephitic exhalations are not conveyed for most of the year to the healthy inhabitants of the town.

If a public hospital is not to become a murderous pit, healthy air for it is one of the first conditions, and when a hospital is founded, this must be one of the prime considerations. Healthy air must be clean but neither too dry nor too humid, and a hospital on a mountain would be as inexpedient, especially for chest patients, as in the valley, e.g., for scrofulous and other cachectic patients. The most salutary place is a healthy, completely free, and somewhat raised site where no obstacle impedes the free circulation of the air and where no mephitic exhalations contaminate it. Therefore high houses and mountains, tall trees and forests, swamps and stagnant waters, churchyards, knacker's yards and factories, which latter stink as much as the former, do not belong in the vicinity of a hospital.

The second requirement that must be taken into account is good and sufficient water. It does not suffice, therefore, merely to examine the soil to learn whether it contains abundant and clear springs so that good wells can be dug. There must also be running water nearby which can be conducted into the institute at small cost. Water is just as indispensable as air, and is required in abundant amounts and good quality not only for drinking but also for cooking, brewing, washing, bathing, etc. If it has to be brought in pipes from afar, it not only raises the costs, it also easily causes shortage of water in case of accident to the machinery. For instance, the Hôtel Dieu at Rouen obtains the water it requires through pipes from a distance one hour away, which consumes a not inconsiderable proportion of the hospital's income. — Rivers close to which a hospital is being built and from which it obtains its water supply, must not be unclean nor shallow, and must not be liable either to dry up or to overflow.

In addition to this, the soil, the region, the quiet position of the hospital, require to be taken into account. Good soil is that which can be easily cultivated and which yields fruits abundantly; it will supply the hospital with cheap and good produce. A friendly and pleasant region has a beneficial effect on sick and convalescent people, and for this reason lunatic asylums were also built in them. But other unfortunates deserve equal consideration, and where the locality permits, this should not be overlooked. A quiet position is all the more necessary, in that the patients need refreshing sleep and beneficial rest for their recovery. Noisy workshops, which even turn part of the night into day, frequented highways, taverns, dance halls, etc., do not belong in the vicinity of hospitals.

If a hospital has such a fortunate locality, care should be taken that it maintains it: therefore nobody is to be permitted to settle near it. The Hôtel Dieu in Paris once had a very favorable position, when the capital was still called Lutetia. It was free on all sides and the water of the neighboring Seine was suitable for its requirements. But since Paris has grown, since building proceeded on all sides around the Hôtel, and the river has been made unhealthy by the impurities of the city, its situation cannot be held to be advantageous anymore.

Finally, the site where a hospital is to be built must be so large that the hospital can have a spacious yard, a relatively large garden, a distant place for drying the laundry, and that a cemetery, at least half an hour distant, can be allotted to it.

§3

The size of a general hospital is determined by the number of the patients to be treated there, but it cannot be put into an accurate arithmetic in proportion to the people's requirements. The mere possibility that an epidemic will increase the number of the sick three- or fourfold, makes it desirable to plan a hospital rather too large than too small. If not all the rooms have to be fully occupied at all times, it has the invaluable advantage that the rooms can be properly alternated, that each of them in turn can be properly aired, cleaned, and whitewashed several times every year.* I shall refer to this later on and show how indispensable this is. However, size also must have its limits, and there is no doubt that the state invests its capital at much higher interest if instead of one large hospital it builds several smaller ones for the requirements of large and populous cities. The larger the towns, the greater is mortality,** and thus mortality, too, is in direct proportion to the size of the hospital.† Even if the required number of physicians, sufficient medicines, attention, etc., are provided, nevertheless it can not be prevented that the large amount of noxious exhalations from many patients lying close quickly contaminates the air, so that

* Fauken, l.c., p. 38, is of the same opinion, and the military hospital in Strasbourg has so many rooms that the sick are put in others as often as seems necessary, and the emptied rooms are in the meantime aired. J. Aikin ("Thoughts on Hospitals," London 1771. Almost completely translated in the collections of selected treatises for the use of practical physicians. Vol. III. 1783, pp. 218 ff.) even wants (obviously too much) the sick to be allotted other rooms during the day.
** S. Home, "Attempt at the History of Mankind," Vol. I, Book 2. Attempt 11, on London.
† M. Stoll, "On the Equipment of Public Hospitals," published by G. A. v. Beekhen. Vienna, 1788, pp. 5–7.

often all the means of cleaning the air fail and no large hospital can be prevented from having its peculiar illnesses.* Can there be a greater contradiction than a hospital disease? A disease which one acquires at the place where one intends to get rid of one's own disease? Yet this is the consequence of immense hospitals where even the greatest efforts to heal are of no avail. Besides, the extraordinary size of such an institute makes supervision extremely difficult, and makes it impossible to prevent disorders of all kinds, fraud, etc.,** so that an experienced writer said openly: "A large hospital without disorders is an impossible thing."† As mentioned before, in Vienna there were in the past several smaller hospitals which were fused into one general hospital. In this way an immense institute originated which was almost unmanageable, in which disorders occurred that had previously been unknown. On one occasion I proposed that the former hospitals be restored, i.e., four in the eight suburbs, each with about 300 beds, and another small one in the capital,†† and even today I am firmly convinced of the great advantage of this course.‡ A few thalers more or less cannot possibly matter to the treasury if they can save the lives of many people, and it is not even certain that the building and administration of two small hospitals, which can accommodate as many patients as one large one, cost more than the large one. But even if it were not so, it is much better not to have a hospital than to have an inappropriate one; but for a good hospital it is essential that it accommodates only a moderate number of patients.

What I have said elsewhere concerning the disadvantage of tall buildings also

---

* The Hôpital Général in Paris gave the scabies to almost every sick person who was admitted. Cf. "Tableau de l'humanité des charités, qui se font à Paris," p. 13. Samml. a. Abh. Tom. cit. p. 211, 218, 219.

** A terrible example of this kind was the Hôtel Dieu in Paris, whereas smaller hospitals such as the Charité, St. Sulpice, Salpétrière, Hôtel des Invalides and others were found in good order. Whoever wants to obtain more information on the subject, is advised to refer to the following works: "Abrégé historique des hôpitaux. Contenant leur origine, les différentes espèces d'hôpitaux etc. etc. par Mr. l'Abbé de Recalde," Paris, 1784. "Traité sur les abus, qui subsistent dans les hôpitaux du royaume, et les moyens propres à les réformer par le même 1786. Idées sur les secours à donner aux pauvres malades dans une grande ville (par Dupont)," Philadelphie, et se trouve à Paris 1786. Extrait des registres de l'académie d. Sc. du 22. Novbr. 1786. Rapport des Commissaires chargés par l'académie, de l'examen d'un projet d'un nouvel Hôtel Dieu. Imprimé par ordre du Roi. Paris, 1787.

† Dupont, l.c.

†† A similar proposal was made by the commissioners of the Academy in Paris when the Hôtel Dieu was to be reformed, and the intention was that instead of one large, four smaller hospitals be built, each for 1200 patients and situated in the corners of Paris. Cf. "Extrait des registres," l.c. This proposal also met approval, as can be seen from the "Essai historique sur l'Hôtel Dieu de Paris, ou tableau chronologique de sa fondation etc. Dédié à tous les citoyens qui ont souscrit en faveur des quatre nouveaux hôpitaux." Par Rodonneau de la Motte, à Paris, 1787.

‡ A respectable writer, C. F. L. Wildberg ("System of Medical Legislation," Berlin, 1820, p. 413. §§849, 850), is of a different opinion and undoubtedly prefers a large hospital to several small ones. However, had he had experience and knew the difficulties that obstruct daily, nay hourly, the efficient equipping and continuous supervision, he would not have remained without doubts!

applies to hospitals, and it is more advisable to extend them in the plan than to give them great height. Weak patients and convalescents, whose state permits and requires them to enjoy fresh air and movement in the open, are unable to climb many stairs. And when everything required, and even sick and dead persons, have to be carried back and forth and so high, it makes hospital service so much more difficult and requires stronger servants. But even more consideration must be given to the fact that the upper rooms in hospitals are unhealthier than the lower rooms, and for this reason alone a hospital should never be higher than two stories.

§4

As regards the most efficient shape that hospitals should have, many quarrels have been conducted and as many mistakes been made. If the physician's voice had been paid more heed than the builder's voice, such an important matter that has repercussions on the well-being of many thousands of the present and the future population would not have been decided by petty considerations and misplaced parsimony. Hospitals would not have failed so often to fulfill their purpose, and mortality would not be as terrible in some hospitals as is unfortunately the case. Such institutions would not be called dishonorable names and avoided by the ordinary people as houses where sick persons are locked up so as to exterminate them all the more quickly.* Thus, fruitless attempts at improvements, intended to make amends for old mistakes, would not devour much larger sums than the builder thought he gained by saving on building materials and by herding as many sick into a narrow space as was at all possible, or by lowering the standard of architectural taste.—The point is here to provide the hospital with such a shape that it nowhere impedes access of free air, that, on the contrary, the air can everywhere circulate without hindrance and carry off the evil exhalations. Therefore, corners and closed off spaces are to be avoided. The rectangle or square, which is the shape of so many hospitals, does not satisfy the above intentions at all: it encloses a space where the air is not sufficiently changed; the air stagnates at the sides of the building, predominantly in the four corners and it becomes contaminated all the more certainly, the more sickrooms open onto the enclosed spaces.** This drawback, and the ensuing disadvantages could not remain undetected for long, and they were partly remedied by splitting the four wings and leaving an empty space in the four corners which are the most dangerous points; this was undoubtedly a very effective improvement.† Things

---

* In the previously mentioned "Traité sur les abus," etc., great shortcomings of the Hôtel Dieu in Paris are freely revealed. It is said there that among the populace the opinion is held that a special disease, maladie de l'Hôtel Dieu, carries people off.

** Ludwig (in his translation of J. Howard's "Reports on the Foremost Hospitals and Plague Hospitals in Europe," Lpz., 1791, p. 438) and J. Aikin (l.c., p. 207 and 218 ff.) rightly harshly criticize this shape.

† This is the way St. Bartholomew's Hospital in London is built.

were less fortunate where one side of a quadrangle was removed,* and if the above disadvantages are to be avoided, it should be seen to it that the lateral wings are much shorter than the front and that the entrance is not blocked by trees, a wall, etc., so that the wind can take effect without hindrance.

A. Petit** wants to see hospitals built in the shape of a star, the center being occupied by the chapel; next to it are the dwellings of the servants, the pharmacy, etc.; the sickrooms should be situated in the rays of the star.—Although at first sight this plan seems to have much to recommend it, its implementation has its doubtful aspects. How contaminated would be the air in the chapel and in the dwellings closest to it! The rays would act like a street closed at one end (dead end) in which, as everybody knows, the air is not sufficiently moved and cleansed. It is approximately the same with the T-shape which was given to the three right-angled wings of the municipal hospital in St. Petersburg. Even more similar is Poyet's proposal† of a circular building of 136 toisen†† diameter. In the center there would be a courtyard of 45 toisen diameter, and the buildings would radiate in 16 rays toward the circumference.— It is easy to see that this proposal is even less likely to be realized if the building is to serve its purpose.—Finally Maret‡ suggests the ellipse; thus, there is no lack of variety in opinions and proposals.

All these men proceeded from the intention of accommodating comfortably as many patients as possible in one room, while not neglecting architectural beauty. However, the latter is not the prime consideration in a public hospital, and as we have seen, the well-being of the sick does not depend in any way on the size of the building. A hospital for 300–400 patients can very well be built in a straight line, without lateral wings, and this shape is undoubtedly the most efficient. Free from all sides, the atmospheric air can have its beneficient effect everywhere, and it will require little effort and preparations always to provide such a building with good air. However, if the hospital is to accommodate more patients and if it must consist of several buildings, the whole can always be given a rectangular shape, or the individual buildings can be situated in a row, but care must be taken that they are not

---

* The Charité in Berlin is built in the shape of a Greek π. Cf. E. Horn, "Public Account of My Twelve Years' Service," etc., Berlin, 1818, p. 2.—Similar to this is the hospital in Rouen where one side of the quadrangle was left open. Cf. J. Hunczowsky, "Medical and Surgical Observations on His Travels Through England and France," Vienna, 1783, p. 155. Or the Middlesex Hospital in London which has the shape of an H.

** Mémoire sur la meilleure manière de construire un hôpital des malades," Paris, 1774. Diction. des Sciences méd. T. XXI, p. 432 ff.

† This plan as well as the proposal to transfer the Hôtel Dieu to the Isle des Cygnes were handed by Poyet to the King in a memorandum. It was given to a nominated commission for assessment, and how these men judged the proposal, as well as Poyet's plan, can be found in the previously mentioned "Extrait des Registres de l'académie," etc., etc.

†† [1 toise = 1.949 m.]

‡ Cf. "Nouveaux Mémoires de l'académie de Dijon," I. Semestre 1782.

too close together and that large courtyards remain between them. For instance
the Vienna General Hospital consists of many more or less long rectangular two-
storied buildings with proper space, and seven large courtyards between them. If
these spaces are kept clean so that rubbish and dirt of all kind do not accumulate
there and enhance the vile exhalations, everything has been done in this respect to
ensure clean air. The Paris Academy also proposed bringing together several smaller
buildings on one site, without joining them together. The advantages of this arrangement have become manifest at the Bartholomew Hospital in London, since its corners
were pierced and this plan may thus be recommended for every large hospital, without
thereby making service more difficult or creating other disadvantages.

* * *

§14

Sickrooms

For our climate the healthiest position of sickrooms undoubtedly is when they
face east or south. Rooms into which the sun does not penetrate all the year round
are damp and unhealthy; and the sick are deprived of much if the sunrays do not
reach them. In every creature, the urge to seek the sunlight dominates; even the plant
pales and becomes stunted when it does not receive sunlight. This urge is even stronger
in sick and convalescent persons, and the gentle sight of the sun affects them like a
great medicine. We can much more easily protect ourselves against the great heat
of the sun than replace it with some means. If the rooms are high and spacious
and arranged in such a way that the air can be renewed, and provided with blinds
toward the south, they will never be so hot in summer that they will hurt somebody.*
Even if such rooms are more difficult to heat in winter, they are, nevertheless, even
then somewhat heated by the sun, and they are thus always less cold than rooms
facing north; moreover, here, where the well-being of patients is concerned, a somewhat increased consumption of fuel must not be taken into account. The position
facing west is not advisable, and, because of the many moist and enfeebling winds
of this direction, unhealthy. Thus the directions east and south remain, as for instance
in the hospital at Bamberg, which are preferable to all others. If the hospital consists
of several individual buildings arranged in a square (see §4 above), it has the
invaluable advantage that not all the hospital rooms have their windows opening
upon the hospital yard which, no matter how large and practically arranged, will
always be largely an enclosed space.

What I said above (§3) about the disadvantage of large hospitals, also applies
on the whole to large sickrooms, and there is nothing more detrimental and nothing
more contrary to the noble purpose of pious foundations than large rooms in which
many patients are placed together.** In winter they cannot be sufficiently heated,

* In Italy and France there are many hospitals which are built like cathedrals or churches. I found that
   their rooms were cool even in hot summer.
** Aikin ["Thoughts on Hospitals," London. 1771.]

yet all the year round the worst air accumulates in them because the air is spoilt more quickly and more often than it can be improved. It is impossible to maintain cleanliness, and equally impossible to effect the necessary separation of the sick. One is forced to bring together the most varied patients, and thus the rooms become veritable reservoirs of the most pestilential exhalations on which hospital fever and gangrene of this name thrive.* If one asks the universal teacher, namely experience, and if one compares the mortality in large sickrooms, as they exist mostly abroad, with the smaller rooms, which are found mostly in this country, there cannot be any doubt which of them is preferable.

It is important, therefore, to determine first how many sick may be put together in one room. For those who suffer it would of course be best if each of them, according to Hoffmann's proposal,** could be allotted a separate room, and in every well appointed hospital a commensurate number of small rooms for one or two persons must be provided for, in which insane, violently delirious, hydrophobics, patients suffering from very badly smelling, malignant and infectious diseases, trepanned, etc., can be placed so that they are separated from the others; but it would be far beyond the capacity of charitable foundations if such consideration were to be accorded every patient, and it would also be unnecessary.

Thus the rooms, except for single patients and for sick prisoners, can be of equal size, so that in one of them ten chronic or acute sick of the ordinary kind, or five or six very acute and dangerous internal and external cases can be placed.

* * *

§23
Clean air

Among the most important things which have to be taken into account in hospitals in the first place is clean air. Clean air is an indispensable condition of maintaining healthy life which requires it every instant. How beneficial it is for the sick can be seen from the fact that gravely ill persons who, as in wartime, are often transported for miles in the open, frequently recover without medicines, whereas their sick comrades within the walls of a badly ventilated hospital expire miserably. However, the integrity of the air in a public hospital becomes all the more the object of the greatest care, the more it tends to absorb all the miasmas which have a deleterious

* After the hospital at Brest had burned down in 1777, the sick were put for one winter into a rope manufactury in which were rooms that could hold as many as 600 beds. The accumulation of people increased mortality so much that this institute was called among the people the grave of the sailors. J. Hunczowsky, "Medico-surgical Observations on his Travels through England and France, Especially about Hospitals," Vienna, 1783.

** C. L. Hoffmann, "On the Necessity of Giving each Patient in a Hospital His Own Room and Bed," and "Confirmation of the Necessity, etc.," Mainz, 1788 and 1789.

effect on the animal body, and more easily to become spoiled by the various exhalations where there are many sick persons together; this is the undoing of those who here seek their salvation.*

The air is moist, mired, and thereby deleterious for the hospital. We can protect ourselves against this by as healthy a position as possible, not using it until it has completely dried out, and keeping it and its environment as clean as possible.— The air is cold, and we oppose to it strong and firm walls, well fitting windows and doors, and efficient heating installations.—The air is hot and depends on the season of the year, but we mitigate it by shutters or venetian blinds, by high rooms which are neither too small nor overcrowded with patients. All these considerations have already been mentioned.—But regardless of this, the air in a hospital is contaminated in other well known ways, and we cleanse it with the aid of mechanics and chemistry.

* * *

† Halleri, "Elementa physiologica," T. 8, p. 150, addenda.

Chapter Three

Admission, distribution, care, duties and release of the sick

§1

Italy gives us a rare example and has many hospitals most of which do the nation honor. There are hospitals in which only native poor persons of both sexes are kept for the rest of their lives, partly free of charge, partly for a small consideration, if by dint of age or feebleness they are unable to provide for themselves. Others are open day and night to alien sick, no matter of what nationality and religion. They need neither attestations nor money to be admitted there and provided for, and when they have been cured, they are transferred to convalescence hospitals in order to recover completely. There are also hospitals for pilgrims and foundations where poor pregnant girls and women can await their time of confinement, hide their pregnancy from the eyes of the world, and give birth. There are homes for foundlings where the unfortunate infants, who either cannot be kept because of the parents' poverty, or are a disgrace before the world and a cause of shame to their mothers, are willingly received, educated, instructed in the arts, kept as long as necessary, and eventually discharged as good craftsmen and housekeepers and as honest persons; foundations where children aged 2 to 4 years, who have been abandoned by their parents, are kept, and hospitals for poor children, orphaned by the death of their parents, are in almost all large cities.*—Other nations, especially the French and English, excel by their special hospitals. There are hospitals for venereal diseases, smallpox, skin, chest, and other diseases, for old persons, for children, for women who have led an evil life,** etc. Germany has its houses for poor relief and foundlings, but fewer special hospitals than general hospitals.

There is no denying that the specialized institutions have advantages over the general ones. Syphilitic, scratching, persons suffering from dry scabs or surgical cases, e.g., heal much more securely in their own hospitals than in those devoted to all sick. It cannot be prevented, however, that someone after a surgical operation, for instance, also falls ill from an internal disease, and if he is not to remain to his

* Letters about Italy in the Deutscher Merkur 1775, Third Quarterly.
** "Collection of selected treatises for practical physicians," l.c., p. 212.

424

detriment with his fellow sufferers, special departments must be made, here, also, if such a state does not permit translocation to another hospital. Moreover, such special hospitals are suitable only for populous cities where there must be more than one hospital in any case, but the number of large cities is small. If a general hospital is well equipped, and if the departments intended for different kinds of diseases are sufficiently separated from each other, however, it also has considerable advantages so that we may forget the special institutions, for these general hospitals virtually include them in themselves.

* * *

§3

The insane

If any unfortunate has a just claim upon mankind, it is the lunatic, a creature who has lost the noblest possession. He requires our help all the more since he, like a dependent child, cannot do anything for himself, and it pleases the philanthropist no end when, to the honor of our century, he sees that the horrifying and repellent scenes in lunatic asylums, where the sick were maltreated like dumb animals,* have been replaced by humaneness. Not so long ago the state did not do anything for the insane except lock them up in order to render them harmless to human society. Now we know and fulfill yet another, a sacred duty: We return the insane to human society as useful members, and this double purpose—securing mankind against the ravings of the insane and curing the latter—has to be the guiding principle in the organization of the insane asylum.**

The soul is never ill, this was reliably established by the research of our psychologists, but the organ is badly attuned, and the insane person has a wrong subjective notion. He is to be distracted from it and guided back to the objective view of life. Therefore, he should never be given time to brood constantly about one subject. He should be placed in a busy atmosphere wherein his habits and inclinations must be regulated according to his mental powers; i.e., all idleness should be banned, and each hour of the day should be filled with a suitable alternation of useful work and fruitful pleasures. To these belong walking, riding, driving, dancing, gymnastic and military games, ball games, skittles, board and card games, optical skills, puppet theater, etc., music and singing, religious service, copying, writing papers, translating,

---

* For how inhumanly the raving mad were sometimes bound and maltreated, see Morgagni, "De sedibus et causis morborum," I. Cap. VIII. Articles 4, 5.—"Relation de la peste de Toulon," p. 228.
** Private asylum for the sick in mind. In Vienna, inaugurated by Dr. L. Goergen. Vienna 1820.— "Remarks on the construction of public hospitals for the cure of mental derangement" by W. Stark. Glasgow 1810—Tuke, "Practical hints on the construction and economie of pauper lunatic asylum," York 1815.—Georget, "De la folie ou alienation mentale," Paris 1823. J. Leupoldt, "Über Leben und Wirken und über psychiatrische Klinik in einer Irrenanstalt" (On Life and Activity and on a Psychiatric Clinic in an Insane Asylum), Nuremberg 1825.

reckoning, drawing, painting, embroidering, various useful work for the requirements of the house such as sewing and knitting, reading exercises, geography and history, geometry, etc., gardening, agricultural work, cardboard work, carpentry, turnery and similar work.

The separation of mentally disturbed persons according to the kind of their illness is usual particularly in England,* but it is not worthy of imitation, and little advantage can be expected from locking up several fools or melancholics together. The example of one lunatic has a healing effect on another if their states are different and form a glaring contradiction. Therefore different insane persons should be brought together in the following order: 1) The department for newly admitted. As long as official reports and medical certificates concerning the individual conditions and former life of a disturbed person, which are indispensable for rational treatment, are not available, or as long as the state is doubtful, even if these certificates have already been obtained, one must confine oneself to observing the suspicious patient, and necessary for that are special admitting rooms which must not be near raving and noisy patients. These preparations should be shortened as much as possible,** and the sick person should be turned over to the suitable department for treatment as soon as his state of health has been ascertained.—2) The department for mild and obedient, not ill-natured patients. They have complete freedom, much comfort and pleasure, carrying out their work almost as if playing.—3) The department for less good-natured and not so obedient patients. Although they also have freedom and amenities, their time for enjoying pleasures is shorter, and the time in which they are made to work is longer.—4) The department for those who have violent attacks. During the paroxysms they are locked up, but in the intervals they enjoy freedom, amusements, and they have work.—5) The department for the worse cases who have short or no intervals. They are unable to work, and have only little or no freedom at all.—6) The department for convalescents who must also have a quiet and friendly stay and complete freedom.

That way it is easy for the physician and attendant to promise the mentally ill person rewards and punishments. The suitable moment is used to show him, even distantly, a better fate which he himself can earn by better behavior. Even better clothes and food are used in order to stimulate a feeling of honor in the patient and to enhance his will power. According to his tractability he is transferred to a better or a worse department. Corporal punishment is of no avail at all,† and must not be

* Tuke, l.c.

** From 9 years' experience of the lunatic asylum in Glasgow ("The Medical Recorder of Medicine and Surgery," Philadelphia 1824. July edition), the best in the whole of Britain, it can be seen that lunatics must receive appropriate treatment as soon as possible, for out of 258 neglected lunatics, only 34 were cured, whereas out of 435 newly admitted and immediately treated patients 226 were released healthy.

† Pinel deserves commendation for having introduced humane treatment of the insane, and it is a fact that the number of raving has decreased very much since violent means of restraint have been abolished. In Gheel, the lunatics walk about freely in the streets and fields without anybody seeming to be watching

applied in future. The usual means of constraint* such as shackles, strait jacket, restraining chair, should be used only as mechanical means of tranquilizing, in order to render the lunatics harmless.

The aforementioned departments are to be viewed as parts of a whole which, however, must also be suitable for being merged if necessary. As mentioned earlier, rooms are small and pleasant, but large communal halls and premises must also be provided. Each department has its garden and place of amusement** with covered galleries, so that patients can stay there and be employed even in bad weather.

There is no doubt that such an institute can very well be combined with a general hospital, and that such a combination may yield considerable advantages, but it must be located in a distant part, partly so that other patients are not affected by the life which spreads around the lunatics and must often spread, partly so that the latter are not endangered by the proximity of the former. The same applies to the lying-in ward.

The lying-in ward

The lying-in ward here has no connection whatsoever with the hospital. Nobody can see from here into the lying-in ward and its inhabitants have even less to fear the exhalations of the sick.—The lying-in ward should have three departments: 1) For pregnant women. It is unsuitable to have pregnant women and women in childbed in the same room, as is done in some maternity homes; the pregnant women who need their strength and health for the coming ordeal should not be disquieted by the crying of babies or endangered by the exhalations of the lochia, etc.—2) For women giving birth. Those who must be assisted surgically in giving birth cannot remain in the common labor room, except if there are no other women in labor present. The sight of such artificial births, the cries of the woman about to be operated on would have the most deleterious effect on other women in labor. Thus, this department, too, must consist of several rooms.—3) For women in childbed. Only 2 or 3 should lie in one room, for nobody exhales more strongly than the woman in childbed, and her child must also be taken into account to a certain extent.

No additional rooms for the sick are necessary because pregnant women and

---

them. Even the shackled ones are used in agriculture. The insance are never teased or stared at by curious onlookers. The inhabitants are not afraid even of those who rave most; they guide them like children. Therefore, mishaps are unknown, and every year 12 to 15 lunatics are discharged as cured. S. Esquirol's report on the lunatic asylum at Gheel near Antwerp in Volume VII of the "Revue médicale française et étrangère," pp. 137–154.

* Credit is due to Horn, Hayner, and Hollaren for mechanical remedies. See "Med. prakt. Adversarien," Fascicle 2, i.e., Draft of a cure against psychic diseases, by Dr. P. J. Schneider. Tübingen 1824.

** The Institute at Vauvres near Paris, established by Falseret and Voisin, can probably compare with that at Gheel. It is designed for 30 lunatics, has large meadows and gardens in which the lunatics plant and do similar work, and in the garden there is a fenced-in pond, 2 feet deep, on which improved patients can go boating.

women in childbed are transferred to the hospital if their illness is something more than a passing indisposition. But for women who want to give birth here in secrecy and pay for it, several rooms must always be held in readiness. The Vienna home has for this purpose a special gate which is constantly guarded by a gatekeeper. Persons who do not want to be seen and recognized are admitted here at any time, covered by veils or masks. Nobody asks their names; they may even ask for a physician or priest from town, or even bring their domestic servants with them in order to be served by them. Only one duty is imposed on such a person, namely to provide a Christian name and surname in a sealed envelope. On the outside of the envelope the number of the room and the bed assigned to her are noted, and then the envelope is returned to her. When she leaves the home, she takes the letter unopened with her; but it provides information about her, in case she dies at the home. Every person here is protected during her stay against any attack from outside, and even against the courts of justice, and the service personnel are instructed to maintain the strictest secrecy.

* * *

§6

Therapeutic principles

The principles according to which we determine food for the sick also guide us, at least in general, in the choice of medicines. If it befits the rational physician, when curing a disease, to search for its causes and to modify his treatment accordingly, he cannot fail to notice that most diseases of the lowest class of people are brought about by a way of life connected with a lack of the basic necessities. The poor man has spent all day doing heavy labor, has filled his stomach insufficiently with coarse bread, and has warmed his blood with a glass of sometimes adulterated brandy. He does not have enough left to protect his bare body against the cold; he wears his only shirt so long that it drops in rags from his body. He enters his miserable hut: To keep the cold air out no window is being opened there; his hungry children, whom he cannot feed sufficiently because his feeble strength is not up to it, cry out to him and assault his fatherly heart. The dinner, if he gets any at all, is bad; he has no bed on which his tired limbs can find rest—he succumbs and is admitted to the house of charity. His body is cleansed of dirt and vermin, he is revived by a lukewarm bath, his skin is refreshed by a fresh shirt; his tired limbs find rest on a comfortable bed, he is in a warm and friendly room, and he sees with shuddering snugness, rain and snow which can no longer penetrate through his torn clothes to his body. His shriveled and cold stomach is revived by nourishing soup, he enjoys the quiet and care of which he had been deprived for so long, and which everybody needs— and lo and behold, he is already half on the way to recovery even before he has received any medicines! From this follows that at least in a public hospital, the therapeutic method may be as simple and economical as possible, and that nowhere else is the expectation method more often applicable than here.

Progress made in medical science has simplified our Materia medica, and has exchanged expensive foreign remedies for cheaper domestic ones. It is precisely the latter that should be used in hospital practice. In isolated cases, it would not bring any gain if the cheaper remedies were preferred against irreplaceable and more expensive remedies, if the latter would cure the disease more rapidly than the former; thus, it would even be against economy and humaneness if musk, Castoreum, Chinese salts, etc., were not applied because of their expense. The best remedy is the one that cures most quickly, with the greatest certainty, and most durably, and it is, thus, also the cheapest, so that it and none other should be chosen. Yet in the majority of cases we can always apply domestic remedies and achieve the required effect, and several great hospital physicians have already remarked that in hospitals where many costly medicines are used, mortality is not at all lower.* Among the remedies that are not indispensable in a hospital are also the so-called Roborantia [tonics]. Once the illness has been overcome and the machinery has been put in order again, which must be achieved by other than these means, the inclination to eat will also return, and good food, to which beer and wine belong, will then do the rest. Even the way in which a medicine is given can make it more expensive or cheaper. Therefore, tinctures, pills, decoctions, etc., should be listed for use after powders, tisanes, etc., if the latter can be used. The cheapness also depends on the time of preparation, and in preparing a nosocomial dispensatory a skilled apothecary should be consulted to give proper information. The dispensatory is a guide both for the physician and the apothecary, and just as the latter need stock only the prescribed medicines, prepared by certain methods, the physician should not prescribe any others. This rule, too, has its exceptions, however, and if the physician deems a new medicine advisable, one that is not stocked, and if the hospital administration approves it, the apothecary is obliged to purchase it. But the pharmacopeia must be revised from time to time and improved, as required; this is a task for the administrator, not for the individual.

No less caution is required in administering and applying the medicines. The external ones, especially ointments, have the unpleasant trait of soiling the linen. Their application must be very much limited. Another dark side are the frauds and misappropriations which cannot be sufficiently suppressed in a hospital. Horn found that in the Berlin Charité, the consumption of wine vinegar was enormous, until he had it adulterated with vermouth. The attendants also stole opium and other tinctures, so that these had to be replaced by other medicines.—The remainders of the previous day must be effectively utilized, empty glasses, boxes, and cases must be conscientiously returned.

* * *

* Horn, "Public Account," l.c., p. 154.

Chapter Four

Of the staff required for hospital administration and their duties

* * *

§3

Hospital director

If the great wheels are to turn smoothly, everything in a public hospital must be arranged according to certain rules and with the utmost care, and one man must be at the head to keep the entire machinery in motion. This man, the director, should be a man of comprehensive knowledge, of indefatigable activity, of proven integrity, and of acknowledged humanitarianism. He puts each person where he belongs, and he must not forget that unexpected events sometimes may multiply the affairs to be dealt with. Therefore, he should not allot to each subordinate more work than can be done with moderate effort; he never demands anything useless or superfluous; he should acquaint everybody with his duties; he should take an overall view; he must demand strict and uncompromising punctuality and obedience, and he should lend his support where necessary.—The director must be given a free hand and he must be entitled to act according to his own judgment in unforeseen cases. He must be informed daily of all the occurrences and matters concerning the hospital, but he will also see to matters himself, in order that the suffering of the sick may be mitigated as quickly as possible, and their recovery expedited. He must be able to apply all the advantages of the institution, and he will reward what is good and punish what is bad. The entire staff of the hospital is to a certain extent dependent on him, but his real sphere of action is with medical affairs. It is his business to see to the quality of the grain, the flour, etc., to discuss with the apothecary the purchase of drugs, etc., but he cannot be expected to himself purchase what the hospital needs. In cases where there is doubt, he will do well not to take decisions by himself, and to avoid all partiality, he should call together the senior physicians, the apothecary and the economic inspector, to deliberate jointly with them as to what is of advantage to the institution, and then to issue his orders.

No matter how well a hospital is run, there will always be complaints by dissatisfied people, which cannot always be avoided even with the best will in the world. Many people believe that in hospital they have to be treated splendidly; some even go to hospital only because they will be fed there; many demand from the physician a better diet than he can permit. The complaints are often due to the caprice of the sick, often to bad taste and malevolence—and all these complaints are directed more or less at the director. He will ignore that, knowing that he fulfilled his duties; the public will do well not to pay heed; the government should justly protect him against such wrongs and confer on him the authority which he needs in order to control a rough crowd.—The government must also let him have his say in choosing a hospital employee and permit him to voice his objections and reasons for his reluctance to employ someone. He must be permitted to test the medical person to be employed, and to give his opinion on his or her ability. If he submits to the government proof of the physical and moral unsuitability of such persons, the government must pay heed and reconsider its choice. The director, not the government, has to live with a subordinate and use him, but how can he do that when favoritism decides instead of merit?—The government likewise must be always ready to heed his representations, to examine them, and to eliminate shortcomings that have been pointed out. But then the director is likewise responsible for everything.

* * *

§5

Hospital physicians

The medical and surgical personnel working at the sickbed are directly subordinate to the director. For this work are employed only men who are well versed in the entire field of their art and who are also knowledgeable in the preparatory and auxiliary sciences, not trained in routines, but scientifically educated, experienced men, i.e., true physicians and surgeons to whose care sick persons can be entrusted. Experience profits art and science very little when it is grounded on deficient theoretical knowledge. In the first instance, the foregoing men are necessary as hospital physicians because 1) they have the role of physicians who are responsible for the sick not only to their conscience, but also to the authorities; 2) they enrich science and art, because the large number of sick in their care permits comparisons; the great variety [of sick] induces all kinds of experiments; the simple method of treatment and the certainty that everything is done as prescribed, which leads to certain results and that nothing forbidden has been administered; the rare cases which occur in hospitals; the post mortem examinations which are not opposed—facilitate observations and have great scientific value; 3) they appear in the role of teachers of younger and less experienced colleagues. In the general hospital each chief physician has a paid and an unpaid assistant physician and a surgical practitioner at his disposal. Likewise each chief surgeon has an assistant surgeon and three surgical practitioners at his disposal one of whom, however, is assigned alternately to the chief physician. This arrangement has a number of advantages: if a chief physician falls ill, an assistant physician takes his place, etc. In addition, the assistants and practitioners assist the chief physicians, look after minor affairs, and daily they have the best opportunity to improve their knowledge of their art. On the other hand, the state thereby gains efficient and good physicians and surgeons for town and country. The positions of assistant physicians and practitioners are filled every two years by new individuals, but the chief surgeons may remain as long as they fulfill their duties and are willing to serve the hospital. Hospital service entails much that is peculiar and that can be learned only in the course of time; however, since it is the chief physicians in particular who direct the treatment of the sick, and the benefit bestowed by the institution depends primarily on them, their frequent replacement can only be deleterious. They are, therefore, entitled to a decent salary and free lodgings in the hospital; the unpaid assistant physicians should also receive free food in addition to free lodgings. One of the physicians has to make an inspection every day, i.e., he has to examine the newly arrived sick, assign a room to them (Chapter 3, par. 2) and be ready for extraordinary cases day and night.—In addition to intellect as a first preference, the hospital physician must have good health, courage, and patience in his arduous work.

The number of physicians and surgeons must be in a suitable ratio to the number of patients. Stoll suggests no more than one physician for 200 acute or 300 chronic patients, and for 20 surgical patients one surgeon. Fauken assigns to each physician 230 patients, in some seasons several more. But if a physician is to visit 200 acute patients, some of them twice, he cannot devote the attention and calm deliberation required by each of them. The time is too short, his spirit will falter under the effort, his zeal will cool, and sloppiness will replace the ever alert and brisk activity. What is to happen to the other duties of the physician? The drug list arrives too late at the pharmacy, the diet slip too late in the kitchen; the prescribed drugs from the pharmacy and the required meals from the kitchen do not arrive at the specified time, etc. The hospital physician is no post horse; his difficult duties deserve to be alleviated; his health is endangered by excessively long sojourn in the atmosphere of disease; he should have leisure for studying his science, and should have to look after only so many patients that in times of emergency he can take over a few more.— I therefore consider it a matter of conscience if a physician is given more than 100 acute or 200 chronic patients for treatment. He himself must treat the grave cases among them, but leave the lighter and convalescent patients to his assistants, and only now and then examines whether they are properly looked after. If the surgeon also leaves the lighter cases and simple bandages to his assistants, he can treat 30 patients, for experience shows that the majority of surgical patients are not grave cases, and that a surgeon does not have to operate every day.

* * *

§15

Administrative director

The medical authority faces another administration which deals with economy, policy, and finances. However, since economy, security, and cleanliness in a public hospital touch upon medical interests, and since the administration of which we are speaking here has to provide the support necessary for healing the sick, it is easy to understand why and to what extent it has to be dependent on the medical management. The physician cannot be required to search the house for defects and see to their repair, or go to the granaries and stores to see whether they are filled with cheap and good stocks, and whether these are well stored. It is his concern, however, when linen and bandages are supplied dirty and torn, when the sick receive bad beer and bread instead of good, when the meat is hard, the vegetables tasteless and indigestible, when windowpanes remain broken, when the privies smell, etc. All these and many more are his concern; he must make demands on the supervisor in these matters and require his obedience. Therefore, an economic inspector should be chosen, to be subordinate to the government and dependent on the director and the chief physicians and surgeons insofar as his business concerns the feeding of the sick and has an effect on their cure. He is an important person and can save the institution considerable sums; being a great administrator, he must have comprehensive economic knowledge; he must be no less faithful and honest, and he must be tidy and punctilious down to the least detail. He should also be a determined man who metes out strict justice, and is everywhere active and attentive, for his subordinates do not all belong to the educated class. In addition to the head warden and subordinate wardens, they include: 1) the hospital scribes, 2) the overseer of the clothes and linen stores, 3) the kitchen personnel, 4)–6) the baker, the brewer, and the butcher with their assistants, 7) the washerwomen, 8) the bath attendants, 9) the porters who also serve as chair bearers and grave-diggers, 10) the house maids, 11) the watchmen, and 12) the gatekeepers. All these people are his subordinates, have to obey his orders, and may expect reward and punishment from him. His sphere of activity includes the interior and exterior of the hospital; he has to see to economic matters of the house and supervise its policy.

* * *

II

MEASURES AGAINST INFECTIOUS DISEASES OF MAN

INTRODUCTION

From ancient times until the present innumerable epidemics, causing terrible destruction, have afflicted nations and have left terrifying traces. Entire countries were depopulated, and sometimes all of mankind was threatened with terrible ruin.

* * *

After giving numerous examples from the field of epidemiology, Frank continues:

All these and many more cases were not sufficient to instruct us as to the causes and the nature of such epidemics; innumerable investigations on the corpses of such diseased persons, and all the experiments made with the living have failed to yield the expected results. We need not take refuge with the supernatural, the stars, the sepsis of the air, the irregularities of the seasons, in order to explain the origin of contagion. We need not see the reason, as the Turks do, in Providence for we know the contagium as a poison sui generis which is produced in the sick organism, and which is transmitted by this organism or by inanimate intermediaries upon contact. But we cannot pride ourselves in being able to heal most of these diseased products; on the contrary, as soon as contagious fever is mentioned, we must admit that this is an obscure field, crisscrossed by contradiction and delusion, and that the art is in its childhood. Yet it will exchange its child's clothing for worthy adornment, the industrious efforts of the physicians will succeed in protecting us from humiliation, and humanity from such great misery! Are we not able to mitigate and heal the venereal disease which was as devastating in its effect as the plague? Did not the immortal Jenner succeed in finding the proper remedy for the smallpox contagion, and thus save the world millions of healthy inhabitants? Can we not expect much from belladonna, which heals the deadly scarlet fever, also as a remedy against this epidemic?—Why should we not hope to be able to find true remedies also for the plague, yellow fever, and other contagious diseases! The art progresses with sure but slow strides, and as long as it is not able to cure the terrible epidemics, it is doubly the sacred duty of the state administration not to stand by idly with folded hands* when mankind can be spared so much misery and distress and so many citizens can be saved for the state, when the murderous, and so far, incurable, but eradicable epidemics can be controlled by suitably chosen and well-applied remedies, nipped in the bud, and completely rooted out from the face of the earth. Despite their fright-fulness, the contagious diseases are best suited for that, and the key to this mystery is supplied by Medical Police.

§2

It is an ancient custom, and it is intrinsic in human reason to protect oneself primarily against diseases which one does not know how to cure, and at times when there was no trace of an art of healing, the greatest legislators distinguished themselves by such ordinances. It was not unknown to the ancients that certain diseases are able to communicate themselves to healthy persons, and they even had knowledge of contagion through intermediaries. They usually ascribed the effect to the diseased exhalations and to the nausea which such sick and often terribly disfigured persons cause to the healthy, and therefore, the preventive measures consisted not only in the isolation and washing of the sick, but also in cleansing their effects with water and fire, as well as cleansing the atmosphere with fire and fumigation. The oldest contagious disease of which an accurate description has been preserved is leprosy, and the oldest measures used against contagious diseases relate to this malady and are preserved in the Scriptures. Everybody who was suspect of having leprosy had to submit to the thorough examination by the Neokoros, and even doubtful cases had to submit to being locked up for 7 days or more. If a person was found to really have leprosy, he was completely isolated from the healthy persons, and a special and remote place was allotted for him.

* * *

§4

The police measures against contagious fever and especially against the plague, although the latter is one of the oldest and most devastating diseases, have been taken only recently. That they were not taken sooner was due to misunderstood dogmas, superstition, and ignorance of the causes and the character of the plague. The gullible ones all the more defend the thesis that this disease was sent by God, since they believe that they find proof of it in the Scriptures. The pest mentioned

---

* Useful and innocent persons in the thousands, who could perhaps be saved at slight expense, are left by the state without defense while no criminal is abandoned without defense. J.Ch. Reil, "On the Recognition and Cure of Fever," Halle, 1815. Vol. V, §30, p. 144.

several times is there as a scourge which Heaven used in order to punish the disobedience and wickedness of mortals, but nothing is said of any quarantine against the plague. This misinterpretation of God's word, that a disease must not be prevented because such measures are not prescribed by the Scriptures, as in the case of leprosy, kept the nations' reason captive up to the fourteenth century, and to this day it ties the hands of the sultan. It is not unconcern and ignorance, as is usually assumed, which is the reason that the Turks do not do anything to combat the plague. The reason is that Mohammed taught: "All that happens in this world comes from God, and it is the greatest crime to oppose God's will." This is the assurance with which the Turk remains among persons suffering from the plague. Due to his religion and the dogma of predestination, he is obliged to disdain and condemn as sinful behavior the measures which the Europeans in the Orient use against this terrible scourge. Hieronymus Mercurialis* explained at great length that the plague is caused by malice and sorcery, and there is also a widespread view that the plague is due to the influence of the stars, that it is produced and spread by the air, and that, therefore, there is no defense against this disease. Yet one sees that persons in contact with those suffering from the plague, also caught it, whereas others, who avoided such contact, remained unharmed by the plague. When people began to observe more closely the course of contagious epidemics, the plague, smallpox, yellow fever, scarlet fever, measles, etc., they found that these contagious diseases did not spread further as soon as contact with infected persons and objects was avoided. Samoilowitz and Valli observed, each at a different place, namely in Moscow and in Smyrna, that those who isolated themselves completely from the sick, were spared the terrible plague which those two men described. Palloni observed the same in connection with the yellow fever epidemic in Livorno, and it is no less known of other contagions, as will be explained later. After such observations made in former times, the conviction soon prevailed that persons who came from plague regions and had conversed with plague-stricken people had to be separated and kept under observation for some time. It was thought that forty days, the longest period for a feverish disease to take its course, was deemed sufficient for deciding the question whether a suspect person had been infected by the plague or not. The name of this institution, Quarantaine [in German] (une quarantaine de jours, i.e., 40 days) already indicates that it originated from the French who were the first to need it in the Mediterranean ports because of the heavy traffic to and from the East. The first proper institutions of this kind were established at the beginning of the seventeenth century in Marseilles**, Toulon, Livorno, etc.; however, such institutions, though less perfect, existed as

* "Med. pract.," pp. 804, 805.—On 6 October 1812, I was told by the Countess Jaroszynska from Podolia, where the plague had broken out in 1796, that the common people there personified the plague and believed that it appeared now in the guise of a horse, now as some other animal, and, therefore, that when such an animal is seen in a village, the alarm bells are sounded.
** "Dictionn. d. sc. med.," T. XXVII, p. 367.

early as the fifteenth century on Majorca and at Venice.* Since then, the excellent institute, e.g., in Marseilles, has attained its present perfection, the plague and yellow fever have always been nipped in the bud, and this city, which was so often depopulated by the plague previously, has been spared this scourge since 1720. Credit for this must be given exclusively to the vigilance of the health officers and the quarantine institutions. The same can be said of the institutions in other countries, and the Austrian states, into which the contagion was so often brought from the neighboring Turkish Empire: it is only their excellent institutions which keep great harm at bay. There is no doubt now that this is the surest means of breaking the violence of the contagions as soon as all states will be inspired by the same philanthropy.

It seems, therefore, to be of no small importance to become acquainted with means, approved by experience, against the spreading of contagious epidemics from the sick to the healthy, and to assist the authorities by word and deed, so that they prevail over the scourge of devastating contagions, and repulse or at least mitigate them. But before I deal more in detail with such an important subject, it seems required and proper to stipulate some general concepts, so that statesmen, without being physicians, may understand what contagious diseases are, how they spread among mankind, and how we can protect ourselves against them and banish them from the face of the earth.

---

* J. Howard, "Histoire des principaux lazarets de l'Europe etc.," traduite de l'Angl. par Th.P. Bertin. Paris, 1801, p. 35.

Chapter One

Epidemics, miasmas, contagions

§1

If the cause of a disease affects only individuals belonging to human society and leaves the others unaffected, sporadic diseases occur. Their cause is, like that of every disease, either external and accidental, which can and must smite only individual persons, or it is within the individuals themselves, and thus every disease, from violent injury to contagious fever, may occur sporadically. It is not unknown that even contagious epidemics at the beginning make a sporadic appearance, and not rarely at that. But if the disease without violent cause attacks simultaneously within a certain time a large number of persons who live together in one region, it is called pandemic. If these pandemic ills are indigenous, stationary, confined to a certain region, they are called endemic, and they are merely local epidemics which were made permanent by causes surrounding us, such as accepted customs and ways of life, the peculiar quality of foods and drinks, unhealthy soil, climate, etc. But if these diseases hold sway for only a certain time and then disappear again, after having afflicted an unusually large number of persons in one region, while perhaps beginning to ravage another region, and if they return again, often after many years, and just as often sooner, they are epidemic diseases.

All these diseases, and thus also the epidemic ones, are in certain cases contagious, in other cases they are not.* But it is of great importance to the health police to know whether a contagious disease is epidemic or infectious, because the measures it has to take in one case are quite different from measures required by the other case. Already it has often happened that a simple epidemic has been confused with a contagious one; this error is all the more easily possible because the general external

* Epidemic is here taken as genus, infection as species, a distinction that is particularly desirable in Medical Police, for it protects against various misunderstandings. If contagious diseases also occur epidemically, a fact that probably nobody will doubt, epidemic cannot be the opposite of infectious or contagious. Foderé, who has given much attention to this subject recently, also subordinates the contagious to the epidemic. See "Leçons sur les épidémies et l'hygiène publique," par F. E. Foderé, Paris et Strasb. 1822–1824. T. I–IV, Chap. VI.

438

cause of the simple epidemic may cause many persons to fall ill simultaneously and in a similar way, and the contagions also occur epidemically. The dispute over the nature of the yellow fever, which is conducted with such fervor, proves how difficult it sometimes is to decide in this matter. But the basis of the infectiousness or noninfectiousness of an epidemic lies in the causes bringing it about, and it is worth the effort to seek these out and investigate them more closely.

§2

The causes of epidemics lie outside people; they have a general effect and are transient. By affecting the outside of the organism of many persons living together in one district, they convert the inner side of the organism; if there is a propensity to it, they give the ability to be effective an alien trend and produce the so-called epidemic diseases. For epidemics to occur, there need not be a certain kind of disease, the important thing is the external cause and the propensity of many individuals, and most disease may hold epidemic sway. This cause, unless it lies in fear, worry, and distress, or in evil morals, bad life, in famine, or in bad or spoilt foodstuffs and beverages, etc., requires a common medium situated outside the human body, which in most cases is the atmosphere. This may really produce epidemic diseases. Cold nights following after warm autumn days cause dysenteries, and the so-called fall dysenteries occur easily and become epidemic in consequence of such quality of the air. Catarrhal and inflamed affections and pure inflammations occur when it is very cold; intermittent and mucus fever (Febris mucosa) are due to humid air in spring; saburra, gall, and putrid fever occur epidemically when it is very hot. If suddenly there is an abrupt change of temperature from cold to warm, or vice versa, and rapid change in the atmosphere from dryness to humidity this affects the outer and inner surface of persons, and in the sensitive, weakly and sickly, whose number is never small, it gives an alien direction to the sensitivity and the ability to be effective, thus the well known winter, summer, fall, and spring epidemics originate. Thus not spoilt air and not the atmosphere is the cause of most diseases, as was wrongly believed. Those that are caused by the atmosphere, the atmospheric epidemics, are slight compared with the host of physical ills from which mankind suffers. Atmospheric epidemics are not contagious, i.e., they are not transmitted from individual to individual, and the pathological matter produced in the body of such persons suffering from the disease cannot again produce the same disease. For the prevention of these atmospheric epidemics, the Medical Police has only a limited sphere of activity, for the police would have to be able to command the elements. The atmosphere can take up the tinder of the disease and spread it. In that case the atmosphere is only the carrier: it receives spoilt exhalations and effluvia causing disease, i.e., miasmas, and conducts them often, without amalgamating with them, for a long time and over great distances, and thus originate the simple, i.e., the miasmatic epidemics. But what are miasmas?

§3

Miasmas are poisonous, volatile vapors which develop 1) from healthy and sick animal bodies. The miasmas which develop from human bodies confined in a narrow space are terrible. Jail and ship fever are proof of that. In 1597, several criminals were tried at a court in Oxford. These persons had been in jail for a long time and brought such bad air from there into the small room where the judges awaited them that these and almost all those present were immediately attacked by the most malignant illnesses and died of them. These prisoners were not ill and did not fall ill, but in the narrow jail that was inaccessible to fresh air, the air had been so poisoned by the animal exhalations and the clothes, and the entire bodies of the prisoners were so steeped in it, that they were fatal to those who came near them. — The human exhalations become even more terrible when the individuals who live together in a narrow and confined room are ill. Who does not know the devastating scourge of hospital fever, hospital infection, and typhoid epidemics which have their origin here! These very volatile animal products escape from the sick organism by way of breath, saliva, sweat, urine and excrement, or rather all the excretions are mixed with miasmas; they have the most devastating effect on the live organism and produce terrible general epidemics. — Miasmas develop from 2) rotting animal and vegetable substances. Unburied or not deeply enough buried human and animal bodies, animal waste in slaughterhouses, butchers' stalls, tanneries, soap works, in factories producing gut strings, etc., latrines, manure pools, peat bogs, flax and hemp roasting, etc., are the sources of such poisonous vapors. The cathedral at Dijon was once so poisoned by the effluvia of corpses that it became the cause of a murderous epidemic. The deleterious miasmas were received by the atmosphere and spread their nefarious effect over mankind. The Cemetery of the Innocents in Paris received about 3000 corpses in that year. In 1779, a pit 50 feet deep had been filled with 1500 corpses; however, the year after that, all the cellars in the neighborhood were so poisoned that everybody who only passed by their ventilation holes was immediately seized by the most terrible illnesses. — The blood and animal wastes of 100,000 pieces of cattle that are slaughtered for the British fleet in Cork, Ireland, are put into a large pit. When there are rains, this quagmire overflows, and as long as the slaughtering lasts, malignant fevers hold sway. — The miasmas develop from 3) stagnant waters or swamps (in which plants also rot), mines, sand pits, etc.* The most insidious swamp miasma is malaria. It rises mostly from rice fields, from

* Nacquart understands by miasmas only those exhalations that come from the sick human body, and he distinguishes them from the effluvies (swamp miasmas) and emanations putrides (rotting animal tissues). "Dictionn. d. sc. med.," T. XXIV, article: infection, p. 442 ff. and T. XXXIII, article: miasmes, p. 354. We shall not deal with this distinction because it is of no importance as regards Medical Police. Only the source of miasmas is different, but their effect on the human body, from which they also develop when the body is healthy, is the same at least insofar as no miasma induces like diseases that propagate from one individual to another.

low-lying marshy soil, as well as from every swamp and stagnant water, no matter how small, in larger or smaller quantity. It consists of a fine vapor, mostly discernible by its odor, which in warm weather rises upward and is often carried very far by air currents. Malaria does not sink down again, and people are safe in the valley while the mountain tops are surrounded by poisoned air. Malaria overtakes people insidiously at night while they are asleep; it even lulls its intended victim to sleep, and is then all the more certain of its prey.* The miasmas which develop in pits, mines, smelting plants, etc., emerge partly from the minerals, and take the life or health of those who inhale them. Many cachexias, which are caused by this, and especially miner's phthisis, are epidemic among miners.**

§4

Thus the miasmas are not the result of a peculiar secretion or a peculiar illness, they are the product of simple fermentation, putrid, mephitic, highly dangerous exhalations which chemistry has so far tried in vain to analyze. They spread into the atmosphere, fly about in it for a long time, remain undecomposed for a long time, especially in stagnant, enclosed air, and thereby gain in intensity. Their effect not only depends on this, but also on the disease from which they developed, and from the state of the atmosphere which receives them. As poisonous exhalations they are not visible to the eye for they leave the air untainted, only sometimes they cause the air to become opaque, but they have a repugnant sweet and stinking-rotten smell. They cling to every surface, but they can spread to human beings only in the dissolved, vaporlike state, and only through the skin, through the respiration and deglutitive organs. They easily combine with humid air, and heat makes them more volatile and effective. In this state they easily affect man and make him sick, but their poisonous sting injures only once: the miasmas can never produce themselves, they have to be produced.

§5

The characteristic trait in the effect of the miasmas on the human organism consists of the following:

1) The miasma stimulates the human organism differently and causes some disease in one man and another disease in someone else. The mephitic exhalations of persons confined to a narrow space cause jail and hospital fever and similar diseases, and

---

* Captain William Smith, about Sicily.—"Dello stato fisico del suolo di Roma etc." di G. Bracchi.— "Con un Discorso sulla condizione dell'aria di Roma negli antichi tempi," Roma 1821.—Histoire des marais et des maladies causées par les émanations des eaux stagnantes," par J. B. Monfalcon. Paris 1824.—"On Marsh Poison" by Ferguson.—Froriep's "Notizen für Natur- und Heilkunde," No. 169.237.

** J. G. C. Ackermann and B. Ramazzini, "Treatise of the Illnesses of Artists and Craftsmen." Stendal, 1780.

also scurvy, gangrene, inflammation of the eyes, etc.—The rotten exhalations of dead animals cause typhoid, putrid fever, carbuncles, and also gastric and gall fevers and other cachexias.—Marsh miasma usually causes intermittent fever, but there are different types of it; it also causes scrofulas, constipation of the intestines, rheumatic diseases and others.

2) The miasma developing from a body afflicted by such a disease cannot transmit the same disease to a healthy person. The exhalations of those afflicted with intermittent and recurring fever and with vascular fever do not give these ills to the healthy. The exhalations of the person suffering from miasmic typhoid do not give typhoid; of the gangrenous they do not give gangrene. Though these exhalations may affect the healthy and make him ill, this illness is of a different kind, or there is some chance involved. All diseases produce miasmas, but these are different, both in character and in effectiveness: they lack a specific poison to reproduce themselves. An animal that had died of anthrax gave to the veterinary surgeon who dissected the carcass, typhoid; on another occasion, it caused local inflammation but no anthrax.

3) Miasmic sick affect the healthy not by contact, not from individual to individual, but through their exhalations which spread into the atmosphere. The miasmas are inhaled, swallowed, or penetrate through the skin covering (through wounds) into the body. Let the patient suffering from dysentery be brought into a room provided with fresh air, touch him from head to foot, and you will not fall ill. But go to him in the room which is filled with the miasma escaped from his sick body, use the night-stool which still contains the evil-smelling excretions of the dysentery patient, and you will leave the room sick if your body is predisposed to the miasma. For precisely this miasma, which escaped from its poisonous source, is received by the atmospheric air. The air is the vehicle, the carrier, it conducts, often from afar, the poisonous vapors to the human body, and through this common external cause, and through such general media, it becomes possible that several similar and simultaneous diseases in one region, i.e., true and not infectious epidemics occur.

§6

But if the external cause induces such a disease which has the ability to spread to healthy individuals through direct touch or through inanimate objects which were in touch with the sick, so that these persons suffer from the same disease and that the same seed, by which this disease was induced, is produced and thus reproduced ad infinitum, then it is a contagious disease. If such a poison touches, affects and thus makes many persons living in one region similarly ill in quick succession, an infectious, i.e., contagious, epidemic originates. The cause is always a specific poison which we call contagion. If it successfully affects the human body, we call it contagion, whereas the effect of miasmas is called infection. It was not rare that these two concepts were confused in pathology, and they still are not accurately enough distinguished from each other, although there is a big difference between them. To the detriment of mankind, most cause to this confusion was given by miasmic and contagious typhoid epidemics, and again in recent times by yellow fever.

* * *

§9

Concluding remark

There are a thousand things in the world with which man is in contact and which, though they are situated outside man, either make him sick outright or put his organism or part of it into such a state that he becomes accessible to morbid matter. The principal external thing is the atmosphere. It has an unlimited range of action which we only partly know, everything in nature is subject to its influence, and it determines the fate of innumerable individuals. On one, it has a fatal effect; it can make the healthy sick and the sick healthy; it can develop or suppress the germ of sickness, depending on whether its composition is favorable or unfavorable, and in both cases it can be proved that in the former case it promoted the spread of contagion, and in the latter case prevented it. If, as was explained above, it is able to produce diseases, suppress sporadic ills, or change them into epidemics, it must be even easier for it to give existing diseases more emphasis, to provide them with more scope and a certain direction, and the question arises, what influence the atmosphere may have on miasmas and on contagions.

If we draw a sharp dividing line between the two sources of diseases, and let this side be the contagious, and on the far side the miasmic fevers in a certain order, the latter only lack some characteristic symptoms, the malignance and contagious power, otherwise they would be identical with the former. The disease this side is mirrored, as it were, in the disease on the other side, like the pest in typhoid fever, smallpox in varicella, yellow fever in bilious fever, cholera morbus in mild cholera, scarlet fever in prickly heat, contagious typhoid in typhus, contagious dysentery in benign autumn illness of this name;—whereas contagious diseases originated at the center of gravity of nature, the miasmic diseases exist only on a reduced scale. But if it can be proved that the latter diseases are only feeble reproductions of the former, that under certain circumstances the latter change into the former, that contagions can arise from miasmas, then the dispute about the origin of the plague, the yellow fever, scarlet fever, and their contagiousness is decided for good, and we then know whence the contagions come.

I may be permitted to make a comparison [between the two] that miasmas have their roots in the plant kingdom, the contagions belong to the animal kingdom. The contagions are on a higher level of perfection than the miasmas, they have an independence that the miasmas lack. The human organism bends under the force of the contagions, they impregnate the entire body, be it ever so healthy, and give its vitality a certain alien direction. The organism apparently plays a subordinate role here; it is unable to modulate the hostile force attacking it, therefore the effect of contagions is constant; therefore, they are able to maintain their independence in their reproduction, and therefore, they are equal to the animal and develop only from the living sick organism.—The miasmas, on the other hand, can excite only the diseased, the weak, the sensitive side of the organism. They subordinate their effect to the individual, and the success of miasmic influences is not determined by them but by the disposition of the affected individual. This also explains why one subject suffers from quartan fever, another from quotidian fever, a third from a glandular disease, and a fourth from a liver or a bilious ailment, although the cause in all these cases was the same. Here the miasma plays a subordinate role, it is unable to force the organism into a certain alien direction; on the contrary, it is modulated by the organism, and therefore it lacks the ability to reproduce. Therefore, it dies during its first act of procreation; thus, it is lower than the animal and develops from vegetables and dead substances.

If the miasma is to be raised to the highest level of pathological potency, if it is to be animalised and raised to the level of contagion, it must pass through the human organism, perhaps several times, and it must be hatched and brought to maturity by confined air, heated by the atmosphere. The strongest and most dangerous miasmas are those which develop from the bodies of sick persons who are crowded into a narrow space. They are much more dangerous than the miasmas which owe their existence to swamps and rotting and fermenting substances, for their nature has incorporated something animal-like, and it accepts increasingly of it, the more often they pass through the organism, so that they finally gain the infectious ability which contagions have. If the exhalations of such miasmatically sick are protected from access by atmospheric air, they cannot be decomposed or dissipated: they concentrate very soon and assume a contagious nature.

* * *

§14

Everything that comes into contact with contagious sick and such convalescents, or comes within their miasma orbit, be they living beings or inanimate objects

If the sickroom is so much filled with contagions, they adhere not only to the walls of the room, penetrate not only into the corners and gaps, but they also infect all the effects and utensils and adhere to everything that the sick person used and was in contact with him and with his miasma range. Therefore, if rooms in which contagious sick lay, or such convalescents live, are not aired properly and long enough, cleaned and whitewashed, the poison remains for years, and may communicate the disease to later inhabitants. A bricklayer in Ofen, who suffered from the plague in 1713 hid in the wall of his house a rag that had been polluted with the pus from his bubo, and closed this hole with a wooden wedge. A full year later, he repaired his house, opened that hole in which the rag still lay, and was immediately attacked again by the plague which then again spread through Ofen (Stocker). Hospitals, prisons, poor-houses, and ships yield sufficient opportunity for such observations. It is exactly the same with tools on and in which the contagion adheres. If they are not thoroughly cleaned and aired, they preserve the contagion, and transfer it at the first opportunity to healthy persons who come into contact with these objects, and are receptive to the poison. A man who took away an implement that had served a plague patient in order to burn it, was immediately infected by it; and in Hermann-stadt, says Chenot, the plague was resurrected when a pillow that had served a plague patient was put into use again after seven months.—Wool and cotton, furs, feathers, silk, linen, or cloth and clothes made from them, are the most suitable carriers of contagions; they preserve them for many years if they are protected against the access of atmospheric air, and can be transported over hundreds of miles without losing their infectious properties.* It was wool with which the plague contagion was brought to Toulon,** cotton with which it was brought from Smyrna and Algiers to Amsterdam in 1663,† and it came to Marseilles with several bales of goods.†† Such bales may pass through many countries, without doing any harm; the contagion is bound, latent. But it awakens and shows its pernicious effect as soon as the bale is opened. A bale of cloth, steeped in plague poison, spread the plague in Toulon only after it had been spread out, following its having remained tightly packed for a long time without doing any harm. Von Hildenbrand packed his black coat, in which in Vienna he had visited a patient suffering from scarlet fever, into his traveling trunk and went to Podolia. When he put on the said coat for the first time 18 months later, he was immediately attacked by scarlet fever which he spread in this region where there were no such sick persons. The clothing of such persons, who were with contagious patients, not only preserves the contagious substance for a long time, it is also thought to be even more contagious than the contagious patient himself.‡

* * *

* Diemerbroeck, "De peste," l. IV. Amstel. 1663. Van Swieten, "Comment.," T. V. §1382 and 1409. J. J. Kuntz, "Diss., inaugur. de peste," Giessae 1683, p. 11, §12.
** "Relation de la peste de Toulon," p. 100, 105, 106.
† Bohn, "Progr. ad diss. de morb. endem.," 1694.
†† "Traité de la peste," p. 7.
‡ Biblioth. Brit. T. XVI, p. 370. "Physical-Economic Excerpts," Vol. 5, pp. 7, 8. Chenot, p. 48, 49.

Chapter Three

Prevention of contagion

§1

The surest prevention of contagious diseases is doubtlessly achieved by exterminating the contagions and by destroying the receptiveness of the human body for such poisons. As regards the latter, so far, we have been successful only with smallpox, which thereby can be completely eliminated from human society. But the former could be achieved with certainty only at the spot where the contagions develop spontaneously. Their mode of origin must be investigated thoroughly, therefore, and to a greater extent, their sources must be blocked, as far as this is within man's power, and thus the contagions exterminated. However, since superstition, ignorance, and unconcern of certain nations make this hope still very remote, and since the contagions in question are not produced on European soil but are brought here from foreign countries, we can protect ourselves against them only by keeping them away from our soil, and if despite that, they reach the country, to endeavor as quickly as possible to destroy them and render them harmless. The present chapter is to show how this is to be achieved.

§2

It is one of the foremost tasks of the state to prevent persons or animals, goods, and all objects to which or whom contagions cling, from entering the country, and there is no doubt that governments are entitled to use all suitable means that do not contravene international law in order to achieve this. Provincial governments, therefore, must conclude conventions with each other to inform each other at the first suspicion of a contagious epidemic in their own or in other countries, and as long as this does not become general, every prudent state administration will obtain the quickest information on such a danger, and then immediately close the borders. This measure, which is known by the name of quarantine, is the first condition of preventing contagious diseases, if efficiently designed and strictly and well administered. Quarantine institutions are necessary not only at the borders of those countries in which contagious diseases rage in the form of epidemics, and which engage in

446

mutual traffic, they are also necessary at coasts and in ports which have trade connections with such countries. The best institutions of this kind are in Austria and France, and it is thanks to these nations that great trouble was several times averted, and we may even have to thank them for our very preservation. The greatest gain would be obtained if the Turks and the Egyptians followed our example.

* * *

England has very efficient quarantine laws.* Every ship bringing persons and goods from regions whence the government fears contagion is to be quarantined at a place, in the manner and for the time as ordered and made known by proclamation and through the London newspapers, and everything that is closely or distantly related to it is subject to the same laws. The quarantine court for the Thames is Standgate Creek. If a plague-like disease is discovered on a ship that is north of Cape Finisterre, the captain must sail without delay to St. Helen's Roads near the Scilly Islands or wherever else he is ordered, and inform a customs officer of his misfortune. The customs officer immediately reports it at the customs of some nearby port whence it is directly reported to the Royal Secretary of State, and the ship must await royal orders at the station. However, if the ship was carried into one of the channels, it is forbidden to enter a port, it must remain in the open roadstead and no man is permitted to land under threat of capital punishment. If there is plague somewhere, and if the order for quarantine has been given, then, when a ship arrives in a port, the highest customs official must go with those ordered for quarantine inspection, and ask from a proper distance what the name of the ship and the commander is, where it took on cargo, which places it touched on the way, whether any of the crew is infected, how long it had been on the way, who had died and of what, to which ships somebody of the crew transferred on the way, where these ships sailed, what kind of goods are on board, etc. If there is any sign of contagion, the ship must leave for a certain place of quarantine, or if necessary be taken there by force.—Keeping the infection secret is a capital crime, as is the refusal to obey the laws and the orders received.—When a ship has arrived at the quarantine, the commander must submit the health attestation, which must have been issued by some British consul, and his diary and log, to the chief of the quarantine commission; otherwise he is liable to a fine of 500 pounds. It is also forbidden under pain of high fines, to land goods at different times and places from those stipulated; also the messenger must no longer leave the ship. Even a person who has not been infected, once he or she has entered a place of quarantine, must not leave, and must remain there for the [quarantine] stipulated time. The conscientious and complete termination of the quarantine must finally be affirmed by the customs officer on the basis

* The main laws concerning this are: 2 Gro. II. 6 and 29. K; 12 Gro. III. 57. 29. K. 34 and 38. K. 33.—
  See "23rd report of the Finance Committee of the House of Commons, and Appendix," Vols. 7–9.

of a sworn statement by the skipper and two members of the crew, or two witnesses. After the necessary medical and other attestations have been produced, the authorities must issue the required certificate to the skipper and the crew. All kinds of forgeries under significant circumstances hereby are punishable by death; the same applies to those who secretly take letters or goods from a ship that has not yet passed the test.—If anywhere within or outside the Empire, the plague breaks out, then according to royal proclamation, no small vessel under 20 tons is permitted to leave a port unless it has deposited 300 pounds for fines against its sailing to any of the suspect places, or allowing any of the crew to transfer at sea to another ship, and undertaking not to take on board cargo from another ship. If a ship leaves without such security, it is confiscated, and the skipper is liable to an additional fine. According to the foregoing regulations, a quarantine officer is thus entitled to ask every arriving ship's commander the following questions: whether his ship touched the island of Rhodos, Morea, the African coasts, the Levant, or the Port of Mogador, or whether on the way back it was in touch with a ship coming from any of those ports, what pilots or other persons from the English coasts had been on board, or otherwise had any communication with the crew, and what diseases altogether had been observed on the ship.—All these regulations do not apply solely to the plague, but to all similar contagious diseases.*

§3

Thus a place of quarantine is a completely isolated institution which is so equipped that persons, animals, and goods, coming from countries where contagious feverish diseases rage, or having been near them, are received, cleaned, and disinfected, and observed and kept as long as is necessary in order that [the receiving country is] convinced of their healthy state. The place where such institutions are established must be removed from human habitations, must be high-lying and dry, and so roomy that the necessary departments can be adequately distant from each other. Among these is a house for the officials where, simultaneously, their requirements can be stored. Another house is that into which the suspect persons are locked. A third and fourth is for the sick and convalescents. There must be separate sties for suspect, sick, and recovering cattle, and a spacious place with sheds where suspect goods and effects are aired, cleaned, disinfected, and stored, and a cemetery. The whole is surrounded by a high wall which in turn is circled by a wide, deep, and distant moat.

Such institutions are necessary not only at sea but also on dry land. No port can dispense with them if it wants to make sure that epidemics are prevented, and they are equally necessary in the country at the frontiers, or if in some province or other contagious diseases rage. Austria has very many and excellently equipped, country quarantine institutions, especially on the Turkish border. Among the sea

* P. Colquhoun, "The Police of London," Leipzig, Part 2, p. 301 ff.—"Remarks on the British Quarantine Laws and the So-Called Sanitary Laws, etc.," by Ch. Maclean. London, 1823.

quarantine institutions, the best among those known in the world is doubtlessly the one at Marseilles, to which the city's extremely favorable position contributes.* As soon as a confirmed report is received that a contagious feverish disease has broken out in a neighboring state or in a distant country with which we are in contact, the ports are closed and feluccas cruise along the coasts. Watch posts are mounted, on land the frontiers are occupied by a military line, and the quarantines are actuated. When everybody at his station does his duty, when these institutions are administered with the greatest strictness and extreme punctiliousness, it is not easily possible for the disease to be brought into the country. It is necessary, therefore, that all quarantine officials be of proven integrity and have a decided liking for their occupation. The highest administration of the quarantine institutions must be in the hands of respected civil servants or such citizens who are impossible to bribe. Also required are a director and a physician, the former for economic and police matters, the latter for medical matters, and other male and female attendants for serving travelers who have been admitted, for cleaning the goods, etc. Every ship, and all persons, as soon as they approach the quarantine, are examined at some distance, and their health passes examined, etc., as described above; at the slightest suspicion they must be kept in quarantine before they are permitted to enter the country. It is cruel to refuse ships with sick crews which present themselves voluntarily for quarantine. Marseilles never does that, it admits every needy person, feeds and cleans such persons, disinfects ships and goods, as will be indicated below, against a certain compensation, and releases the healthy and cleaned, provided with new passes. It even received the sick army of 9,000 men upon its return from Egypt, and gave it comfort!

Lady von Freygang describes the quarantine institution to which she had to submit in December 1812 upon her return journey from Georgia, which had been infected by the plague. This occurred at Restow, called the St. Dmitri Fortress, on the river Don, near Nakhichevan, Arai, Novocherkassk and Taganrog. "At that place, one has to be provided with a certificate by the Governor General which confirms what the state of the country is, whence one comes, and whether the plague rages there or not. This paper is received by a man who wears tarred clothes and gloves. Then one is led into a shower where all effects are put down; one must separate those that one needs for the night and put them aside so that they are immediately fumigated with hydrochloric acid according to Guyton Morveau's method. Until this is done, one must put on the clothing that one is given. Then one goes to the inspection room. Here the women are examined by a woman who must state that

---

* "Dictionnaire d. sc. medicales," T. XXVII, p. 366 ff. Fischer's treatise on the quarantine institution at Marseilles, in his travel to Hyères. This work is also obtainable as a special printing. But since, in the meantime, Aubin-Louis Millin ("Voyage dans les départements du midi de la France," Paris 1807 and 1808. T. III, p. 218–243) gave some of this information in a better way, Mr. Fischer makes up for these amendments in Kopp, "Jahrb. der Staatsarzk.," 1st annual set, pp. 401–410.

she did not find the slightest sign of plague, whereupon one puts on the fumigated clothes. When the time of quarantine is over, one receives a certificate with which one is admitted to the country of the Don Cossacks."

As a rule, the duration of quarantine is, without exception, 40 days; in the meantime, it has been realized that in many cases this period is too long. In order to be certain that among the foreigners who arrived there is no infected one, not exactly 40 days are required.

* * *

After reporting on various preventive measures against infectious diseases (fresh air, acids, fumigation), he deals in the subsequent paragraphs with the great achievement of the 18th century: Edward Jenner's introduction of [cowpox] vaccination.

§12

Otherwise, conditions in reference to human smallpox are different. This is a general pest to which, except for a few cases, everyone is subject once, but only once. The means of protection is a salutary surrogate which, by inducing a mild illness that is absolutely harmless, although similar to the original illness, forever extinguishes the hereditary disposition of the animal organism. Vaccination, for only this can be meant here, is undoubtedly the greatest and most important discovery ever made for Medical Police, and it depends only on energetically applying the effective teachings of this science to remove forever epidemic smallpox from the face of the earth. To attain this final aim, the following is needed:

1) that the vaccine be generally introduced in all states, and
2) that the correct procedure in its application always be observed.

In that case, not only will smallpox, varioloid, varicella be completely eliminated and exterminated, but we soon will no longer even need vaccination. But so long as large states, even European ones, treat this matter halfheartedly and superficially, so long as clergymen and physicians declare themselves against the good cause, and so long as midwives, school teachers, escaped barber-surgeon apprentices, and persons who know little of vaccination and nothing of cowpox vaccine, themselves have permission to undertake this, and do so, we cannot dispense with the vaccine and we must clear it of the stain with which unauthorized hands have soiled it.

§13

The vaccination laws which have been enacted by various states so far intend mainly to induce people voluntarily or to impose indirect compulsion. When at the end of the last century Jenner made his great discovery known, societies and institutes were soon founded in various places which had the intention of promoting and spreading vaccination. Physicians who undertook this humanitarian activity were publicly decorated and rewarded by governments, and public physicians were employed who vaccinated every volunteer free of charge. The beneficial effect of the new invention was preached from the pulpit, it was made everybody's duty not to be against the matter, princes gave the best example and, like physicians, had their children vaccinated. The reasonable part of the nation followed suit, but this part was by far the smallest. One became convinced that this way vaccines would spread very slowly, and every day one saw victims of smallpox fall who could have been saved so easily. Stricter measures were therefore taken. Recipients of charity were refused any assistance if their children were not vaccinated, admission to an elementary school could not take place until the vaccination certificate had been produced. The same law applied to the apprentice who wanted to be apprenticed without payment to a master. Sick persons who had found charitable admission and cure in public hospitals were not permitted to be discharged unvaccinated, if they had not yet had smallpox.* Houses in which smallpox patients dwelt were marked with public warning notices, etc.

Despite these and similar regulations, we have not yet advanced so far as to be able to say that vaccination is generally widespread, and there are still enough parents who absolutely refuse to recognize their duty to safeguard their children against smallpox by a sufficiently proven means. Now, when Jenner's discovery is almost thirty years old, we still hear of killing smallpox epidemics in civilized states, and we are still far from the final aim of the vaccine, i.e., the complete extermination of smallpox. It is truly admirable what forbearance the governments display in such an extremely important matter, where the lives and health of millions are at stake, do not have recourse to the only, most certain, most efficient and most rapid means, and even hesitate to order general vaccination.

* * *

Universal vaccination, to which everybody has to submit who is not prevented from it by illness, is the only and the surest means of preventing an outbreak of smallpox and of stamping it out completely. There can no longer be any question whether a government is entitled to order universal vaccination; the government is entitled to do so. It has to protect dependent children against the folly and the ill will of their parents and not permit sensible and obedient citizens to suffer and incur danger because of the stupidity and obstinancy of a single individual.—Such universal vaccination is preceded by an enlistment in order to find out who has had smallpox, who is vaccinated, and who is not. Those who do it, go from house to house and make the house-owners responsible for not concealing any individual. Everybody who has not yet had smallpox and is not sick in bed is vaccinated. The costs are borne by the state. Every six months, possibly in spring and fall, the public

---

* Captain J. G. Stedman ("Voyage à Surinam et dans l'intérieur de la Guiane," traduit de l'Ang. par P. F. Henry, Paris an VII. T. I. p. 7) wisely proposes to vaccinate all persons destined for the army and the navy before they are posted.

vaccination is repeated, and everybody who has not had his children vaccinated by the time they are two years old is to be severely punished. Of course, everybody is free to choose whether to have his children vaccinated at the expense of the state by a physician employed for that purpose, or at his own expense by other physicians. In either case, the child to be vaccinated is kept under control, and if the defense pox develops normally, he receives a vaccination certificate which protects him from further penalty. Weak children can always be vaccinated; only real illness is a reason for postponement.

* * *

BIBLIOGRAPHY

ACKERKNECHT, E. H. Medizin der Aufklärung (Medicine of the Enlightenment).—*Schweiz. med. Wschr.*, Vol. 89, pp. 20–22. 1959.

ACKERKNECHT, E. H. *Kurze Geschichte der Medizin* (Brief History of Medicine). Stuttgart. 1967.

AUSPITZ, H. J. P. Franks Experimente über die Schutzkraft der Vaccine (J. P. Frank's Experiments with the Protective Power of Vaccines).—*Arch. Derm. Syph.*, Vol. 5, pp. 83–102. 1873.

BALLESTRASSE, F. Influenza del Brownismo in Italia: La Lettera ad un amico di Giuseppe Frank.—*Scientia Veterum*, Vol. 124, pp. 1–50. 1968.

BAMBERGER, H. VON. Zur Erinnerung an J. P. Frank (To the Memory of J. P. Frank).—*Wien. med. Jahrb.*, n.s., Vol. 1, pp. 97–116. 1886.

BARNARD, C. C. The Epistola Invitatoria of J. P. Frank.—*Janus*, Vol. 39, pp. 149–164. 1935.

BARNARD, C. C. Christian Rickmann (1741–1772) a Forgotten Pioneer of Social Medicine.—*Med. Hist.*, Vol. 1, pp. 226–236. 1957.

BAUMGARTNER, L. and E. M. RAMSEY. Johann Peter Frank and His "System einer vollständigen Medicinischen Polizey".—*Ann. Med. Hist.*, n.s., Vol. 5, pp. 525–532. 1933; Vol. 6, pp. 69–90. 1934.

BELLONI, L. La Medicina a Milano dal Settecento al 1915.—In: *Storia di Milano*, Vol. 16, Part 17, pp. 933–1028. Milano. 1962.

BERTEAUX, J. *Un pervers de génie J.-J. Rousseau. Essai de synthèse medico-psychologique.* Thèse pour le doctorat en médecine année scolaire, 1938–1939, No. 65. Lille. 1939.

BRANDT, R. *Rousseaus Philosophie der Gesellschaft* (Rousseau's Philosophy of Society). Stuttgart-Bad Cannstatt. 1973. (Problemata 16)

BREITENECKER, L. Die Bedeutung J. P. Franks für die Entwicklung der Hygiene in Österreich (The Importance of J. P. Frank for the Development of Hygiene in Austria).—WikliWo, Vol. 71, pp. 165–167. 1959.

BUCHER, H. W. *Tissot und sein Traité des nerfs. Ein Beitrag zur Medizingeschichte der schweizerischen Aufklärung* (Tissot and His Traité des nerfs. A Contribution to the History of Medicine of the Swiss Enlightenment).—*Zürch. med.-gesch. Abh.*, n.S., Vol. 1. Zürich. 1958.

CASTELLI, G. *Figure dell'Ottocento alla "Cà Grande".* Milano. 1940.

DIEPGEN, P. J. P. Frank im Lichte der Gegenwart (J. P. Frank in the Light of the Present).—*Klin. Wschr.*, Vol. 19, pp. 534–536. 1944.

DOLL, K. *Dr. Johann Peter Frank, 1745–1821. Der Begründer der Medizinalpolizei und der Hygiene als Wissenschaften. Ein Lebensbild* (Dr. Johann Peter Frank. 1745–1821. The Founder of the Medical Police and of Hygiene as Sciences. Description of His Life). Karlsruhe. 1909.

DUKA-ZÓLYOMI, N. and H. ROTTER. J. P. Franks Grundkonzept der Bekämpfung des Alko-
holismus (J. P. Frank's Basic Concept of Fighting Alcoholism).—WMW, Vol. 114, pp.
266–268. 1964.

DUKA-ZÓLYOMI, N. *Zacharias Gottlieb Hussty. 1754–1803. Mitbegründer der modernen Sozial-
hygiene* (Zacharias Gottlieb Hussty, 1754–1803. Co-Founder of Modern Social Hygiene).
Bratislava. 1972.

DURKHEIM, E. *Montesquieu and Rousseau, Forerunners of Sociology.* Translated by Ralph
Manheim.—Ann Arbor. 1960.

EBSTEIN, E. Über den Kliniker J. P. Frank in Pavia (The Clinician J. P. Frank in Pavia).—
Arch. stor. Sci., Vol. 4, pp. 326–330. 1923.

FISCHER, A. Zum Gedächtnis des Erscheinungsjahres (1779) von J. P. Franks Medicinischer
Polizey (To the Memory of the Year of Publication (1779) of J. P. Frank's Medical Police).—
SozHyg. Mitt., Vol. 13, pp. 74–80. 1929.

FISCHER, A. Natürliche und verschuldete Krankheiten (Natural and Man-Made Diseases).—
SozHyg. Mitt., Vol. 16, pp. 45–50. 1932.

FISCHER, A. *Geschichte des deutschen Gesundheitswesens* (History of German Public Health),
Vol. 2. Berlin. 1933.

FRACCARO, P. *L'università di Pavia.*—Küssnacht am Rigi. [n.d.]

FRANK, JOHANN PETER. *Biographie des Dr. Johann Peter Frank. Von ihm selbst geschrieben*
(Biography of Dr. Johann Peter Frank. Written by Himself). Wien. 1802.

FRANK, JOHANN PETER. *System einer vollständigen medicinischen Polizey* (A System of Complete Medical Police). 3rd Revised Edition. Wien. 1786–1817.

FRANK, JOHANN PETER. *Supplement-Bände zur medicinischen Polizey* (Supplementary Volumes
to the Medical Police), Vol. 1. Tübingen. 1812. 2nd and 3rd Vols. Published by G. Chr.
G. Voigt. Leipzig. 1825.

FRANK, JOHANN PETER. *Akademische Rede vom Volkselend als der Mutter der Krankheiten
(Pavia 1790).* Eingeleitet, ins Deutsche übertragen und mit Erklärungen versehen von
Erna Lesky (Academic Speech on The People's Misery—Mother of Diseases (Pavia. 1790).
Introduced, Translated into the German and Provided with Explanations by Erna Lesky).—
Sudhoffs Klassiker der Medizin, Vol. 34. Leipzig. 1960.

FRANK, JOHANN PETER. *Seine Selbstbiographie.* Hrsg., eingeleitet und mit Erläuterungen
versehen von Erna Lesky (His Autobiography. Edited, Introduced and Provided with
Explanations by Erna Lesky).—Hubers Klassiker der Medizin und der Naturwissenschaften,
Vol. 12. Bern-Stuttgart. 1969.

FRANK, JOHANN PETER. *La Biografia.* Edited by Pier Luigi Mondani, Translated by Francesco
Tantini.—Scientia Veterum, Vol. 133. Pisa. 1969.

GAUTIER, L. *La Médecine à Genève jusqu'à la fin du XVIIIe siècle.* Genève. 1906.

GREEN, F. C. *Jean-Jacques Rousseau. A Critical Study of His Life and Writings.* Cambridge.
1955.

GUHRAUER, G. E. Aus den ungedruckten Denkwürdigkeiten der Aerzte Johann Peter und
Jos. Frank (From the Unprinted Reminiscences of the Physicians Johann Peter and Jos.
Frank).—*Dtsch. Museum,* Vol. 2, pp. 15–35. Leipzig. 1852.

HAAG, F. E. Bernhard Christoph Faust und Johann Peter Frank (Bernhard Christoph
Faust and Johann Peter Frank).—MMW, Vol. 87, pp. 1031–1033. 1940.

HARMS, B. Die Vorgänger J. P. Franks (The Predecessors of J. P. Frank).—*Wiss. Z. Karl-Marx-Univ. Lpz.*, Mathematisch. naturwiss. Reihe, Vol. 5, pp. 81–86. 1955–1956.

HAUBOLD, H. *Johann Peter Frank, der Gesundheits- und Rassenpolitiker des 18. Jahrhunderts* (Johann Peter Frank, the Health and Race Politician of the 18th Century). München-Berlin. 1939.

HAUBOLD, H. J. P. Frank bereitet die Herausgabe seiner Medicinischen Polizey vor (J. P. Frank Prepares the Publication of His Medical Police).—*Sudhoffs Arch. Gesch. Med. Naturw.*, Vol. 32, pp. 314–316. 1939.

HAUBOLD, H. Wie J. P. Frank aus Wien vertrieben wurde (How J. P. Frank was Driven from Vienna).—MMW, Vol. 86, pp. 1125–1128. 1939.

HELLER, R. J. P. Frank's "De morbis pecudum".—*Bull. Hist. Med.* [in press].

HIRSCH, A., E. GURLT, and A. WERNICH. *Biographisches Lexikon der hervorragenden Ärzte aller Zeiten und Völker* (Biographical Lexicon of the Outstanding Physicians of All Times and Nations). 3rd Edition, Edited by V. Haberling, F. Hübotter, K. Vierordt. 6 Volumes. München-Berlin. 1962.

HOFFMANN, K. F. J. P. Frank, der Begründer der Hygiene (J. P. Frank, the Founder of Hygiene).—MMW, Vol. 93, p. 1750. 1951.

KING, L. S. *The Road to Medical Enlightenment, 1650–1695*. London-New York. 1970.

KING, L. S. Friedrich Hoffmann and Some Medical Aspects of Witchcraft.—*Clio Med.*, Vol. 9, pp. 299–309. 1974.

KING, L. S. Witchcraft and Medicine. Conflicts in the Early Eighteenth Century.—In: *Circa Tiliam. Studia Historiae Medicinae. Gerrit Arie Lindeboom septuagenario oblata*, pp. 122–139. Leiden. 1974.

KOELSCH, F. Zum Gedenken an Johann Peter Frank, den Begründer der deutschen Sozialmedizin (To the Memory of Johann Peter Frank, the Founder of German Social Medicine). —MMW, Vol. 107, pp. 1958–1959. 1965.

KOELSCH, F. Johann Peter Frank—seine Bedeutung für die Arbeitsmedizin (Johann Peter Frank—His Importance for Labor Medicine).—*Dtsch. Ärztebl.*, Vol. 63. 1735–1737, 1777–1781, 1812–1813, 1855–1887. 1966.

KRATTER, J. Über J. P. Frank und seine Bedeutung für die Entwicklung der Gesundheitspflege (On J. P. Frank and His Importance for the Development of Hygiene).—*Österr. Sanitätsbeamte*, Nos. 1/3, p. 33. 1888.

LESKY, E. Johann Peter Frank als Organisator des medizinischen Unterrichts (Johann Peter Frank as Organizer of Medical Teaching).—*Sudhoffs Arch. Gesch. Med. Naturw.*, Vol. 39, pp. 1–29. 1955.

LESKY, E. *Österreichisches Gesundheitswesen im Zeitalter des aufgeklärten Absolutismus* (Austrian Hygiene in the Period of Enlightened Absolutism).—Arch. f. österr. Gesch., 122/1. Published by Österr. Akad. d. Wiss. Wien. 1959.

LESKY, E. Von der Staatsarzneikunde zur Hygiene (From State Medicine to Hygiene).—WilkiWo, Vol. 71, pp. 168–171. 1959

LESKY, E. Johann Peter Frank.—In: *Neue Deutsche Biographie*, Vol. 5, pp. 341–342. Berlin. 1961.

LESKY, E. *Die Wiener medizinische Schule im 19. Jahrhundert*. Studien zur Geschichte der Universität Wien (The Vienna Medical School in the 19th Century. Studies Pertaining to the History of the Vienna University), Vol. 6. Graz-Köln. 1965.

LESKY, E. Johann Peter Frank.—In: *Die berühmten Ärzte,* pp. 148–150. Edited by R. Dumesnil and H. Schadewaldt. Köln. 1966.

LESKY, E. Medizin im Zeitalter der Aufklärung (Medicine in the Period of the Enlightenment). —In: *Lessing und die Aufklärung,* pp. 77–99. Veröffentl. d. Joachim Jungius-Gesellschaft d. Wissenschaften Hamburg. Göttingen. 1968.

LIPPICH, F. W. *De Maximiliani Stoll et Joannis Petri Frank. Vita praecipuisque meritis in praesentem medicinae statum.* Wien. 1845.

MAIWALD, K. H. Johann Peter Frank 1745–1821. Sein Beitrag zur Kenntniss des Diabetes mellitus (Johann Peter Frank, 1745–1821. His Contribution to the Knowledge of Diabetes Mellitus).—*Die Therapie des Monats,* No. 10/1, pp. 14–20. 1960.

MERBACH, [P. M.]. J. P. Frank als Begründer der medizinischen Polizei und öffentlichen Gesundheitspflege in Deutschland (J. P. Frank as the Founder of the Medical Police and Public Health Service in Germany).—*Jber. Ges. Natur-a Heilk.* Dresden 1880–1881, pp. 66–71. 1881.

METZE, M.-G. *J. P. Frank und seine Beziehungen zur Arbeitshygiene* (J. P. Frank and His Relationship to Labor Hygiene).—Med. Diss. Erlangen. 1948. [Typescript]

MIDELFORT, E. H. C. *Witch Hunting in Southwestern Germany, 1562–1684. The Social and Intellectual Foundations.* Stanford, California. 1972.

MÜLLER-DIETZ, H. J. P. Frank und die Reform des medizinischen Studiums in Petersburg (J. P. Frank and the Reform of Medical Study in Petersburg).—*Verhandl. XX. Internat. Kongr. Gesch. Med. Berlin,* 98–102. Hildesheim. 1968.

NEUBERGER, M. J. P. Frank als Begründer der Rückenmarkspathologie (J. P. Frank as the Founder of the Pathology of the Spinal Cord).—WikliWo, Vol. 22, pp. 1341–1343. 1909.

NEUBURGER, M. Ein neurologisches Konsilium P. Franks (A Neurological Consilium by P. Frank).—WMW, Vol. 62, pp. 2439–2440. 1912.

NEUBURGER, M. J. P. Frank und die Neuropathologie (J. P. Frank and Neuropathology).— WikliWo, Vol. 26, pp. 627–631. 1913.

NEUBURGER, M. *Das alte medizinische Wien in zeitgenössischen Schilderungen* (The Old Medical Vienna in Contemporary Descriptions). Wien-Leipzig. 1921.

NEUBURGER, M. Die Begründung der öffentlichen Hygiene als Wissenschaft durch J. P. Frank (The Founding of Public Hygiene as a Science by J. P. Frank).—*Mitt. Volksgesundh-Amts, Wien,* No. 12, pp. 114–118. 1930.

PROBST, CH. Johann Peter Frank als Arzt am Krankenbett (Johann Peter Frank as Physician at the Sickbed).—*Sudhoffs Arch. Gesch. Med. Naturw.,* Vol. 59, pp. 20–53. 1975.

PUSCHMANN, TH. *Die Medicin in Wien während der letzten 100 Jahre* (Medicine in Vienna during the Last 100 Years). Wien. 1884.

QUADT, M. *Materialien zur Beurteilung der Beziehungen J.-J. Rousseaus zur Heilkunde seiner Zeit* (Materials for Judging the Relation of J. J. Rousseau to Medicine of His Time).— Med. Diss. Berlin. 1944. [Typescript].

RANG, M. *Rousseaus Lehre vom Menschen* (Rousseau's Teaching on Man). 2nd Edition. Göttingen. 1965.

ROHLFS, H. Johann Peter Frank, der Begründer der Medicinalpolizei (Johann Peter Frank, the Founder of the Medical Police).—In: *Die medicinischen Classiker Deutschlands,* Sec. 2, pp. 127–211. Stuttgart. 1880 (with Bibliography of Frank's works).

ROSEN, G. What is Social Medicine? A Genetic Analysis of the Concept.—*Bull.' Hist. Med.,* Vol. 3, pp. 11–46, 279–314. 1948.

ROSEN, G. Cameralism and the Concept of Medical Police.—*Bull. Hist. Med.,* Vol. 27, pp. 21–42. 1953.

ROSEN, G. Hospitals, Medical Care and Social Policy.—*Bull. Hist. Med.,* Vol. 30, pp. 124–149. 1956.

ROSEN, G. The Fate of the Concept of Medical Police.—*Centaurus,* Vol. 5, pp. 97–113. 1957.

ROSEN, G. *A History of Public Health.* New York. 1957.

Rousseau, Jean-Jacques et son oeuvre. Problèmes et recherches.—Commémoration et colloque de Paris, 16–20 Oct. 1962. Paris. 1964. (Actes et colloques 2).

RUDOLF, G. Jean-Jacques Rousseau (1712–1778) und die Medizin (Jean-Jacques Rousseau (1712–1778) and Medicine).—*Sudhoffs Arch. Gesch. Med. Naturw.,* Vol. 53, pp. 30–67. 1969.

SABINE, J. C. The Civil Administrator—Most Successful Physician.—*Bull. Hist. Med.,* Vol. 16, pp. 289–318. 1944.

SCHILLER, F. Health Aspects of the Noble Savage. Origin, Definition, and Subgroups: Noble, Holy, Metaphorical and Real Savages.—*Clio Medica,* Vol. 6, pp. 253–273. 1971.

SCHMITZ, K. E. F. *Die Bedeutung Johann Peter Franks für die Entwicklung der sozialen Hygiene* (Johann Peter Frank's Importance for the Development of Social Hygiene), Vol. 6, No. 7.— Veröffentl. a. d. Geb. d. Medizinalverwaltung. Berlin. 1917.

SCHNELLER, J. *Rede zum Andenken Peter Frank's. Gehalten am 5. Juni 1852* (Speech in Memory of Peter Frank. Held on 5 June 1852). Wien. 1852.

SEILER, H. *Peter Frank (geb. 1745, gest. zu Wien 1821) zu seinem 150 jährigen Geburtstage den 14. März 1895 nach den eigenen Aufzeichnungen desselben* (Peter Frank (Born 1745, Died in Vienna 1821) to His 150th Birthday on 14 March 1895 According to His Own Notes). Dresden. 1895.

SHKLAR, J. N. *Men and Citizens. A Study of Rousseau's Social Theory.* Cambridge Studies in the History and Theory of Politics. Cambridge. 1969.

SHRYOCK, R. H. *The Development of Modern Medicine: an Interpretation of the Social and Scientific Factors Involved.*—Univ. of Pa. Press, Philadelphia. 1936. Revised Edition: New York. 1947. English Edition: Oxford Univ. Press. London. 1948.

SIGERIST, H. E. The People's Misery: Mother of Diseases, an Address Delivered in 1790 by J. P. Frank, Translated from the Latin, with an Introduction by H. E. Sigerist.—*Bull. Hist. Med.,* Vol. 9, pp. 81–100. 1941.

SIGERIST, H. E. *Landmarks in the History of Hygiene,* pp. 47–63.—Oxford Univ. Press. London. 1956.

SIGERIST, H. E. Johann Peter Frank.—In: *Grosse Ärzte. Eine Geschichte der Heilkunde in Lebensbildern.* 4th Revised and Enlarged Edition, pp. 217–229. München. 1959.

STÜBLER, E. *Geschichte der medizinischen Fakultät Heidelberg 1386–1925.* (History of the Medical Faculty Heidelberg. 1386–1925). Heidelberg. 1926.

TREUE, W. *Mit den Augen ihrer Leibärzte* (With the Eyes of Their Physicians-in-Ordinary), pp. 97–100. Düsseldorf. 1955.

TRZEBIŃSKI, ST. Dwa listy Dr. de Carro w sprawie pamiętników Józéfa Franka.—*Archwm. Hist. Filoz. Med.,* Vol. 4, pp. 313–316. 1926.

Trzebiński, St. *Des Mémoires de Jean-Pierre et Joseph Frank rédigés par ce dernier* (Manuscrit de la Société de Médecine de Wilno). Wilno. 1928–1929.

Vaccari, P. *Storia della Università di Pavia.* Pavia. 1957.

Valsecchi, F. *L'assolutismo illuminato in Austria e in Lombardia.* 2 Vols. Bologna. 1931–1934.

Vaughan, C. E. *The Political Writings of Jean-Jacques Rousseau.* 2 Vols. Cambridge. 1915.

Vetter, R. *Die medizinischen Fakultäten in Leipzig und Strassburg zu Goethes Studienzeit* (The Medical Faculties in Leipzig and Strasbourg at the Time of Goethe's Studies).—Med. Diss. Bonn. 1950.

Wandruszka, A. *Leopold II., Erzherzog von Österreich, Grossherzog von Toskana, König von Ungarn und Böhmen, Römischer Kaiser* (Leopold II, Archduke of Austria, Grand Duke of Toscana, King of Hungary and Bohemia, Roman Emperor), 2 Vols. München-Wien. 1963–1965.

Wieger, F. *Geschichte der Medizin und ihrer Lehranstalten in Strassburg* (History of Medicine and Its Schools in Strasbourg). Strasbourg. 1885.

Wurzbach, C. von. *Biographisches Lexikon des Kaiserthums Österreich* (Biographical Lexicon of the Austrian Empire), 60 Vols. Wien. 1856–1891. 1 Reg.—Vol. 1923.

Zeiss, H. Deutsche Ärzte in Russland (German Physicians in Russia).—AGM, Vol. 31, pp. 219–246. 1938.

Zeiss, H. J. P. Franks Tätigkeit in St. Petersburg (J. P. Frank's Activity in St. Petersburg).—*Klin. Wschr.,* Vol. 12, pp. 353–356. 1939.

INDEX OF PERSONAL NAMES

Aesculapius, 303
Albinus, Bernhard Siegfried, 360
Alexander I., ix, xiii
Astruc, Jean, 360
Augustus, 57
Bacon, Francis, 253, 391
Baumer, Johann Wilhelm, 13
Becher, Johann Joachim, xv
Borelli, Giovanni Alfonso, 278
Brown, John, 317
Cabanis, Pierre Jean Georges, 314f.
Citois (Citesius), François, 294
Constantine, 57, 223, 250
Cook, James, 184, 297
Daniel, Christian Friedrich, 285
Eberhard, Johann, 285
Eller, Johann Theodor, 291
Empedocles, 294
Esquirol, Jean-Etienne-Dominique, 426
Fothergill, John, 278f.
Frank, Johann Peter, vii–xxiii
Frank, Joseph, 387
Franz II, xiii
Frederick I, of Prussia, 306
Gassner, Johann, xxif., 252, 258f.
Gilibert, Jean-Emanuel, 317, 389
Gregory, John, 337
Gruner, Christian Gottfried, 285
Guyton-Morreau, Louis Bernard, 290, 449
de Haen, Anton, 244
Haller, Albrecht von, 54, 256, 423
Heister, Lorenz, 38, 304
Hensler, Philipp Gabriel, 291
Hoffmann, Christoph Ludwig, 422
Homer, 295
Hörnigk, Philipp Wilhelm von, xv
Horn, Ernst, 429

Jenner, Edward, 291, 434, 450
Joseph II, ix, xif., xvf., xixf., 179, 199, 216, 227, 279, 291, 342, 382
Justi, Heinrich Gottlob von, xv
Krünitz, Johann Georg, 231f.
Lancisi, Giovanni Maria, 293, 331
Leake, John, 357, 359f.
Leopold II, xiii, 85, 224
Locke, John, 129
Mai, Franz Anton, xxii, 259
Maret, Hugues, 420
Maria Theresa, xv
Marsilius, Ficinus, 351
Mercurialis, Hieronymus, 257, 436
Mirabeau, Victor de Riqueti, 106
Mohammed, 436
Montaigne, Michel de, 129
Morgagni, Giovanni Battista, 425
Müller, Peter, 38
Muratori, Ludovico Antonio, 290
Napoleon I, ix, xiv
Palloni, Gaetano, 436
Petit, Marc-Antoine, 420
Pinel, Philippe, 426
Poyet, Bernard, 420
Ramazzini, Bernardino, 126, 185, 294, 441
Rauen, Wolfgang Thomas, 15
Reimarus, Johann Albrecht Henrich, 307
Rickmann, Christian, 15
Roederer, Johann Georg, 360
Röschlaub, Andreas, 354
Rousseau, Jean Jacques, xvif., 10, 17–20, 64, 106, 112, 154, 214, 302
Ruysch, Fredrik, 360
Sacombe, Jean-Francois, 359
Samoilowitz, 436
Scarpa, Antonio, 298

Scherf, Johann Christian Friedrich, 287
Sennert, Daniel, 244, 257
Smyth, James Carmichael, 290
Sonnenfels, Joseph von, xv, 85, 116, 196, 287
Spe, Friedrich von, 253ff.
Sprengel, Kurt, 316
Stifft, Joseph Andreas, xiii
Stoll, Johann, 286f., 389
Stoll, Maximilian, 432
Süssmilch, Johann Peter, 33, 44, 54, 97, 158, 240, 298
Swieten, Gerard van, xiii, 56, 73, 84, 194, 293
Sydenham, Thomas, 392
Tissot, Simon André, 83, 129, 241, 344

Tronchin, Théodore, 291
Tuke, Daniel Hack, 425f.
Uden, Konrad Friedrich, 140
Unzer, Johann August, 265, 309
Valli, Eusebio, 436
Voigt, Georg Christian Gotthilf, 389, 406
Weyer, Johann, xxi, 244, 251, 253, 256, 293
Willis, Thomas, 257
Wolff, Christian, xvi
Wrabez, Joachim, 381
Zacchias, Paolo, 194
Zacutus, Lusitanus, 250
Zimmermann, Johann Georg, 180, 192, 243, 259

INDEX OF SUBJECTS AND PLACES

Abdominal paracentesis, 303.
Abortion, 96, 102–107.
Accident, definition of, 207f.
Accidents, xix, 13, 203–206, 209–217;
  of children, 109–111.
Accoucheur, 81f., 357–360.
Aggression, 228f., 235–238.
Air
  cleanliness of, 118, 411, 422f.
  in foundling hospitals, 118.
  in hospitals, 411, 416, 419f., 422f.
  in human habitations, 177.
  pollution of, 177ff., 185, 194f.
Alcoholism, 18, 156, 157f.
America, 179.
Amsterdam, Holland, 178, 445.
Amulets, 249f.
Amusements, 168–174;
  bullfights, 223f.
  music, 173f.
  psychological aspects of, 168f., 223.
  theater plays, 171f.
Anatomy
  beginnings of, 331.
  high degree of perfection of, 331.
  teaching of, 317f.
Animal fights, 223f.
Animal magnetism, 307.
Apoplexy, 156.
Apothecaries, 301f., 306, 398, 429.
Apparent death, 13, 217–280, 298, 303;
  definition of, 273.
  instruction of physicians on, 275.
  reanimation measures, 274f.
Army, 49f.
Assistants
  duties of, 350.

in hospitals, 431.
Astrology, 247, 436.
Austria, 28;
  fertility, 56.
  hospitals, 392.
  post-mortem examinations, 334.
  quarantine institutions, 437, 447f.
  universities, 392.
Authorities, 57f., 68.

Bachelors, see Secular celibacy;
  taxing of, 34f.
Baptism treats, 158f.
Bedside teaching, xii, 299, 318f., 339–352, 372f.,
  392;
  by the Socratic method, 351.
  examination of the sick, 347–349.
  in surgery, 355.
Beggar, 127, 302.
Behavior
  aggressive, of human beings, 228f.
  in traffic, 214–217.
  of common people concerning medicine, 308f.
  of dying persons, 263.
  of hunters, 221, 226f.
  of nations, 168f.
  of physicians, 302f.
  of pregnant women, 72f., 102.
  of students toward different classes, 313.
  of the poor, 428.
Berlin, xiv;
  hospitals, 116, 420, 429.
  inoculation, 291.
  mortality of newborn infants, 116.
  suicide, 240.
Birth
  city women giving, 65.

Birth (cont.)
  peasant women giving, 65.
  statistics, 115.
Birth control, *see* Conception.
Blindness, 187.
Boredom, 169.
Botanical gardens, 14, 382.
Brawls, 236f.
Brothels, 98–101.
Bruchsal, Germany, x, 258, 381.
Burying alive, 265–267.

Cameralism, xv.
Castration, 58.
Catholic Church, 6f., 28f., 173, 263f.
Cattle diseases
  magic cures for, 251f.
Case history, 349f.
Celibacy, 6f., 241;
  clerical, 27–31.
  military, 49f.
  secular, 32–35.
Charlatans, 304, 306f., 308.
Chemical laboratories, 221.
Chemistry, 301, 306.
Child
  care, 110f.
  labor, xviii, 50, 121, 126f.
  murder, 92, 103–107, 114.
  neglect, 116.
Childbed, 79–85.
Children
  abandoning of, 103ff., 114ff.
  accidents of, 109–111.
  amulets worn by, 249.
  as beggars, 127.
  diseases of, caused by witches, 257.
  illegitimate, 97f., 114.
  mortality of, 98.
  nutrition of, 112f.
Cleanliness, public, 183–196;
  of nations, 183.
  of rivers, 184.
  of streets, 186–190.
Climate, 21, 180.
Clinical schools, 299, 339–352;
  lack of patients with various diseases, 373.
  necessary doubling of the clinic and its teachers, 343f.

St. Petersburg, 332.
Vilna, 332.
Clothing, 68f.;
  effects of fashions, 163.
  effects of, on sex appeal, 162.
  general considerations of healthy, 161f.
Conception
  prevention of, 96, 115f.
Confession, 263f.
Consilia medica, 351f.
Contagious diseases, 434–452;
  causes of, 439f.
  in foundling hospitals, 119.
  in hospitals, 411.
Convent education, 66f.
Cooks, 159.
Corset, 68f., 165f.
Creator, *see* God.
Croup, 294.

Dances, 67f., 132f.
Death
  differences from life, 266.
Death penalty, 105f.
Debauchery, 18, 32, 50, 58, 92, 95, 154, 156, 313.
Degeneration, xvii, 12, 134;
  of peasants, 49f.
Dietary laws, 146f.
Diseases
  as punishment, 436.
  division of, 353.
  duration of, economic considerations, 302.
  incurable, 411.
  suitable for admittance into hospitals, 411ff.
Dispensatory, 429.
Dissection, *see* Anatomy, Morbid anatomy.
District physicians, 397f., 409.
Divorce, 59f.
Drinking water, 150–152.
Dropsy, 303.
Drugs
  administration of, 301.
Dwellings, 175–180;
  construction of, 181.
Dying persons, 262–264;
  behavior of, 263.
  psychological treatment of, 263f.
  spiritual succor for, 262f.

Ecology, *see* Pollution.
Edinburgh, Scotland
    bedside teaching, 299, 341.
    three clinical teachers, 343.
Education, 122–135;
    effects of theater on, 171.
    general rules of, 122f.
    health, 64–69, 128f.
    in foundling hospitals, 120.
    monastic, 66f., 135.
    of civil servants concerning health, 330.
    of people concerning health, 309.
    of physicians on how to proceed with the apparently dead, 275.
    scholastic, 369.
England
    accidents, 205.
    behavior, 169.
    hospitals, 424.
    lunatic asylums, 426.
    midwifery, 360.
    quarantine laws, 447.
    suicide, 240.
    theater plays, 172.
Enlightenment, 244, 257f.;
    function of priest in, 275.
    function of schoolteacher in, 275.
    lack of, 308.
    social changes due to, 322.
Epidemics, 290, 294, 398, 434–452.
Epileptics, 412.
Excitability, 336f.
Exorcism, xxf., 252, 258.

Fashion, 163;
    in hairdressing, 164.
    in make-up, 165f.
Fecundity, *see* Fertility.
Fertility, 53ff.;
    female, 54.
Feudalism, xviii–xx.
Fever
    hospital, 412.
    intermittent, 301, 412.
    miasmatic, 443f.
    scarlet, 412.
Fiber, 336f.
Fire, 219f.
Floods, 218f.

Foodstuffs
    animal, 146f.
    examination of, 145, 399.
    grain, 148.
    in general, 144f.
    shortage of, 139f., 148f.
    vegetable, 148f.
Forceps, 301, 358.
Forensic medicine, 5, 11, 140, 285, 304, 394.
Forests
    influences on health, 21.
Foundling hospitals, 114–121;
    in Coimbra, 120.
    in Grenoble, 117.
    in London, 117.
    in Montpellier, 117.
    in Paris, 115, 118f.
    mortality in, 116f.
    number of foundlings in, 115.
France
    behavior, 169.
    celibacy, 28.
    hospitals, 422.
    marriage, 62.
    medical curriculum, 339.
    population, 16.
    suicide, 239.
    swamps, 179.
    theater, 170, 172
    treatment of dying persons, 263f.
    treatment of pregnant women, 75.
Freedom, 33, 63, 199, 312, 313.
Freiburg/Breisgau, Germany, xiv, 271.

Germany
    behavior, 169.
    charlatans, 306f.
    climate, 21.
    fashion, 163.
    health conditions, 176.
    hospitals, 424.
    hunting, 220f.
    intemperance, 157.
    post-mortem examinations, 332.
    sorcery, 245.
    suicide, 239.
    surgeons, 314.
    theater, 172.
Gheel, Belgium, 426f.

God, 25, 38, 47, 79, 91, 144, 153, 161, 165, 246, 436.
Göttingen, Germany, xi, 337.
Gout, 156, 303.
Gymnastics, 128–131, 296.

Hamburg, Germany
    reanimation mandate, 274f.
    street regulations, 187.
Hangman
    as physician, 306.
Health education, *see* Education.
Heidelberg, Germany, ixf.
Herniotomy, 58.
Hippocratic medicine, 295f., 316, 391.
Holland, 183, 218.
Hospitals, 409–414;
    administration of, 433.
    admittance into, 411ff.
    air in, 416, 421f.
    as schools for physicians, 339, 341–352, 410.
    Charité, Berlin, 116, 420, 429.
    criticism of, 139.
    director of, 430f.
    disorders in large, 418.
    foundations of, 13f.
    General Hospital, Vienna, xi, 383, 405, 411.
    in Bruchsal, 381.
    in England, 424.
    in La Rochelle, 117.
    in London, 419f., 421.
    in Paris, 418f.
    in Vienna, 117.
    mortality in, 409.
    number of physicians in, 432.
    paying patients in, 410f.
    physicians in, 431f.
    shape of, 419f.
    special, 424f.
    type of construction, location of, 415ff.
Hospital fever, 409, 412, 419, 422, 444.
Hungary
    climate of, 21.
Hunger, 148.
Hunting, xixf.;
    accidents, 220f.
    dangers for peasants, 226f.
Hydrochloric gas, 290.
Hysteria, 258, 412.

Illegitimate birth, 94.

Indian medicine, 296.
Injuries
    caused by animals, 109f.
    on the street (to pedestrians), 188f.
Inoculation, 291, 380.
Insanity, 425–428.
Intemperance, 153, 160;
    diseases caused by, 156.
Internal medicine, 299;
    necessary doubling of the clinic and its teacher,
        343ff.
    professor of, and director of hospital, 342.
    teaching of, 338. *See* Bedside teaching.
Isolation, 413, 422
Italy
    climate, 21.
    hospitals, 424.
    murders, 235f.
    nocturnal noise, 224f.
    poisoning, 233.
    poor relief, 424.
    population, 16.
    walking on foot, 20.

Jesuits, 30, 199, 369.
Jews, 63;
    dietary laws of, 146f.
    evaluation of pregnancy among, 70.
    hygiene of, 142.

Kalmuks, 250.

Latrines, 191f.
Lead colic, 294.
Leipzig, Germany
    accidents, 203.
    suicide, 240.
Leprosy, 435f.
Leyden, Holland
    bedside teaching, 299, 341.
License for medical practice, 372–375, 397.
Life
    invisible, 266, 273.
    visible, 266.
Lists
    of births, 398.
    of deaths, 398.
    of pregnant women, 75f.
Livorno, Italy, 436.

Lombardy, xii, xviii, 199, 212, 342, 375.
London
  accidents, 203f.
  alcoholism, 157.
  cleanliness (dirty streets), 183f., 186, 188.
  hospitals, 419, 421.
  smog, 196.
  traffic, 215.
Love, 61.
Lunatic asylums, 417, 425–427;
  in Paris, 427.
  in Vienna, 425.
Lunatics, 425–427;
  admission in asylums, 426.
  treatment of, 425f.
Luxury, xvii, 17, 20, 134, 145, 156, 181, 407, 415.

Magic, xx–xxii, 244–261;
  cures for cattle diseases, 251f.
  medical tricks, 250.
Make-up, 165f.
Malaria, 441.
Malta, 187.
Marriage, 36–52;
  fertility of, 41.
  free choice, 62.
  impediments to, 46–52.
  love in, 61.
  prohibition of, 49f.
  promotion of, 34f., 49, 61.
  purpose of, 40, 53.
  quarrells in, 57f.
  time for, 36ff.
Marseille, France, 436f., 445, 449.
Masturbation, 241, 292.
Maternity hospitals, 14, 427f.
Medical associations, 299.
Medical board, 394;
  Supreme Medical Board, 396–399.
Medical Curriculum, xii;
  must be conducted by good teachers, 314.
  of France, 339.
  of Pavia, 327, 334, 355.
  principles of, 317–322.
Medical education, 311;
  by demonstration of objects, 318–320.
  by teaching to doubt everything, 321.
  principles of, 317–322.
  time required for, 320.

Medical ethics, 302f., 305f., 324.
Medical examinations, 365;
  causes of the failure of, 366–370.
  number of examiners, 368f.
Medical journals, 299.
Medical Police
  apology for, 140ff.
  concept of, x, 287.
  contents of, 90.
  continuation of, 199f., 271f., 285f., 379.
  criticism of, 286f.
  definition of, xvi, 12f., 287f.
  freedom and, 10f., 141.
  influence on the states, 291, 388.
  preparatory work of, 3.
  purpose of, 4f., 8, 11, 23, 89.
  terminology of, 285.
Medical research, 410.
Medical schools, 311–410;
  fundamental instruction at, 327.
  postgraduate studies at, 328.
  practical instruction at, 318f.
  seat of, 312.
Medical topography, 180, 398.
Medicine
  based on experience, 316, 391.
  causes of the inefficiencies of, 307f.
  defense of, against charges, 153f.
  definition of, 390.
  division of, 289, 295.
  history of, 295.
  importance of, for the state, 391.
  progress in, 297.
  specialization of, 295.
  theoretical, 391f.
  unification of, with surgery, 353–355.
  utility of, 289–305.
Melancholy, 169, 172, 241. 409.
Mental disorder,
  philosophy of, 316.
Mercury, 301, 412;
  salivation caused by, 412.
Miasmas, 440–443.
Midwifery, x, 72, 80f., 300, 357–361;
  appreciation of, 357.
Mines, 212;
  miners' diseases, 441.
Miracles, 252f., 260.
Misery, see Poverty.

Morbid anatomy, 14, 331–335;
    museum of, xii, 319f., 334f., 381, 398; *see* Post-
    mortem examinations.
Mortality rate
    caused by alcoholism, 157f.
    during childbed, 298, 300, 357.
    in foundling hospitals, 116f.
    in hospitals, 409.
    in large cities, 153, 181.
    of children, 128.
    smallpox, 291.
    venereal diseases, 297.
Moscow, 436.
Murder, 235f.
Music, xiii, 171f., 173f.

Nations
    behavior of, 169.
    cleanliness of, 183.
Natural history, 330.
Natural philosophy, 306f., 316.
Nature, 37, 61, 64, 108, 144, 153, 161, 165, 181, 257,
    302.
Nervous diseases, 19, 156, 297.
Nile, 185.
Nobility, 30, 133f.;
    behavior of, 221, 226f., 230f.
    education of, 66.
    intemperance of, 157.
    post-mortem examinations of, 332.
    sterility of, 55.
Noise, 224f.
Nosology, 339.
Nutrition, 139–160;
    of newborn infants, 112f., 118.
    shortage of foodstuffs, 139f.

Obstetrics, 81f., 300, 357–361.
Occupational diseases, 19, 126, 131f., 164, 294, 441.
Outpatients' departments, 341.
Oxygen, breathing of, 279.

Paederasty, 57.
Paramedical phenomena, 258f.
Paris, xiv;
    accidents, 215.
    carriages, 134.
    cemeteries, 440.
    child murder, 114.

cleanliness of the streets (dirty streets), 186, 188.
    exposure of children, 115.
    fashion of clothing, 163.
    hospitals, 418.
    Hôtel Dieu, 417, 419.
    lunatic asylums, 427.
    number of foundlings, 115.
    poisoning, 233.
    police regulations, 7, 141.
Pathological anatomy, *see* Morbid anatomy.
Patient, examination of, 347f.
Pavia, Italy, vii, xif., xviii, 199, 236, 259;
    bedside teaching, 299, 341, 344f.
    medical curriculum, 317, 327, 334, 374f., 382.
    pathological museum, 334.
Pellagra, 303.
Peruvian bark, 301.
Petersburg, Russia, xiiif., 383;
    bedside teaching, 345.
    clinical school, lack of post-mortem examina-
    tions, 332.
    hospitals, 420.
    pathological museum, 335.
Pharmacopeia, 429.
Philanthropy, 15, 23, 50, 84, 90ff., 105f., 114, 180,
    224, 265, 324, 332, 380, 389, 428.
Philosophy, 315, 391;
    when outside its boundaries, a mental disorder,
    316.
Physician
    as guardian of public health, 290ff.
    criticism of young, 299.
    duties of, 305.
    instruction of, on apparent death, 275.
    obligation of, to a dying person, 263f.
    quality of a good, 169, 323f.
Physicians
    and magic, 251, 260.
    and witchcraft, 256.
    Army, 392.
    assistant, 431f.
    chief, 431f.
    country, 392.
    disproportionate increase of, 322.
    distribution of, in the country, 354.
    hospital, 431f.
Physiology, 336f.
Plague, 291f., 305, 380, 393, 435f., 437, 444f.
Planned recreation, 168–174.

Poisoning, 230–234.
Poisonous plants, 149, 399.
Poland
  climate, 21.
  population, 16.
Police, 222f.
Pollution
  caused by dung heaps and liquid manure pits, 188.
  caused by hemp and flax, 185.
  caused by trades and crafts, 192–196.
  of air, 177f., 412f.
  of environment, 182.
  of town moats, 185.
  of water, 178f.
Polygamy, 53f., 71, 96.
Poor-relief, 75, 85, 114, 407ff., 424.
Poppy-juice, 169, 260.
Population
  and army, 49f.
  calculation of, 25.
  concept of, 12f.
  relation of, to state, 15f.
Postgraduate education, 320, 328, 340, 375.
Post-mortem examinations, 296, 298, 332ff., 352, 381.
Poverty, in relation to health, 17f., 22, 75, 85, 109f., 114, 127, 139f., 313, 407ff., 428.
Pregnancy, 70–78;
  appreciation of, 70, 79, 93, 358.
  care during, xix, 73f.
  dancing during, 132, 141f.
  psychological change during, 102.
Pregnant women
  imagination of, 72f.
  in lying-in wards, 427f.
  lists of, 75f.
  treatment of, 71f., 398.
Preventive medicine, 290f., 393f.
Private apartments, see Latrines.
Procreation
  decline of, 42f.
  extramarital, 93–101.
  free choice, 61f.
  healthy, 292.
  influence of religion on, 24.
  lust for, 25, 36f., 91.
  purpose of, 53.
Prostitution, 92, 95.

Prussia
  medical examinations, 367f.
  population, 16.
Psychology
  in medical examinations, 368.
  in politics, 169.
  on insanity, 425.
  word memory, 368f.
Public women, see Prostitution.

Quarantine, 436f., 446–450.

Rabies, 292, 422.
Races, 131f.
Rack, 254f.
Reanimation, 274–280, 298;
  breathing in air from mouth to mouth, 278f.
  by oxygen, 279.
Resuscitation, 13.
Rights of mankind, 92, 94, 116, 199, 226, 230.
Rivers, 18, 178.
  pollution of, 184f.
Rome
  accidents, 209f.
  animal fights, 223.
  cloaca maxima, 189, 192.
  games, 169.
  laws, 222.
  murders, 236.
  paederasty, 57.
  poisoning, 230f.
  pregnancy, 70.
  regulations of marriages, 42.
  suicide, 239.
Russia
  salary of professors, 315.
  serfdom, 322.

Safety
  definition of, 201f.
  of children, 110f.
  of mines, 212.
  of vehicles, 213f.
  road, 212f.
Scabies, 412, 418.
Scarlet fever, 412, 434, 445.
Scholastic instruction, 369.
Scurvy, 297f.
Secret medicines, 306, 398.

Security, *see* Safety.

Semiotics, 339.

Sensitiveness, 129, 170.

Serfdom, xviii, 322.

Sexual intercourse, 46, 53f., 61, 97.

Sexuality, 25, 32, 46, 61, 95–101.

Sick rooms, 346, 411f., 421f.

Skin diseases, 119.

Slaughterhouses, 192f.

Smallpox, 291, 393, 450–452.

Smog, 196.

Social medicine, vii, xv, xviii.

Social status
 of bachelors, 35.
 of married people, 35.
 of midwives, 360f.
 of surgeons, 301.
 of women, 57f., 74.

Society
 classification of, 59.
 physician and, 390f.

Sorcery, 244–261, 293, 297, 436.

Spain
 behavior, 169.
 population, 16.

Special pathology, *see* Bedside teaching.

Speyer, Germany, x, 251, 335, 380.

Sport, 128–132.

Springs, 150f.

State
 importance of medicine for, 391.

State medicine, 271, 285, 379.

Statistics, 16f., 56.

Sterility, 55–66.

Strasbourg, France, 381.

Streets, 186–190;
 sluices, 189f.

Students, 313;
 as teachers of children, 314.
 behavior of, 352.
 examinations of, 365–372.
 increased number of, caused by social changes in
  Europe, 322.
 number of, at sickbed, 344, 373.
 of surgery, 355f.
 quality of, 322f.
 social status of, 314.

Study, of medicine
 admission to, 370f.

gratuitous, 370.

Suicide, 169, 238–243, 400f.

Superstition, 13, 244–261, 398.

Surgeons
 in hospitals, 432.
 instruction of, on apparent death, 275.
 magic cures of, 251.
 social status of, 301, 314, 353.

Surgery, 353–356.
 appreciation of, 295, 300f.
 teaching of, 355f., 381.
 unification of, and medicine, 353ff.

Swamps, 179, 293f., 393.

Sweden
 child murder, 106.
 climate, 21.
 female sterility, 55.
 foundling hospitals, 114.
 mortality of pregnant women, 72.
 pollution, 186.
 population, 16

Switzerland
 bachelors, 35.
 fertility, 54.
 floods, 218.
 population, 16.
 suicide, 243.

Symptomatology, 339.

Taverns, 159f.

Teachers
 economic aspects of lectures, 328f.
 qualities of, 314f.

Theater, 171–173.

Therapeutics
 principles of, 428f.
 teaching of, 345f.

Torture, 254ff.

Towns, 175–182;
 accidents in, 203–205, 214–217.
 cleanliness of, 184.
 influences on health, 177, 182.
 large, 22.
 mortality in, 181.
 pollution of, 185, 192–196.
 seat of medical schools, 312.
 social aspects of, 182.

Traffic, 214–217;
 accidents in, 214.

Traffic (cont.)
  regulations, 214f.
Tragedy
  effects of, 171f.
Turks, 436, 447.
Tuscany
  celibacy, 31.
  fighting games, 223f.
  inoculation, 291.
Universities
  constitution of, 365.
  lectures at, 328f.
  structure of, 312.
Unwed mothers, 91f., 114f.

Vaccination, 291, 380, 450–452.
Vampires, 293.
Vehicles, 213;
  examination of, 214.
Venereal diseases, 32f., 48, 95, 99, 117f., 292, 297,
  412, 424.
Venice, Italy, 179, 437.
Veterinary science, 14f.
Vienna, xi–xiv, 140, 271;
  accidents, 203, 216.
  bedside teaching, 299, 341, 344f.
  Civic Hospital, 117.
  General Hospital, 383, 405, 411, 418, 421.
  medical examinations, 367.

  mortality of foundlings, 117.
  pathological museum, 334f.
  revision of medical studies, 330.
  revision of studies, 388.
  sandy streets, 187.
  students as tutors of children, 314.
  Supreme Medical Board, 396–399.
  traffic, 214f.
Vilna, Lithuania, xiii;
  bedside teaching, 345.
  medical school, 332.
  pathological museum, 355.
  post-mortem examinations, 334.
Votive gifts, 252.

Walking, 133f.
Water
  in hospitals, 416.
  pollution of, 178, 194f.
Wax models, 252.
Wells, 150f.
Wet nurses, 112f., 117f.
Wigs, 164.
Witchcraft, xx–xxii, 247–261, 293;
  physical explanation of witch signs, 255, 258.
  symptoms of bewitching, 253f.
  water test, 254, 304.
  witch salve, 256.
  witch trials, 254.